Biofertilizers in Agriculture and Forestry

Revised Third Edition

Biofertilizers in Agriculture and Forestry

Revised Third Edition

NS Subba Rao FNA

Oxford & IBH Publishing Co. Pvt. Ltd.
New Delhi
(*A Unit of* CBS Publishers & Distributors Pvt Ltd)

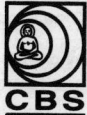

CBS Publishers & Distributors Pvt Ltd

New Delhi • Bengaluru • Chennai • Kochi • Kolkata • Mumbai
Bhopal • Bhubaneswar • Hyderabad • Jharkhand • Nagpur
• Patna • Pune • Uttarakhand • Dhaka (Bangladesh)

Biofertilizers in
Agriculture and Forestry
Revised Third Edition

ISBN-13: 978-81-204-0791-6
ISBN-10: 81-204-0791-1

OXFORD & IBH
New Delhi
(A Unit of CBS Publishers & Distributors Pvt Ltd)

Published by Satish Kumar Jain and produced by Varun Jain for
CBS Publishers & Distributors Pvt Ltd
4819/XI Prahlad Street, 24 Ansari Road, Daryaganj, New Delhi 110 002, India.

Ph: 23289259, 23266861, 23266867   Fax: 011-23243014   Website: www.cbspd.com
e-mail: delhi@cbspd.com; cbspubs@airtelmail.in.
Corporate Office: 204 FIE, Industrial Area, Patparganj, Delhi 110 092
Ph: 4934 4934   Fax: 4934 4935   e-mail: publishing@cbspd.com;
publicity@cbspd.com

Branches

- **Bengaluru:** Seema House 2975, 17th Cross, K.R. Road, Banasankari 2nd Stage, Bengaluru 560 070, Karnataka
  Ph: +91-80-26771678/79   Fax: +91-80-26771680   e-mail: bangalore@cbspd.com
- **Chennai:** 7, Subbaraya Street, Shenoy Nagar, Chennai 600 030, Tamil Nadu
  Ph: +91-44-26260666, 26208620   Fax: +91-44-42032115   e-mail: chennai@cbspd.com
- **Kochi:** 42/1325, 1326, Power House Road, Opp KSEB Power House, Ernakulam 682 018, Kochi, Kerala
  Ph: +91-484-4059061-65   Fax: +91-484-4059065   e-mail: kochi@cbspd.com
- **Kolkata:** No. 6/B, Ground Floor, Rameswar Shaw Road, Kolkata-700014 (West Bengal), India
  Ph: +91-33-2289-1126, 2289-1127, 2289-1128   e-mail: kolkata@cbspd.com
- **Mumbai:** 83-C, Dr E Moses Road, Worli, Mumbai-400018, Maharashtra
  Ph: +91-22-24902340/41   Fax: +91-22-24902342   e-mail: mumbai@cbspd.com

Representatives

Bhopal	0-8319310552	Bhubaneswar	0-9911037372	Hyderabad	0-9885175004
Jharkhand	0-9811541605	Nagpur	0-9021734563	Patna	0-9334159340
Pune	0-9623451994	Uttarakhand	0-9716462459		
Dhaka (Bangladesh)	01912-003485				

Printed at Chaman Enterprises, Daryaganj, New Delhi, India

Preface to the Third Edition

In this edition, the scope of the book has been extended to Forestry and the title of the book has accordingly been changed to *Biofertilizers in Agriculture and Forestry*. The role of mycorrhizal Fungi in conjunction with *Frankia* (For some non-leguminous plants) and *Rhizobium* (For nodulated leguminous plants) to provide the much needed nitrogen and phosphorus to growing seedlings in the nursery stage has been increasingly realized, especially in afforestation practices aimed at recovering barren lands and sites spoiled by mining. In this sense, this new edition adds a fresh dimension to microbial practices advocated to sustain plant growth through renewable sources of fertilizers.

The text provides scientific yet popular insight into crop and tree cultivation by organic inputs. It is invaluable for students, researchers, and administrators in the twin disciplines of agriculture and forestry.

March 1993   N.S. SUBBA RAO

Dr. M.S. Swaminathan, F.R.S. Member,
Planning Commission, Yojana Bhavan,
New Delhi 110001

May 13, 1981

Foreword

During the last two decades, agricultural production has increased in developed and certain developing countries due to the use of high yielding varieties and enhanced consumption of chemical fertilizers and water. The pathway of productivity improvement followed so far has however been accompanied by an exponential increase in the consumption of non-renewable forms of energy. In view of the escalating energy costs, energy will be a key limiting factor for increasing agricultural production in future. Therefore, it is essential for us to evolve and adopt a strategy of integrated nutrient supply by using a judicious combination of chemical fertilizers, organic manures and biofertilizers. Biofertilizers harness atmospheric nitrogen with the help of specialised soil microorganisms. Such nitrogen-fixing microorganisms are either free living in soil or symbiotic with plants and directly or indirectly contribute towards the nitrogen nutrition of plants. Recent reports on the nitrogen fixing capabilities of *Azolla-Anabaena* symbionts show that about 40 kgN/ha along with addition of bulk quantities of organic matter in the form of *Azolla* biomass which increases to about 10 fold in about 30 days, could be realised. Free living bacteria of the genera *Azotobacter, Beijerinckia,* the blue-green algae and *Azospirillum* form important contributors of nitrogen to soil through the non-symbiotic process. It is estimated that addition of blue green algae to rice fields enriches the soil by 40 kg N ha. Thus, biofertilizers can make a significant contribution towards the development of strategies for productivity improvement which do not lead to an exponential rise in the consumption of non-renewable forms of energy.

Dr. N.S. Subba Rao has a very distinguished background in the field of research on biofertilizers and therefore, he is eminently suited to write this book on biofertilizers in agriculture. He has presented in this well-illustrated book an up-to-date account of fundamental as well as applied aspects of research in this field. Dr. Subba Rao has not only critically evaluated the work in progress on biofertilizers in different countries but also indicated the outlook for the future. The publication of this book is indeed timely when we are trying to evolve a new strategy for agricultural production based on an integrated nutrient supply system.

I hope this book will be useful to research workers, teachers and planners in the field of biofertilizers as well as to other agricultural scientists, especially in the developing countries. I also hope that this book will stimulate the widespread development of 'Nitrogen farming' techniques. Our gratitude goes to Dr. Subba Rao for this labour of love on his part.

M.S. SWAMINATHAN

Preface to the First Edition

The term 'biofertilizers' or more appropriately 'microbial inoculants' can be generally defined as preparations containing live or latent cells of efficient strains of nitrogen-fixing, phosphate-solubilizing, or cellulolytic microorganisms used for application to seed, soil, or composting areas with the objective of increasing the numbers of such microorganisms and accelerating certain microbial processes to augment the extent of the availability of nutrients in a form which can be easily assimilated by plants. In a larger sense, the term may be used to include all organic resources (manures) for plant growth which are rendered in an available form for plant absorption through micro-organisms or microorganisms-plant associations or interactions. Such mircrobiological processes may be as complex as that of nitrogenase-mediated reactions in nitrogen-fixing microorganisms which reduce elemental nitrogen into ammonia or as simple as the organic acid secretion by phosphate dissolving bacteria. Complex polysaccharides are broken down by certain fungi and actinomycetes and a variety of nitrogen interconversions take place in soil due to microorganisms involved in the nitrogen cycle. An ideal fertile soil is not only charac-terized by optimum physical properties and chemical constituents conducive for plant growth but also by microbiological processes which are maintained in an equilibrium. These microbiological processes are part of nitrogen, phosphorous and carbon cycles. In fact, wild ecosystems have sustained themselves through centuries by means of such natural inter-conversions of essential elements.

The modern day intensive crop cultivation requires the use of chemical fertilizers but fertilizers are not only in short supply but also expensive in developing countries. Therefore, the current trend is to explore the possibility of supplementing chemical fertilizers with organic ones, more particularly biofertilizers of microbial origin. Microbial processes are not only quick but consume relatively less energy than industrial processes. Secondly, they have the advantage of being diversified into small units to meet the demands of specific problems of location which one is apt to come across in the agricultural practice of nations which have not taken to mechanization of farming. A small or a marginal farmer has to be educated on the ways and means of recycling farm wastes. In soil, myriads of microorganisms are at work in fixing nitrogen, mobilizing other plant nutrients, and degrading ligno-cellulosic wastes. Very often microorganisms are not as efficient in natural surroundings as one would expect them to be and therefore, artificially multiplied cultures of selected microorganisms play a part in accelerating nature's way of recycling organic resources.

The idea of 'inoculation' was indirectly known to our ancestors when they transferred large amounts of soil from areas where leguminous crops were flourishing to areas where they were less luxuriant. In a sense, they were 'inoculating' nodule-forming bacteria from one field to another. The first *Rhizobium* inoculant preparations were provided to farmers as laboratory-grown nodule bacteria on agar media. This was soon replaced by carrier-based cultures which not only improved the shelf life of cultures but also increased the bacterial load on seed. Methods of mass culture and seed inoculation were improved in the United States and Australia which were later adapted to other countries to suit local needs. With the advent of the energy crisis, non-symbiotic nitrogen-fixing microorganisms got their due emphasis and applied research took shape in developing countries. Nitrogen-fixing bacteria and blue-green algae and aquatic *Azolla* containing nitrogen-fixing blue-green alga *Azolla anabaena* were highlighted. Microbiological methods of energy production such as biogas and alcohol came to be recognized as the future hope of mankind.

Applied work relating to biofertilizers has been done in India on a large scale with legumes as well as non-legumes. In many instances, the yield increases due to these biofertilizers may be marginal but poor countries can ill afford to neglect any low cost input which can bring corresponding dividends to the farmer where labour is not as expensive as it is in advanced countries. While the biofertilizer technology appears to be relevant to poor nations, sophisticated basic research involving expertise and money which can improve the ability of crops or microorganisms to get the most out of microbiological processes is being increasingly carried out in the United States, the United Kingdom, and Australia. Genetic engineering research to insert nitrogen-fixing genes into other bacteria and higher plants has received the attention of molecular biologists and likewise, plant physiologists, biochemists, and plant geneticists have been pursuing work towards a clearer understanding of basic mechanisms underlying the innate ability of plants to benefit from microbial associations. Studies on biological nitrogen fixation have thus become a multidisciplinary approach but microbiologists and agronomists are jointly involved in the application of biofertilizer technology at the field level.

The literature on this aspect is not only voluminous but also varied and widely dispersed in journals and reports. The objective of this book is to bring together our knowledge into a small book form. The need for such a book has been felt by the author through numerous inquiries by cultivators and scientists interested in the overall picture of the role of microorganisms in nutrient mobilization into plants. The book has been written to provide brief, basic, relevant information on all aspects of the subject with illustrations and appropriate references. Not all the available literature on the subject has been cited but important ones have not been omitted. The book will serve both biologists and agricultural scientists who are interested in alternative sources of energy on the farm through beneficial microorganisms. Relevant materials from published sources have been drawn which are duly acknowledged at appropriate places.

I am grateful to Dr. M.S. Swaminathan, who has been kind enough to write a foreword to the book, and to Dr. O.P. Gautam, Director General, ICAR, Dr. N.S. Randhawa, Deputy Director General (S), Dr. H.K. Jain, Director, IARI, and my colleagues in the Division of Microbiology for their encouragement.

Indian Agricultural Research Institute N.S. SUBBA RAO
New Delhi

Contents

Contents

1

Introduction

Man began to cultivate land in an organized way for food grains around 8000 B.C. Very soon, he learned that the same land cannot support the growth of plants endlessly and this led him to think about ways to improve the fertility of soil. The earliest records indicate that Romans and Aryans had many manuals for farmers to improve the cultivation of crops. For instance, Columella's treatise *Husbandry* written about 60 A.D. contains descriptions of several agricultural practices which were in use in the Roman empire for many generations. After the fall of the Roman empire, the Arabian culture flourished in the 12th century, when Ibn-al-Awan, a Moorish scholar, wrote a handbook on agriculture. This was followed by 18th century farming practices such as those of Jethro Tull (English) and the Norfolk 'four-course' system developed in Holland by years of experience based on crop rotations.

Meanwhile, many people wondered about the ingredients in soil which nourish plants. In the 16th century, Bernard Pallissy, a potter to the French royalty, argued that plant residues contained the 'salt' or the 'principle' which supported plant growth, while Jan Baptista van Helmont believed that water was the 'principle' capable of supporting the growth of plants. Later, the idea that certain ingredients in soil dissolved in water actually supported plant growth was established by experiments of John Woodward of England. Some others considered 'humus' the supporter of plant growth. However, all conjectures were set aside when the French scientist, Antoine Lavoisier, developed a table of chemical elements in 1794. He also showed that plants and animals used up oxygen by a process of respiration (USDA, 1957).

Soil Fertility

The experiments of J.B. Boussingault, a French agriculturist, in 1834 revealed the important chemical constituents of both plants and soil. This was followed by the work of Justus Von Liebig, a German chemist, who was able to prepare a balance sheet of plant nutrition in relation to soil. By about this time, Boussingault also proposed that legumes fix nitrogen in soil. One of the milestones in the area of soil fertility was the discovery of superphosphate in 1840 by John Bennet Lawes and his associate J.H. Gilbert at the Rothamsted Experimental Station in England. Further researches at Rothamsted led to a greater understanding of the chemistry of soil and the chemical requirements of plants. Boussingault's thinking on the role of legumes in soil fertility was substantiated by the discovery of legume root nodules by Hellreigel in Germany in 1886 and the discovery by Beijerinck, a Dutch scientist, in 1888 that bacteria in root nodules of legumes now called *Rhizobium* are causative agents in the fixation of atmospheric nitrogen.

Chemical fixation of nitrogen was known only several years after our understanding of the implications of biological nitrogen fixation. Fritz Haber, a German chemist, successfully synthesized nitrogen and hydrogen into ammonia during the early years of World War I. No discovery leading to soil fertility has ever equalled that of Haber. In fact, the Haber-Bosch process of ammonia synthesis, requiring temperature up to 800°F, a catalyst, and high pressures above atmospheric pressure has remained, till today, the sole method for the production of nitrogenous fertilizers in the world. Strangely, this very combination of nitrogen and hydrogen could also be accomplished by nitrogen-fixing microorganisms in soil and within the nodular tissues of certain plants at ordinary pressures and temperature mediated by an enzyme known as 'nitrogenase'.

Man-made fertilizers as we know them today, those containing N_2, P_2O_5 and K_2, increase the output of agricultural products and meet the ever increasing demands of the human population, which have been further accentuated by the limited availability of additional fertile farm land. The world's population, food production, and fertilizer consumption have increased gradually. It has been forecast that there will be a further increase in population in the developing countries by about 2.1 million people at the end of 2000 A.D. To guarantee enough food for all, either the population growth has to be stemmed or more fertilizer has to be found to meet the ever increasing demand for protein. The increase in world fertilizer requirement by

2000 A.D. would be approximately three times the rate of current consumption (Table 1).

Table 1: Population, grain production and fertilizer use, and projections for future

Year	Population (millions)	Grain production (million tons)	Fertilizer consumption (million tons)
World			
1980	4374	1575	113
2000	6253	2235	307
Developed countries			
1980	1145	840	83
2000	1317	1221	197
Developing countries			
1980	3229	735	30
2000	4936	1032	110
India			
1980	694	130	5.60
2000	1059	175	18.90

Source: Verghese, 1977.

Chemically Fixed Nitrogen versus Biologically Fixed Nitrogen

Fertilizer nitrogen will continue to serve for increasing grain production into the foreseeable future but efforts should also be oriented towards augmenting biological nitrogen fixation mediated by microorganisms. An average acre of grain legumes like soybeans, beans, or peas provides sufficient protein for 1000–2000 days for one person, whereas an average acre of plant materials converted to animal protein like beef and poultry provides only for 75–250 days (Burns and Hardy, 1975). As the per capita income increases the demand on animal protein also increases accompanied by a several-fold decrease in the intake of vegetable protein. Therefore, in the affluent nations, where the per capita income is high, the demand for fixed nitrogen for conversion into animal protein is higher than that of less affluent nations where the per capita income is low and consequently, the intake of vegetable protein is more pronounced.

Accurate estimates of annual turnover of nitrogen in the biosphere vary from 100 to 200 million tons (Delwiche, 1970; Burns and Hardy, 1975; Burris, 1977; Subba Rao, 1977). The ratio between chemically fixed nitrogen and biologically fixed nitrogen ranges approximately from 1:4 to 1:2.5 and within biological fixation, the legume fixation is equivalent to or at least half that of industrial fixation (Table 2). The amounts of kg N_2 fixed/ha/yr for individual legumes has been roughly estimated as follows: 125–335 for alfalfa, 85–190 for red clover, 80–150 for peas, 65–115 for soybean, 65–130 for cowpea, and 90–155 for vetch (Alexander, 1977).

Table 2: Estimates of annual biological nitrogen fixation on earth

Systems	$\dfrac{kg\,N_2\,fixed}{(ha \times yr)}$	Metric tons/yr $\times 10^{-6}$
Legumes	140 (80)	35 (20)
Non-legumes	35	9
Permanent grassland	15 (8)	45 (24)
Forest and woodland	10 (5)	40 (20)
Unused land	2	10
Total land		139 (83)
Sea	1 (0.5)	36 (18)
Total		175 (101)

Note: Fertilizer from chemical N_2 fixation was 40×10^{-6} metric tons/yr in 1976. Data extracted from Burris (1977), who has incorporated the estimates of Burns and Hardy (1975); the figures in parentheses indicate values assigned by experts at a meeting in Uppsala, Sweden, 1976.

Accurate estimates of the amounts of N_2 fixed by grain legumes have been made by the International Atomic Energy Agency (IAEA), Vienna, using labelled nitrogenous fertilizers. Some of the results obtained by the collaborating scientists in the agency's network of experiments in different countries are shown in Table 3. These values appear to be rather realistic but nervertheless do not minimize the value of legumes in the nitrogen economy of cultivated plants.

The demand for chemically fixed nitrogen is bound to be on the increase and the nitrogen gap gets doubled by 1995 (Table 4). Such a gap would be difficult to bridge in the wake of the energy crisis. Furthermore, in the area of chemical fixation, no major break-through is yet visible to minimize the energy requirements of the conventional Haber-Bosch process for the production of ammonia. In developing countries, the construction of new nitrogen fertilizer plants is not only expensive but time consuming. Farmers in many parts of Africa do not use inorganic nitrogenous fertilizers because they are imported and expensive. Therefore, the strategy for improving agricultural production in developing countries should take into account inexpensive, realistic, and pragmatic programmes to augment biological nitrogen fixation.

Table 3: Accurate estimates of symbiotic N_2 fixation by different legumes by the isotope dilution method — results of field trials using labelled ($^{15}NH_4$)$_2$ SO_4

Country	Legume	Year	Total amount of N_2 fixation (kg/ha)
New Delhi, India (IARI) (Mean of 3 Years' field experiments)	Chick-pea (Cicer arietinum)	1979–1982	61.6
Larisa, Greece	Medicago sativa	1980	72.8
Faisalabad, Pakistan	Mung bean (Vigna radiata)	1981	45.3
Piracicaba, Brazil	Phaseolus beans	1980	37.0
Egypt	Faba beans (Phaseolus vulgaris)	1980	101.0

Source: IAEA Reports, Vienna, Austria.

Table 4: The world's demand for N (million tons) in coming years which clearly shows the need for renewed efforts to augment our resource

	1980	1985	1990	1995	2000
Developed countries	37.5	47.6	58.9	71.4	85.1
Developing countries	18.1	25.4	33.9	43.6	54.5
World	55.6	73.0	92.8	115.0	139.6

Source: Verghese, 1977.

How to Augment Biological Nitrogen Fixation

There are both novel and conventional approaches to this problem (Subba Rao, 1976a, 1976b, 1977, 1979). Conventionally, attempts should be made: (1) to increase the area under cultivation of grain legumes by the introduction of legumes in inter-, multiple, and relay cropping; (2) to provide efficient strains of rhizobia for inoculating legumes and other non-symbiotic nitrogen fixers for inoculating cereals; (3) to evolve a technology enabling the newly introduced nitrogen fixers to successfully compete with the strains of nitrogen-fixing microorganisms already present in soil; (4) to evolve varieties of plants responsive to both biologically and industrially fixed nitrogen; (5) to overcome the inhibition of fertilizer nitrogen on biological fixation of nitrogen; (6) to define agronomic practices leading to better fixation and conservation of nitrogen on the farm; (7) to discover inexpensive nitrification inhibitors such as neem cake; and (8) to evolve simple practices to conserve water on the farm because optimum moisture is needed for successful nodulation and hence biological nitrogen fixation in legumes.

There is no limit to speculation in the unconventional approaches, which are indeed receiving considerable attention in recent years. Some of the considerations are: (1) to extend nitrogen fixation to cereals by inducing the formation of nodules on root; (2) to transfer genes from nitrogen-fixing bacteria to non-nitrogen-fixing bacteria by transformation, transduction, and conjugation; (3) to implant nitrogen fixation capacity from nitrogen-fixing bacteria into crop plants by protoplast fusion and tissue culture methods; (4) to overcome barriers in intergeneric hybridization between nodulating legumes and cereals, both at the floral level in intact plants and at the cellular level, in cell cultures; (5) to synthesize 'nitrogenase', the enzyme responsible for converting N_2 to NH_3, and harness it for use in nitrogen fixation as a catalyst in industrial processes; and (6) to extend research into new nitrogen-fixing associations among plants and harness them to agriculture.

Exciting discoveries have been made in recent decades which bring an optimistic note to many of the speculations cited above. The *nif* operon (a cluster of nitrogen-fixing genes) has been transferred from a nitrogen-fixing bacterium, *Klebsiella pneumoniae*, into a common enteric bacterium, *Escherichia coli*. At the cellular level, cultured plant tissues and cells have been made to take up nitrogen-fixing bacteria and fix atmospheric nitrogen. Roots of rice and rape plants have been made to produce nodules which seem to fix elemental nitrogen. These experiments have paved the way for eventual release of plants capable of growing without the need for chemical fertilizers. Studies on detection, isolation, and characterization of plasmids in nitrogen-fixing bacteria are in progress in many laboratories with a view to using plamids as 'vectors' in transferring *nif* genes into higher plants. The parts of the enzyme nitrogenase have been interchanged from one nitrogen-fixing microorganism into another without detriment to the property of nitrogen fixation. Biochemists have unravelled the structure and composition of nitrogenase while microbiologists have identified the existence of more plants bearing nitrogen-fixing nodules. Many fodder grasses and cereals like maize have been found to exhibit associate symbioses with nitrogen-fixing *Azospirillum* bacteria. Legumes have been shown to benefit by the dual action of obligate endophytic fungi in plant roots (endomycorrhizae) and *Rhizobium* in root nodules; the endomycorrhizal fungi appear to influence the uptake of phosphorus which helps in better fixation of nitrogen in root nodules. The biochemical basis for specificity in the legume-*Rhizobium* symbiosis has been explained as an interaction on the root surface involving the two symbionts mediated by carbohydrate-binding proteins called 'lectins'. The magnitude of loss of energy by hydrogen evolution along with N_2 reduction in nodules formed by hydrogenase-negative strains of rhizobia has been shown to be greater than that induced by hydrogenase-positive strains; field experiments have shown that hydrogenase-positive strains proved to be better inocula and helped in increasing soybean yields when compared to inocula produced by hydrogenase-negative strains. Such observations serve to point out that hydrogenase-positive strains conserve energy within the nitrogenase reactions (Dunican *et al.*, 1976; Dobereiner, 1977; Dazzo, 1980; Evans *et al.*, 1980; Islam *et al.*, 1980; Cocking *et al.*, 1990). However, at the moment it is not clear whether such research findings could be of agronomic importance to improve crop yields by better nitrogen fertilization.

Development of Inoculant Research and Industry

Microbial inoculants are carrier-based preparations containing beneficial microorganisms in a viable state intended for seed or soil application and designed to improve soil fertility and help plant growth by increasing the number and biological activity of desired microorganisms in the root environment. Starting from modest laboratory preparations in the mid-1930s in the United States, rhizobial inoculants (also known as legume inoculants) have become industrial propositions in the United States, Europe, Australia, and India. Following the success of legume inoculants all over the world, carrier-based *Azotobacter* and *Azospirillum* inoculants for non-leguminous crops are becoming increasingly popular in India in recent years. Currently, besides, agricultural research institutes, and universities in India, the agencies also active in supplying biofertilizers are: 1. The MP State Agro Industries Dev. Corp. Ltd., Bhopal, 2. The Maharashtra Agro Industries Dev. Corp. Ltd., Bombay, 3. Department of Agriculture, Madras, (TN), 4. National Agri. Co-op. Mktng. Federation of India Ltd., Indore, 5. Gujarat State Co-op. Mktng. Federation Ltd., Baroda, 6. Gujarat State Fertilizers Co. Ltd.,

Fertilizer Nagar, Dist. Baroda, 7. Micro Bac India, Calcutta, 8. Indian Organic Chemicals Ltd., Bombay, 9. Madras Fertilizers, Madras.

In 1895, Nobbe and Hiltner introduced laboratory-grown cultures of rhizobia called 'Nitragin' grown on a solid medium containing extracts of leguminous plants, gelatin, sugar, and asparagine. In this maiden attempt, 17 different inoculants for important leguminous crops were produced (Fred *et al.*, 1932; Burton, 1967, 1979). In 1920, the situation in the United States was such that besides the U.S. Department of Agriculture and 20 research institutions, 17 commercial concerns were marketing inoculants. The following companies are currently active in North America in supplying *Rhizobium* inoculants: *Lipha Tech*, 3101 W. Custer Ave., Milwaukee, WI 53209, USA, ph (414) 462-7600; *Philom Bios Inc.*, 104–110 Research Drive, Saskatoon, Sask., Canada S7N 3R3, fax 306-975-1215; *Micro BioRhizogen*, Bay 5–116 103rd St. East, Saskatoon, Sask., Canada, fax 306-374-8510; *ESSO-Biologicals Canada*, 15-401 Innovation Blvd., Saskatoon, Sask., Canada S7N 2X2 fax 306-975-3750; *Titre Inc.*, 361 Rothiemay, Rd., Ryegate, MT 59074, USA or Box 220, Beachville, Ontario NOJ 1AO, Canada; *Urbana Laboratories*, P.O. Box 1393, St. Joseph, MO, 64502, USA, ph 1-800-821-7666.

In Russia and Poland non-symbiotic nitrogen-fixing bacteria of the genus *Azotobacter* gained importance in the early part of this century. A product under the trade name 'Azotobakterin' was used for soil and seed treatment and spectacular benefits were recorded on the yield of vegetables and cereals.

Reviewing the work on *Azotobacter*, Martin Alexander (1961) of Cornell University, USA, said that 'careful analysis of the Soviet experiments is difficult because of the scarcity of statistical evaluations. It is possible that the *Azotobacter* effects are not real and may be accounted for by the normal variability of field experimentation. The greater yields are difficult to reconcile with rapid decline of *Azotobacter* in inoculated soil and with the absence of the specialized structure (nodule) that permits the *Rhizobium*-legume symbiosis to operate so efficiently. For the present, therefore, reports of benefits arising from *Azotobacter* inoculation must be considered as equivocal'.

In summarizing the same work, two well-known soil microbiologists of Russia said that 'an increase in the yield of field crops of not more than 10 per cent in an agricultural experiment is not regarded as exceeding the limits of experimental error. As to the positive action of *Azotobacter*, it can only be said that statistical analysis repeatedly demonstrates the reliability of the results' (Mishustin and Shilnikova, 1969).

Field experiments have also been carried out in India on *Azotobacter chroococcum* inoculation of wheat, rice, onion, brinjal, tomato, and cabbage. Yield increases have been rather variable from simple general increases to significant increases in rice, cabbage, and brinjal (Sundara Rao *et al.,* 1963; Sundara Rao, 1964; Lehri and Mehrotra, 1968, 1972; Mehrotra and Lehri, 1971; Joi and Shinde, 1976). *Azotobacter* inoculants are popular in India because they can be applied to many non-leguminous crops and promote seed germination and initial vigour of plants due to growth substances produced by the organism (Shende *et al.,* 1977).

Blue-green algae play a role in the nitrogen economy of tropical rice soils (De, 1939; Singh, 1961; Subramanyam and Sahay, 1964; Venkataraman, 1972). The nitrogen-fixing algae can be cultured in open-air tanks and used for rice cultivation. The results obtained by algal inoculation of rice fields in India have shown the possibility of using blue-green algae as biofertilizer in rice cultivation.

Microorganisms convert bound phosphates such as superphosphate and rock phosphate into forms which are easily assimilated by plants (Gerretsen, 1948; Sperber, 1957; Sethi and Subba Rao, 1968; Sundara Rao, 1968). The Russian microbiologists introduced a product called 'phosphobakterin' containing cells of *Bacillus megatherium* var. *phosphaticum* for soil and seed application. Since then, other microorganisms have been tested in India and the results are quite promising.

Cellulose is the main component of organic matter in plant residues. Numerous microorganisms in soil degrade cellulose to different degrees and the products containing either the cells of cellulolytic microorganisms or their enzymic extracts are being produced in Europe and the United States and marketed for quick composting of agricultural wastes. Some of the brand names of such products from Europe are 'Cofuna', 'Agromax', and 'Eokomit'. In India, similar products are yet to be produced and marketed although considerable research on cellulolytic and lignolytic microorganisms has been done.

Thiobacilli (sulphur-dissolving bacteria) were used in the preparation of 'biosuper' in Australia by mixing rock phosphate and sulphur. The suphuric acid produced in the mixture dissolves the rock phosphate and thereby enhances phosphorus nutrition of plants. Whether this kind of biofertilizer is worthwhile and economical in India depends on the availability of sulphur and rock phosphate for this purpose and the utility of the product on the farm for increasing yields of crop plants.

The re-discovery of *Azospirillum brasilense* in Brazil (Dobereiner *et al.*, 1976) led to field testings of Indian isolates of the bacterium on a large scale in India (Subba Rao *et al.*, 1979a, 1979b) which have shown beneficial inoculation effects of this organism on ragi, bajra, sorghum, maize, barley, and oats. Field trials point out significant increase in yields of crops in many locations and also indicate savings on the application of inorganic nitrogenous fertilizers from 20 to 30 kg N/ha, depending on the crop and location.

The future for the inoculant industry in developing countries is bright. In the whole of Africa, there are very few places where fertilizer factories exist and the average farmer scarcely uses fertilizer nitrogen for crop production. Therefore, agronomists all over the world should take cognizance of developments in the area of organic fertilization of soil, especially biofertilizers.

The energy crisis has necessitated the search for renewable resources for nitrogen inputs in crop cultivation. One way to achieve partial self-sufficiency is to recycle animal and plant residues by scientific methods of composting. Using sunlight, which is abundant in the tropics, the cultivation of tiny water-borne *Azolla* ferns in aquatic nurseries on the farm has been continuously practised in Thailand, Vietnam, and China with the object of using the biomass as a nitrogen-rich green manure in rice cultivation. The *Azolla* fern, which has the nitrogen-fixing blue-green alga *Anabaena azollae* in its fronds, grows profusely as a floating plant in flooded rice fields and can fix 100–150 kg N/ha/yr in approximately 40–60 t biomass. The tremendous potential of this fern is being harnessed in other countries including India. Next only to nodulating legumes in its N_2-fixing potentialities the *Azolla-Anabaena* association appears to hold promise for the future. It is this kind of technology which can be taken as an example in planning future strategies in agriculture to save on costly inputs which come from non-renewable sources of energy.

Tropical rain forests are fast dwindling at a rate of 142,000 sq km/yr, primarily due to logging. The total area cleared annually is about 12.01 million ha (FAO sources). India alone contributes to this devastation to the extent of 1.5 million ha/yr and the highest is in Indonesia to the extent of 9 million ha/yr. Other factors which diminish forest cover are conversion of land to farming and fuelwood gathering. In fact, felling of trees for cooking energy is inescapable in third world countries and the only solution to stem this decline lies in extensive replanting or afforestation. Scientifically managed nurseries are needed for fast-growing trees. The use of nitrogen-fixing bacteria, especially rhizobia, for nitrogen-fixing leguminous trees in the nursery stage together with inoculation with vesicular-arbuscular mycorrhizal (VAM) fungi to provide facility for greater absorption of phosphorus have been considered desirable microbiological practices all over the world. The application of beneficial nitrogen-fixing and phosphate-mobilizing *Rhizobium* and VAM fungi is an integral part of modern nursery technology. Similarly, inoculation of seedlings of alder (*Alnus* spp.) and *Casuarina* spp. with appropriate *Frankia* cultures has been advocated.

The estimated area under nonforest waste lands in India is around 93,700,000 ha, where limiting factors such as salinity, alkalinity, lack of water, waterlogging, and unknown parameters operate in any programme of afforestation. While we are aware of the soil microbiology of arable soils, we are completely ignorant of the microbiological aspects of wastelands, especially with regard to the ability of these denuded soils to support nitrogen-fixing rhizobia and phosphate-mobilizing mycorrhizae. This knowledge is important since self-propelling nitrogen-fixing tree species are ideal candidates for afforestation of barren lands. The future objectives should be to identify and develop suitable microbial inoculants for selected nitrogen-fixing tree species. Some of the species recommended for planting are shown in Table 5.

Table 5: List of recommended firewood species

For Humid Tropics	
Acacia auriculiformis	*Eucalyptus citriodora*
Albizia lebbek	*Eucalyptus grandis*
Alnus jorullensis	*Eucalyptus microtheca*
Anogeissus latifolia	*Eucalyptus saligna*
Anogeissus leiocarpus	*Eucalyptus tereticornis*
Avicennia spp.	*Gliricidia maculata*
Azadirachta indica	*Gliricidia sepium*
Bruguiera spp.	*Gmelina arborea*
Cajanus cajan	*Grevillea robusta*
Calliandra calothyrsus	*Guazuma ulmifolia*
Cassia siamea	*Inga edulis*
Cassia spectabilis	*Inga vera*
Casuarina cunninghamiana	*Leucaena leucocephala*
Casuarina equisetifolia	*Muntingia calabura*
Casuarina lepidophloia	*Parkinsonia aculeata*
Eucalyptus camaldulensis	*Pithecellobium dulce*
	Pongamia glabra

Table 5 continued

Table 5 Contd.

Rhizophora apiculata
Rhizophora mangle
Rhizophora mucronata
Sesbania grandiflora
Syzygium cummii
Terminalia spp.
Trema guineensis
Trema micrantha
Trema orientalis
Other Trema spp.
For Tropical Highlands
Acacia dealbata
Acacia decurrens
Acacia mearnsii
Alnus glutinosa
Alnus jorullensis
Alnus nepalensis
Alnus rubra
Casuarina cunninghamiana
Casuarina equisetifolia
Casuarina junghuhniana
Casuarina luehmannii
Eucalyptus bicostata
Eucalyptus camaldulensis
Eucalyptus citriodora
Eucalyptus globulus
Eucalyptus gomphocephala
Eucalyptus grandis
Eucalyptus macarthuri
Eucalyptus maidenii
Eucalyptus saligna
Eucalyptus viminalis
Grevillea robusta
Trema orientalis
For Arid and Semiarid Regions
Acacia auriculiformis
Acacia brachystachya
Acacia cambagei
Acacia cyanophylla
Acacia cyclops
Acacia decurrens
Acacia holosericea
Acacia mollissima
Acacia nilotica
Acacia raddiana

Acacia seyal
Acacia tortilis
Albizia lebbek
Anogeissus leiocarpus
Anogeissus pendula
Azadirachta indica
Cajanus cajan
Cassia siamea
Casuarina cristata
Casuarina decaisneana
Casuarina equisetifolia
Casuarina glauca
Casuarina stricta
Colophospermum mopane
Eucalyptus camaldulensis
Eucalyptus citriodora
Eucalyptus gomphocephala
Eucalyptus microtheca
Eucalyptus occidentalis
Eucalyptus tereticornis
Eucalyptus viminalis
Gmelina arborea
Halozylon aphyllum
Halozylon persicum
Parkinsonia aculeata
Pinus brutia
Pinus eldarica
Pinus halepensis
Pithecellobium dulce
Prosopis alba
Prosopis caldenia
Prosopis chilensis
Prosopis cineraria
Prosopis farcta
Prosopis juliflora
Prosopis pallida
Prosopis tarmarugo
Tamarix spp.
Tamarix aphylla
Tamarix articulata
Terminalia glaucescens
Zizyphus jujuba
Zizyphus mauritiana
Zizyphus nummularia
Zizyphus spina-christi

REFERENCES

Alexander, M. (1961). *Introduction to Soil Microbiology*. John Wiley and Sons, New York.

Alexander, M. (1977). *Introduction to Soil Microbiology* (Second Edition). John Wiley and Sons, New York.

Burns, R.C., and Hardy, R.W.F. (1975). *Nitrogen Fixation in Bacteria and Higher Plants*. Springer Verlag, New York.

Burris, R.H. (1977). Overview of nitrogen fixation. In *Genetic Engineering for Nitrogen Fixation*. Ed. A. Hollaender. Plenum Press, New York. pp. 8–18.

Burton, J.C. (1967). *Rhizobium* culture and use. In *Microbial Technology*. Ed. H.J. Peppler, Reinhold Publishing Corporation, New York. pp. 1–29.

Burton, J.C. (1979). New developments in inoculating legumes. In *Recent Advances in Biological Nitrogen Fixation*. Ed. N.S. Subba Rao. Oxford & IBH Publishing Co. Pvt. Ltd., New Delhi. pp. 380–405.

Cocking, E.C., Al-Mallah, M.K., Benson, E., and Davey, M.R. (1990). Nodulation of non-legumes by rhizobia. In *Nitrogen Fixation: Achievements and objectives*. Eds. P.M. Greshoff, L.E. Roth, G. Stacey and W.E. Newton. Chapman and Hall, London.

Dazzo, F.B. (1980). Determinants of host specificity in the *Rhizobium*-clover symbiosis. In *Nitrogen Fixation*, Vol. II. Eds. W.E. Newton and W.H. Orme-Johnson. University Park Press, Baltimore. pp. 165–189.

De, P.K. (1939). The role of blue-green algae in nitrogen fixation in rice fields. *Proc. R. Soc.*, **127** (3), 121–139.

Delwiche, C.C. (1970). The nitrogen cycle. In *The Biosphere*. A Scientific American book. W.H. Freeman and Co., San Francisco. pp. 69–80.

Dobereiner, J. (1977). N_2 fixation associated with non-leguminous plants. In *Genetic Engineering for Nitrogen Fixation*. Ed. A. Hollaender, Plenum Press, New York. pp 451–461.

Dobereiner, J., Marriel, I.E., and Nery, M. (1976). Ecological distribution of *Spirillum lipoferum*, Beijerinck. *Can J. Microbiol.* **22**, 1464–1473.

Dunican, L.K., O'Gara, R., and Tierney, A.B. (1976). Plasmid control of effectiveness in *Rhizobium:* Transfer of nitrogen-fixing genes on a plasmid from *Rhizobium meliloti* to *Klebsiella aerogenes*. In *Symbiotic Nitrogen Fixation in Plants*. Ed. P.S. Nutman. Cambridge University Press, London. pp. 77–90.

Evans, H.J., Emerich, D.W., Ruiz-Argueso, Maier, R.J., and Albrecht, S.L. (1980). Hydrogen metabolism in the legume-*Rhizobium* symbiosis. In *Nitrogen Fixation*, Vol. II. Eds. W.E. Newton and W.H. Orme-Johnson. University Park Press, Baltimore. pp. 69–86.

Fred, E.B., Baldwin, I.L., and McCoy, E. (1932). *Root Nodule Bacteria and Leguminous Plants*, Univ. Wisconsin, Madison, Wisc.

Gerretsen, F.C. (1948). The influence of microorganisms on the phosphate intake by the plant. *Plant and Soil*, **1**, 51–81.

Islam, R., Ayanaba, A., and Sanders, F.E. (1980). Response of cowpea (*Vigna unguiculata*) to inoculation with VA-mycorrhizal fungi and to rock phosphate fertilization in some unsterilized Nigerian soils. *Plant and Soil*, **54**, 107–117.

Joi, M.B., and Shinde, P.A. (1976). Response of onion crop to azotobacterization. *Maharashtra Agric. Universities*, **1** (2–6), 161–162.

Lehri, L.K., and Mehrotra, C.L. (1968). Use of bacterial fertilizers in crop production in U.P. *Curr. Sci.*, **37**, 494–495.

Lehri, L.K., and Mehrotra, C.L. (1972). Effect of *Azotobacter* inoculation on the yields of vegetable crops. *Indian J. Agric. Res.,* 9(3), 201–204.

Mehrotra, C.L., and Lehri, C.K. (1971). Effect of *Azotobacter* inoculation on crop yields. *J. Indian Soc. Soil Sci.,* 19(3), 243–248.

Mishustin, E.N., and Shilnikova, V.K. (1969). Free-living nitrogen fixing bacteria of the genus *Azotobacter*. In *Soil Biology: Reviews of Research,* UNESCO. pp 72–109.

Sethi, R.P., and Subba Rao, N.S. (1968). Solubilization of tricalcium phosphate and calciu phytate by soil fungi. *J. Gen. Appl. Microbiol.,* 14, 329–331.

Shende, S.T., Apte, R.G., and Singh, T. (1977). Influence of *Azotobacter* on germination of rice and cotton seed. *Curr. Sci.,* 46, 675.

Singh, R.N. (1961). *The Role of Blue-green Algae in Nitrogen Economy of Indian Agriculture.* Indian Council of Agricultural Research, New Delhi.

Sperber, J.I. (1957). Solution of mineral phosphates by soil bacteria. *Nature,* Lond., 180, 994–995.

Subba Rao, N.S. (1976a). Field response of legumes in India to inoculation and fertilizer application. In *Symbiotic Nitrogen Fixation in Plants.* Ed. P.S. Nutman. Cambridge Univ. Press, London. pp 255–268.

Subba Rao, N.S. (1976b). Is Nitrogen Deficient? In *A Treatise on Dinitrogen Fixation,* Eds. R.W.F. Hardy and A.H. Gibson, Wiley Interscience, New York. pp. 1–32.

Subba Rao, N.S. (1977). *Soil Microorganisms and Plant Growth,* Oxford & IBH Publishing Co., New Delhi.

Subba Rao, N.S. (1979). Chemically and biologically fixed nitrogen—Potentials and prospects. In *Recent Advances in Biological Nitrogen Fixation.* Ed. N.S. Subba Rao, Oxford & IBH Publishing Co., Pvt. Ltd., New Delhi. pp. 1–7.

Subba Rao, N.S., Tilak, K.V.B.R., Singh, C.S., and Lakshmi Kumari, M. (1979a). Response of a few economic species of graminaceous plants to inoculation with *Azospirillum brasilense. Curr. Sci.,* 48, 133–134.

Subba Rao, N.S., Tilak, K.V.B.R., Lakshmi Kumari, M., and Singh, C.S. (1979b). *Azospirillum*—A new bacterial fertilizer for tropical crops. *Sci. Rep.,* CSIR, (India), 16(10), 690–692.

Subramanyam, R., and Sahay, M.N. (1964). Observation on nitrogen fixation by some blue-green algae and remarks on its potentialities in rice culture. *Proc. Indian Acad. Sci.,* 60B, 145–154.

Sundara Rao, W.V.B. (1964). Soil organic matter and microorganisms. *Bull. INSA,* 26, 221–226.

Sundara Rao, W.V.B. (1968). Phosphorus solubilization by microorganisms, *Proc. All India Symp. on Agricultural Microbiology,* Univ. Agric. Sci. Bangalore, India. pp. 21–29.

Sundara Rao, W.V.B., Mann, H.S., Pal, N.B., and Mathur, R.S. (1963). Bacterial inoculation experiments with special reference to *Azotobacter. Indian J. Agric. Sci.,* 33, 279–290.

Sundara Rao, W.V.B., Mann, H.S., Pal, N.B., and Mathur, S.P. (1966). Bacterial inoculation experiments with special reference to *Azotobacter. Ind. J. Agric. Sci.,* 33, 279–290.

USDA (1957). *The Year Book of Agriculture.* The US Government Printing Office, Washington, DC.

Vekataraman, G.S. (1972). *Algal Biofertilizers and Rice Cultivation.* Today and Tomorrow Printers and Publishers, New Delhi.

Verghese, M.C. (1977). *Issues Facing the World Fertilizer Industry,* Proceedings of the FAI-IFDC Fertilizer Seminar 1977, Trends in Consumption and Production. The Fertilizer Association of India, New Delhi PS-1/1–41.

2

Rhizobium Inoculant

The role of legumes in enriching the fertility of soil was known through the centuries. However, scientific demonstrations of the value of legumes in contributing to the nitrogen nutrition of plants were done only in the latter half of the 19th century by Bousingault, Hellriegel, and Wilfarth (quoted by Fred *et al.*, 1932). The experiments carried out by these scientists conclusively proved that nodules on legume roots are responsible for fixing atmospheric nitrogen.

Leguminous plants are classified into three major botanical subfamilies of the family Leguminoseae — the Ceasalpinioideae, the Mimosoideae, and the Papilionoideae. There are nearly 750 genera and 18,000–19,000 species of leguminous plants of which 500 genera and approximately 10,000 species belong to the subfamily Papilionoideae. Not all leguminous plants bear nodules on their root system and it is known that certain tree species do not possess them at all. Hardly 16–20 per cent of leguminoseae have so far been examined for nodulation, of which 90 per cent of Mimosoideae, 23 per cent of Ceasalpinioideae, and 97 per cent of Papilionoideae possess root nodules.

Apart from legumes nodulated by the genus *Rhizobium*, roots of some plants belonging to diverse families are also nodulated by members of actinomycetales (tentatively classified in the genus *Frankia*) and fix considerable amounts of nitrogen. These plants are equally important in nitrogen fixation and will be discussed elsewhere in the book since inoculants are also produced currently and often used for inoculating such plants.

Isolation of *Rhizobium* from Nodules

Nodules of different legumes are of various sizes and shapes. In the same plant, nodules of all sizes are present. Leguminous plants are carefully uprooted and the root system washed in running water to remove adhering soil particles. The colour of the nodules varies — some are transluscent to white-brown and many others are brown, pink, and green, depending on the state of the pigment in them. In practice, healthy, unbroken, firm, and preferably pink nodules are selected and washed in water. They are immersed in 0.1 per cent acidified $HgCl_2$ for 4–5 minutes. In some laboratories, 3–5 per cent H_2O_2 is used instead of $HgCl_2$. Nodules which are surface-sterilized with $HgCl_2$ are washed repeatedly with sterile water and dipped in 70 per cent ethyl alcohol followed by more washings with sterile water. These practices vary in different laboratories but the critical point is that microorganisms on the surface of the nodule must be killed by a sterilizing agent and the sterilizing agent must also be washed off the nodules before they are used for isolation.

The nodule is crushed in a small aliquot of sterile water with the help of a glass rod. There are two ways by which colonies of rhizobia can be isolated: either serial dilutions are prepared from the nodule extract and aliquots of appropriate dilutions are spread on yeast extract mannitol agar (YEMA) or the fluid from crushed nodules is spread on the surface of YEMA plates with the help of a smooth glass rod. The plates are incubated up to 10 days in an incubator at 26°C. Large gummy colonies of bacteria will emerge within 4–5 days and later, it is likely that smaller colonies will also arise. Not all colonies of bacteria which come up on plates are necessarily rhizobia since bacteria of a related genus *Agrobacterium* may also grow on agar plates along with *Rhizobium*. The entire procedure is schematically shown in Fig. 1.

Identification

The one sure way of identifying rhizobia is to conduct plant tests and see if effective nodules are produced on roots. A plant test is done under bacteriologically controlled conditions with assemblies ranging from small tubes to pots. Before these tests are done for a large number of cultures one may have to carry out certain routine cultural tests (Vincent, 1970).

Growth on media — Rhizobia grow very poorly on peptone glucose agar but grow well on YEMA in the form of watery or white

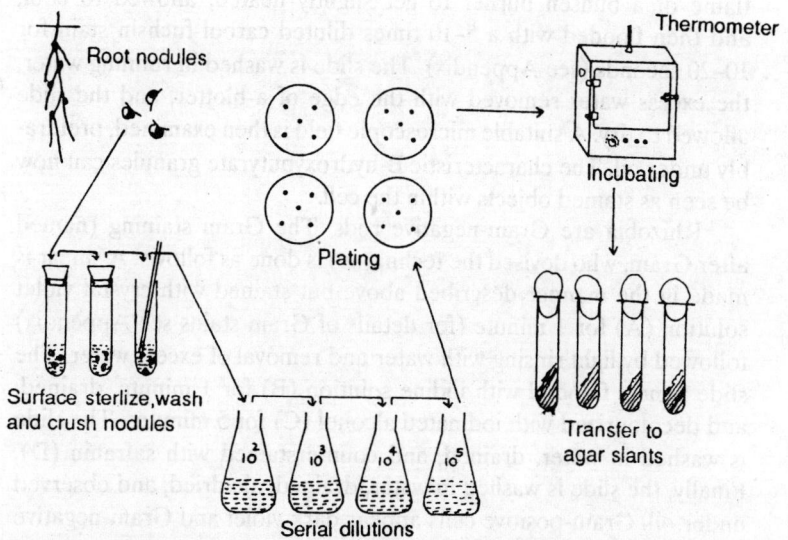

Fig. 1. Schematic representation of procedures recommended for isolation of *Rhizobium* from root nodules.

colonies (see Appendix for medium composition). Most strains produce gum (extracellular polysaccharide) of varying composition.

Microscopy — The reader is advised to go through a standard textbook on microbiology to get acquainted with basic principles of microscopy (Pelczar *et al.*, 1977). Under a phase contrast microscope, rhizobia are discernible even in simple water mounts and show up the presence of characteristic refractile granules of B-hydroxybutyrate within cells. *Rhizobium* cells in clover rhizosphere are small to medium-sized (0.5–0.9×1.2–$3.0\,\mu$). They are motile when young and have bipolar, subpolar, or peritrichous flagella. Under an electron microscope, two membranes averaging 7–$9\,\mu$ in diameter are apparent in *R. trifolii*. The outer membrane is the rigid cell wall and the inner membrane is the protoplasmic lining. In between the two membranes is a regular non-rigid intermembrane area ($50\,\mu$). The *Rhizobium* cell has a large, irregularly shaped nuclear region in the centre surrounded by a narrow region of denser protoplasm (Mosse, 1964).

Smears of bacteria are made as follows: a loopful of a selected bacterium is spread out on a microscope slide in a drop of water and allowed to dry in air. The slide is passed through the top portion of the flame of a bunsen burner to get slightly heated, allowed to cool, and then flooded with a 5–10 times diluted carbol fuchsin stain for 10–20 seconds (see Appendix). The slide is washed in running water, the excess water removed with the edge of a blotter, and the slide allowed to dry. A suitable microscopic field is then examined, preferably under oil. The characteristic B-hydroxybutyrate granules can now be seen as stained objects within the cell.

Rhizobia are Gram-negative rods. The Gram staining (named after Gram, who devised the technique) is done as follows: A smear is made in the manner described above but stained with crystal violet solution (A) for 1 minute (for details of Gram stains see Appendix) followed by light rinsing with water and removal of excess water. The slide is now flooded with iodine solution (B) for 1 minute, drained, and decolourized with iodinated alcohol (C) for 5 minutes. The slide is washed in water, drained, and counterstained with safranin (D). Finally, the slide is washed in water, drained, air-dried, and observed under oil. Gram-positive cells appear dark violet and Gram-negative cells appear clear red.

Congo red test — This test is designed to differentiate rhizobia from agrabacteria. An aliquot of 2.5 ml of a 1 per cent solution of the dye in water is added to a litre of YEMA (for composition see Appendix). On this medium, when suspected strains of nodule bacteria are plated, rhizobia stand out as white, translucent, glistening, elevated, and comparatively small colonies with entire margins in contrast to stained colonies of agrobacteria.

Hofer's alkaline broth test — The test is based on the fact that agrobacteria grow at higher pH levels, while rhizobia are unable to do so. A medium having high pH of 11.0 (see Appendix) is used to screen new isolates of nodule bacteria for this purpose.

Lactose agar — Agrobacteria utilize lactose by the action of the enzyme ketolactase, whereas rhizobia cannot utilize the sugar. This can be detected on agar medium containing lactose at 10 g/l, as follows: Nodule bacteria are grown on lactose agar plates for 4–10 days (depending on the strains) and the plates are flooded with Benedict's reagent (see Appendix). The formation of yellow colouration due to Cu_2O indicates the presence of agrobacteria.

Plant Tests

The ability of *Rhizobium* to infect small-seeded legumes can be tested on nitrogen-free media containing agar, vermiculite, sand, etc.

Examples of small-seeded legumes are berseem clover and lucerne nodulated by *R. trifolii* and *R. meliloti*, respectively. For large-seeded legumes, other methods are available which will be described later in this chapter.

Seedling agar tubes for small seeded legumes — Thornton (1930) and Jensen (1942) used different media for seedling agar (see Appendix for composition). For this purpose, depending on the requirements, various sizes of tubes plugged with cotton have been used in nodulation studies. The volume of agar to be poured into tubes depends on the requirements of a particular study. Gibson (1963) modified the seedling agar by adding several trace elements (see Appendix). Nitrogen controls are usually maintained by adding the required amounts of KNO_3 solution.

Seeds are surface-sterilized to get rid of superficial micro-organisms. There are a number of ways of doing this: (1) The seeds are rinsed in 90 per cent ethyl alcohol and suspended for 3–5 minutes in acidified 0.2 per cent $HgCl_2$. They are then washed repeatedly in sterilized water and planted directly on agar in test tubes. Otherwise, they are initially germinated on water agar in inverted petri plates so as to provide straight roots and subsequently the seedlings are transferred to tubes. (2) Seeds are also surface-sterilized by being suspended for 10 minutes in 3–5 per cent H_2O_2, freshly prepared chlorine water, or hypochlorite solution. Later, the seeds are washed in several changes of sterile water to get rid of the sterilant. (3) Employing dry seeds and dry test tubes, concentrated sulphuric acid could be used for surface-sterilizing hard-coated seeds such as those of berseem and lucerne. The test tubes and seeds are kept for 24 hours in a desiccator over $CaCl_2$ and then used for surface sterilization with concentrated sulphuric acid for 10–20 minutes. The seeds are then washed in quick changes of sterile water to avoid burning of the seed coat.

Nitrogen-free agar is poured into each tube, the open end of which is closed with a loose cotton plug (so as to permit sufficient aeration) and sterilized in an autoclave at 15 lbs pressure (120°C) for 20 minutes (Fig. 2). They are either slanted when slants are required (which is preferable) or retained as such when deep agar is required. The lower portion of the tubes is shielded with black paper to avoid light falling on the root system and the tubes are put into racks for convenience in handling.

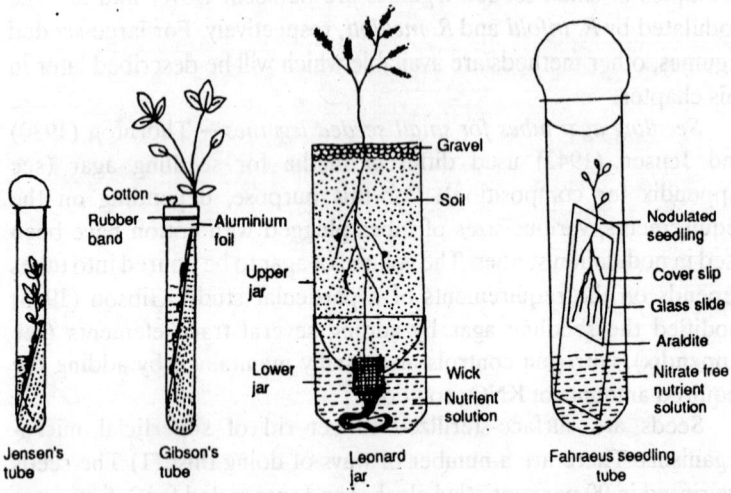

Fig. 2. Different methods for testing *Rhizobium* isolates for nodulation abilities — from left to right: Jensen's seedling agar method showing seedling growing on agar slant; agar seedling method modified by Gibson; Leonard jar assembly for growing large-seeded legumes; and Fahraeus seedling tube for studying infection of roots by rhizobia.

Inoculation of seed or seedlings is done by pouring a suspension of specific *Rhizobium* made from scrapings of growth from 2- to 4-day-old fresh slants. The suspension is poured either into petri dishes containing germinated seeds or mixed in 1/4 strength nitrogen-free nutrient solution without agar and poured into tubes (about 5–10 ml for each tube) so as to bring part of the root system in contact with the solution. When pre-inoculated seeds or seedlings are transferred to agar slants, 1/4 strength nitrogen-free nutrient solution (5–10 ml for each tube) without the rhizobial suspension is poured into tubes. While handling a large number of tubes, some sort of automatic device for transferring exact aliquots of nutrient solution into tubes would be of great help. In fact, all such modifications involving methods of handling tubes, nutrient medium, and seeds or seedlings vary from individual to individual and much depends upon the plant type and the nature of the experiment.

Partly enclosed seedling agar tube — As opposed to completely enclosed seedling agar tubes, this method allows freedom to the shoot system to grow freely in air while the root system is still enclosed in a closed space (Gibson, 1963).

Nitrogen-free agar is poured (approximately 13–15 ml) into tubes (150 x 20 mm), slanted, and allowed to solidify in such a way that the slope of the agar reaches the top of the tube. The top of each tube is covered by a thin circle of aluminium foil and held in place with a rubber band. A small aperture is made on the foil and fitted with cotton wool, which not only affords aeration but also acts as an inlet for replenishing nutrient solution in tubes (Fig. 2). In all these procedures, the usual sterility control must be maintained to prevent contamination. Aseptically grown seedlings are placed in a second hole (opposite to the hole carrying the cotton plug) in such a way that the root system lies on the agar slope and the shoot system comes out of the tube. This is done by using a pair of sterile forceps, care being taken not to injure the seedling while transplanting. The tubes are now covered with larger specimen tubes containing pieces of cotton wetted with sterile water to prevent desiccation of the seedling. The cover tube is removed when the seedlings are well established. The watering hole is used for pouring in sterile liquid medium and for inoculating seedlings at different age levels. The tubes are covered with black or brown paper to prevent light from falling on the root system. It has been claimed that this partly enclosed method of growing seedlings is better than the completely enclosed seedling agar method described earlier.

Leonard bottle-jar assembly (Leonard, 1944; Vincent, 1970) — A wide bottle of 750 ml capacity with its bottom cut and neatly ground is inverted in a glass jar of suitable dimensions in such a way that the neck of the bottle snugly fits in and occupies a position as shown in Fig. 2. A suitable wick (cotton wool or ordinary cotton lamp wick will do) is passed through the narrow end of the bottle in such a manner that it not only trails itself in the nitrate-free nutrient solution in the jar but also touches the uppermost region of the sand substrate in the bottle. The wick is intended to maintain a steady supply of nutrient to the growing plant by the capillary action of the sand. The sand substrate is wetted with 1/4 strength nitrate-free nutrient solution (see Appendix) until the solution begins to drip through the wick at the bottom. The jar at the bottom is also filled with the same nutrient solution and the top portion of the assembly is covered with a petri dish. The assembly (Fig. 2) may be covered with a water-resistant brown paper bag which may be partly retained with the help of rubber bands during the growth of plants to protect the roots from light and contamination with other microorganisms through the junction between the two glass parts. The entire set-up is sterilized in an autoclave at 20 lbs pressure (126°C) for 2 hours and cooled before use.

At this stage, seeds are surface-sterilized, washed with sterilized water, and sown on sand. On germination, the petri dish is removed, seedlings are inoculated with a bacterial suspension, and dry sterilized gravel poured in between the seedlings to prevent aerial contamination. As usual, uninoculated sets and nitrate controls are always maintained for comparison.

Depending upon the size of the plant grown in the jar assembly, the nutrient solution at the bottom jar may have to be changed by separating the two halves of the assembly under aseptic conditions. It is advisable to practise setting up these assemblies for a while before attempting to screen rhizobial strains for efficiency grading.

Pot culture tests — Pot culture tests are done using sand or soil. Fine-grade river sand is washed well in tap water and immersed in acid for 2 days. The acid is decanted and the sand washed in several changes of tap water and distilled water to get rid of the last traces of acid. The sand is neutralized, dried, autoclaved (20 lbs pressure for 20 minutes), and put in plastic or porcelain pots. *Rhizobium*-inoculated seeds are sown and watered with nitrogen-free nutrient solution as and when necessary through a plastic or porcelain saucer placed in the lower end of the pot. Any other suitable material like vermiculite, perlite, or sand could be used instead of sand.

There is, however, no substitute for soil for growing plants although native strains of rhizobia present in soil may interfere with tests intended to determine the efficiency of individual strains. Testing rhizobial strains for their performance in unsterilized soil helps in judging the competitive ability of selected strains against the native population of rhizobia in soil. Soils which are autoclaved are relatively free from native microbial population. By using autoclaved soil (at 20 lbs pressure for 2 hours), it is possible to test strains of a given *Rhizobium* sp. for comparative performance. By following this method, the efficiency of different isolates of *R. japonicum* on soybean has been successfully tested in autoclaved soil at the Microbiology Division, Indian Agricultural Research Institute, for several years. Soil from fallow plots (pH 7.8) is mixed well, sieved, and filled in earthenware pots at the rate of 10 kg per pot. Sterilized river sand watered with nitrate-free mineral medium or sand and soil mixture (1:1) can also be used, depending on the experience of the individual worker. The pots are watered to the level of 50 per cent moisture-holding capacity of the soil and sterilized in a large horizontal autoclave at 20 lbs pressure for 2 hours. The pots are allowed to incubate in a pot culture house for four days and the soil in each pot is loosened and mixed well with the help of a stout glass rod. *Rhizobium*-inoculated seeds are sown and uninoculated as well as nitrogen controls are maintained for comparison.

Many soils contain native strains of *Rhizobium* capable of nodulating a given species. Therefore, the object of strain testing is not only to find out effective strains among myriads of strains isolated from different agroclimatic areas but also to see if a given effective strain can compete with native strains and enhance yield. With this objective, screening is initially done in pots using unsterilized soil and later, some of the selected strains are field-tested in different locations before the strains are recommended for mass production. However, Vincent (1970) advocates soil cores from different places whereby natural sampling of soil can be done so as to retain the physical and chemical properties of soil, and also the spatial distribution of rhizobia *in situ*. These soil cores can be transported and tests done conveniently in one place to determine the efficiency of native rhizobia. Watering is done by boiled and cooled water to eliminate the influence of extraneous rhizobia.

Growth cabinets — Controlling the environmental temperature is the main problem in raising plants in glass houses under Indian conditions, unless the laboratories are situated in high altitudes (5000 feet above see level) where one can expect mild climate for most of the year. For small-scale experiments, the use of growth cabinets which can be cooled by air-conditioners or water coolers is the method of choice for season-bound legumes. Such cabinets or small rooms can be fitted with warm-white fluorescent tubes supplemented with one or two incandescent lamps for each pair of fluorescent lights. The illumination can be lateral; overhead illumination can also serve provided the distances between plants are maintained so as to prevent mutual shading. Suitable reflectors using aluminium foils can be provided to improve the intensity of light. The photoperiod can be adjusted from 12 to 16 hours a day, depending on the nature of the plants, with the help of automatic switches.

Pot culture house — In tropical countries such as India, glass houses are unsuitable since they tend to heat up and expensive coolers are needed to bring down the temperature. Instead, pot culture houses with wire-netting on all sides (to prevent birds from damaging the crᵣ)s) have proved useful for most of the year in warm climates prev ng in India.

Is. lated root culture technique (Raggio *et al.*, 1957; Barrios *et al.*, 1963; Bunting and Horrocks, 1964) — In this method, excised roots are used. The growing root is cut from an actively growing 2- to 4-day-old seedling and the blunt end implanted in a small vial containing organic constituents in solidified agar. The tip of the excised root is suspended in a nitrate-free mineral salt medium in a petri dish or in a test tube into which a suspension of *Rhizobium* is added. In this manner, the organic constituents are provided through the cut end of a root and the growing end receives mineral constituents along with *Rhizobium*. Nodules begin to develop on excised roots within 3 weeks. The composition of the media used in excised root nodulation studies is given in the Appendix. The method may be useful to test the effect of different chemicals on nodulation under controlled conditions, but cannot be recommended for testing rhizobial strains for efficiency.

Callus and cell cultures — Explants of roots, stem, and apical meristem can be grown into an undifferentiated callus mass on a suitable basal medium (for tissue culture medium, see Appendix). From these calli, a well-differentiated plant can emerge which may be transferred to soil and grown until flowering and fruit setting take place. Similarly, suspensions of isolated cells or protoplasts of plant tissues can be grown and multiplied aseptically. In recent years, root calli and cell cultures have been used to study interactions of plant tissues with rhizobia (Holsten *et al.*, 1971; Ranga Rao *et al.*, 1973) and *Azotobacter* with the ultimate object of finding out whether nitrogen-fixation capacity can be transferred from bacteria to higher plants and thereby render all land plants self-sufficient with regard to nitrogen. This approach needs coordinated action among biochemists, geneticists, and microbiologists.

Root hair infection method — Seedlings of small-seeded legumes can be grown on agar slants made up of nitrogen-free medium, fixed in 4 per cent formalin or acrolein at regular intervals, and their roots examined for the presence of infection threads in root hairs and emergence of nodule primordia on roots. Depending on the extent of infection, the strains can be rated for virulence. Fahraeus and Ljunggren (1968) devised a technique for continuous observation of roots which was later modified by Nutman (personal communication). This method consists of overlaying a large cover glass on a microscope slide in such a way that the four corners are mounted over tiny bits of cover glass and sealed with araldite so as to leave enough space between the cover glass and the glass slide. The microscope slide is now inserted in a boiling tube containing 5–10 ml of nitrogen-free nutrient medium. The tube is plugged with cotton wool, autoclaved, cooled, and used for growing seedlings. Soon after germination, the radicles are placed in the space between the slide and the cover glass and the seedling allowed to grow. The shoot system will now grow in the space inside the glass tube and the root system elongates in between the slide and the cover glass. The slide with the intact seedling can be periodically removed and examined under a microscope for infection threads (Fig. 2).

Field trials — The ultimate test for an effective strain of *Rhizobium* is to find out how well it is able to establish and perform under field conditions. Choosing a site for field trials is an important consideration. The first prerequisite is to minimize the interference by native strains of rhizobia and hence, soils with low count of rhizobia and low content of available nitrogen are preferable.

Bell and Nutman (1971) have used a design for field experiment which seems to meet the requirements for field testing of rhizobial strains. The treatments used in the 4 x 4 x 2 factorial design of four randomized blocks were as follows: G — ryegrass; O — uninoculated lucerne; I — lucerne inoculated with ineffective (non-nitrogen-fixing) strain. The nitrogen fertilizer treatments were: N — no fertilizer (0 kg/ha); N_1 — small amount (66 kg/ha) of nitro chalk, a commercial nitrate fertilizer containing 21 per cent N and 18 per cent calcium carbonate; N_2 — medium amount (132 kg/ha) of nitro chalk; and N_3 — large amount (198 kg/ha) of nitro chalk. The soil amelioration treatments were: U — unmodified nutrition (no lime or PK, etc.), and M — with lime and PK, etc., to bring pH to 7.0 and to supply all nutrients other than N such as P, K, Ca, S, or minor elements.

Randomization of G, O, I, and E treatments was restricted by arranging them in strips across each block and keeping the strip order in each block at random. This was done to restrict contamination between inoculated and uninoculated controls. The number of plots for four replications was halved (128 to 64) by confounding some interactions with block and single plot errors. The plan of one block of field experiment is shown in Fig. 3.

Fertilizer and lime were applied before sowing. A heavy inoculum was provided (50,000 bacterial cells/seed) by way of seed inoculation.

Between strips and blocks, 1.0 m wide paths were kept clean by hand weeding or herbicide spraying. The usual precautions to prevent

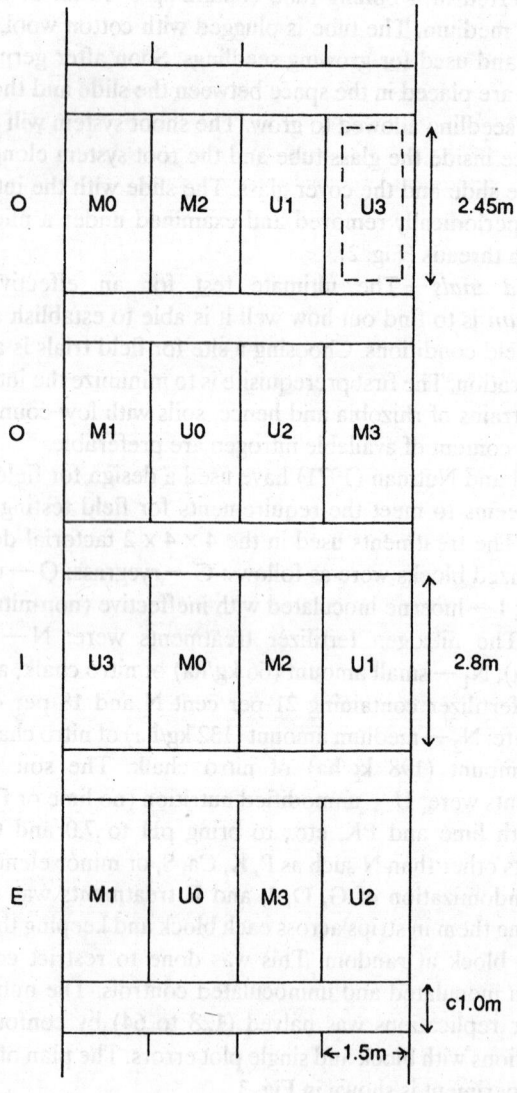

Fig. 3. Plan of one block of field experiment, approximately to scale. Harvest area (– – –) 2.45 m x 0.91 m. Values 0, 1, 0, and 3 indicate N levels. For further details see text (from Bell and Nutman, 1971).

damage by animals and birds were taken. Data were taken at intervals on yield, nodulation, and rhizobial counts.

Measurement of Nitrogen Fixation

The Kjeldahl method has been routinely used for measurement of biologically fixed nitrogen. It serves the purpose when differences are large enough to provide room for errors of sampling and other inherent factors in the procedures followed.

One of the accurate ways to measure N_2 fixation is to quantify the uptake of ^{15}N-enriched N_2 (Burris et al., 1943). It necessitates the use of expensive mass spectrometer and $^{15}N_2$ gas. The natural abundance of this stable isotope is 0.3663 atoms and hence any deviation from this natural abundance can be calculated as under:

$$\% \ ^{15}N \text{ excess} = \text{Atom\% } ^{15}N \text{ (of sample)} - \text{Atom\% } ^{15}N \text{ in control.}$$

Bottles stoppered with rubber serum stoppers or plastic bags can be used to house the suspected N_2-fixing sample, the air evacuated from the bottles, and the bottles gassed with $^{15}N_2$ through a glass syringe piercing the rubber stopper. After exposure to predetermined periods, the samples are inactivated by acid or other means and the gas analysed by injection into a mass spectrometer to ascertain the ^{15}N concentration of the N_2 which was fed into the sample (Fiedler and Proksch, 1975). The sample under test for $^{15}N_2$ fixation is digested by the Kjeldahl method and an aliquot of the ammonia obtained is used for determining the total nitrogen while the remainder is concentrated, converted to N_2 and its $^{15}N_2$ level determined by mass spectrometer. From the data on total nitrogen in the sample, ^{15}N concentration of N_2 gas, and the ^{15}N level of the sample, the amount of $^{15}N_2$ fixed by the test sample can be calculated.

Uniformly labelled nitrogenous fertilizer can be used to measure nitrogen fixation. It is possible to arrive at figures regarding nitrogen derived from fertilizer (Ndff) by knowing the atom% ^{15}N excess of the labelled fertilizer and the isotope analysis of the plant tissue as follows (Legg and Sloger, 1975):

$$\% \text{ Ndff} = \frac{\text{Atom\% } ^{15}N \text{ excess (plant)}}{\text{Atom\% } ^{15}N \text{ excess (fertilizer)}} \times 100$$

Therefore, % nitrogen derived from other sources such as soil or air (Ndof) = 100 − Ndff

$$\text{Then, \% fixed N} = \left[1 - \frac{\text{Atom\% } ^{15}N \text{ excess (plant)}}{\text{Atom\% } ^{15}N \text{ excess (soil)}}\right] \times 100$$

The total amount of nitrogen available for a given plant is known as 'A' value (Fried and Broeshart, 1967). The quantity of symbiotically fixed nitrogen by a legume crop under field conditions can be estimated by simultaneous determination of 'A' value of a control non-legume crop along with the legume crop. The non-leguminous crop is generally a cereal crop but in the case of soybean, a non-nodulating isoline of soybean has also been used. The application of fertilizer is done at a low level to the legume crop so as to allow symbiotic process to go on uninterrupted while the non-legume crop receives a high rate of fertilizer. The 'A' value of non-legume crop reflects only soil nitrogen, whereas the 'A' value of the nodulating crop represents soil as well as symbiotically fixed nitrogen. Therefore, the amount of symbiotically fixed nitrogen expressed in kg N/ha can be calculated by multiplying the difference in 'A' values between the legume and the non-legume crop by the percentage utilization of fertilizer nitrogen by the nodulating legume crop (Fried and Broeshart, 1975).

Nitrogenase, the enzyme which reduces N_2 to NH_3, also reduces acetylene (C_2H_2) to ethylene (C_2H_4). This property has been used to measure the extent of nitrogen fixation by any sample (Dilworth, 1966; Koch and Evans, 1966; Schollhorn and Burris, 1967) and the method has been very popular as the 'acetylene reduction' method. It is simple, sensitive, inexpensive and widely used. Small serum bottles, plastic hypodermic syringes, and intact potted plants in plastic containers, plastic bags, or suitable airtight contraptions can be used to house the test materials. The container is evacuated and C_2H_2 gas admitted by a cylinder or through a hypodermic syringe. Generally, a mixture of C_2H_2, O_2, and argon is used. After incubation to desired periods, samples of the gas from the containers are withdrawn and analysed for C_2H_4 levels by means of gas chromatography. Ethylene standards are used to produce a standard curve from which the C_2H_4 levels of experimental samples are calculated. A conversion factor of 1/3 N_2 reduced per C_2H_2 reduced is generally used to calculate the amount of N_2 fixed, which is based on the fact that C_2H_2 reduction involves a two-electron and N_2 reduction a six-electron transfer reaction. This ratio varies according to experimental conditions and strictly speaking it is desirable to obtain specific factors for each set of experimental conditions so that reliable calculations can be made (Burris, 1974).

Classification

Rhizobium has been classified in Bergey's *Manual of Determinative Bacteriology* in such diverse families as Azotobacteriaceae, Mycobacteriaceae, Myxobacteriaceae, and Pseudomonadaceae. Speciation of *Rhizobium* is based on the cross-inoculation grouping from results obtained by the classical studies of Fred *et al.* (1932). The basis for cross-inoculation grouping lies in the ability of an isolate of *Rhizobium* to form nodules on roots of a limited species of legumes which are related to one another. Based on this principle, rhizobia that can form nodules on roots of certain legumes have been collectively taken as a species. This system of classification has helped in the practical methods of legume inoculation by rhizobia. Under this scheme, seven species are generally recognized (Table 6).

Table 6: Cross-inoculation groups of *Rhizobium*

Rhizobium spp.	*Cross-inoculation grouping*	*Legume types*
R. leguminosarum	Pea group	*Pisum, Vicia, Lens*
R. phaseoli	Bean group	*Phaseolus*
R. trifolii	Clover group	*Trifolium*
R. meliloti	Alfalfa group	*Melilotus, Medicago, Trigonella*
R. lupini	Lupini group	*Lupinus, Orinthopus*
R. japonicum	Soybean group	*Glycine*
Rhizobium sp.	Cowpea group	*Vigna, Arachis*

The system of cross-inoculation grouping of rhizobia is not free from limitations because rhizobia have been often found to cross-infect or interchange between groups. However, there is no better alternative to this system. Therefore, many rhizobiologists have come to regard the cross-inoculation grouping as a convenient and satisfactory way to classify rhizobia into species.

It is also possible to differentiate rhizobia on the basis of growth on a defined substrate, as fast growers and slow growers. Studies have been done on morphological and physiological characters (colonial character, vitamin, carbohydrate and nitrogen nutrition, antibiotic sensitivities, and infective attributes) of rhizobia to find out if a better method of rhizobial classification can be proposed. The results have shown that fast-growing pea and bean rhizobia (*R. trifolii, R. leguminosarum,* and *R. phaseoli*) could be united under a common species name, *R. leguminosarum* Frank (the type species in Bergey's classification) and the fast-growing *R. meliloti* Dangeard could remain a distinctive species. The agrobacteria (*A. radiobacter* and *A. tume-faciens*) could be united as one species, *R. radiobacter* (Beijerinck and Van Delden Lohnis). The slow-growing lupin, soybean, and cowpea rhizobia, *R. lupini, R. japonicum,* and *Rhizobium* sp. (cowpea group) could be designated as a separate genus *Phytomyxa* with a new name *P. japonicum* Kirchner. In this manner, root nodule bacteria could be delimited into the two genera *Rhizobium* and *Phytomyxa*, the former having three species, *R. leguminosarum, R. meliloti,* and *R. radio-bacter*, and the latter with only one species, *P. japonicum* (Graham, 1964).

This proposal has been re-examined by other workers. They came to the conclusion that the genus *Rhizobium* need not be split at the generic level and that *Agrobacterium* need not necessarily be merged with *Rhizobium* (t Mannetje, 1967).

Rhizobia are able to produce acid or alkali on YEMA medium. Based on this criterion, the fast-growing *R. phaseoli, R. trifolii, R. leguminosarum,* and *R. meliloti* could be grouped as acid producers while the slow-growing *R. japonicum, R. lupini,* and *Rhizobium* sp. (cowpea) could be grouped as non-acid producers. The slow-growing, non-acid-producing rhizobia have been considered the ancestral forms of rhizobia, since they are associated with primitive tropical legumes growing in alkaline environment (Vincent, 1970).

The base composition of pure DNA (expressed as molar percentage of guanine and cytosine) of several rhizobia has been analysed and a suggestion has been made to regroup rhizobia as fast-growing peritrichous strains having a low percentage (G + C) composition in the range of 58.6–63.1 per cent which belong to *R. leguminosarum* and *R. meliloti*. On the contrary, it has been suggested that the sub-polarly flagellated, slow-growing strains having a somewhat higher percentage (G + C) mostly in the range of 62.8–65.5 per cent come under *R. japonicum* (De Ley and Russel, 1965). However, more studies are needed in this direction before we can come to any definite conclusions on the use of DNA base composition data in the classification of nodule bacteria.

As per the ninth edition of Bergey's *Manual of Determinative Bacteriology,* the genus *Rhizobium* consists of three reorganized species: *R. leguminosarum,* which will contain three biovars (*trifolii, phaseoli,* and *viceae), R. meliloti,* and *R. loti*. In this reorganization, the earlier three species — *R. leguminosarum, R. trifolii,* and *R. phaseoli* — have come under the common species *R. leguminosarum.* The fast-growing members of the cowpea rhizobia and the earlier *R. lupinus* have been included in *R. loti*. The new genus *Bradyrhizobium* has been created which consists of the species *B. japonicum*. This new genus encompasses all the slow-growing members of the cowpea rhizobia and the earlier species of *R. japonicum*.

The newly proposed classification is as follows (from Elkan, 1984):

Genus I: *Rhizobium*

Rhizobium leguminosarum (biovars *trifolii, phaseoli, viceae*), *R. meliloti, R. loti* — fast-growing, sub-polar flagellated strains from *Lotus* and *Lupinus* with strong affinity for *L. corniculatus, L. densiflorus,* and *Anthyllis vulneraria* (but also nodulates *Orinthopus sativum*). Includes the fast-growing strains nodulating *Cicer, Sesbania, Leucaena, Mimosa,* and *Lablab*.

Genus II: *Bradyrhizobium*

Slow-growing, polar, or sub-polar flagellated strains nodulating soybean, *Lotus uliginosus, L. pendulatus,* and *Vigna*. Includes those slow-growing strains nodulating *Cicer, Sesbania, Leucaena, Mimosa, Lablab* and *Acacia*. The possibility exists that other species will eventually be defined within the genus, but for the present it is suggested that, other than *B. japonicum* (the type species), the various cultures be designated as *Bradyrhizobium* sp. (*Vigna*), *Bradyrhizobium* sp. (*Cicer*), etc.

Serological methods have helped in distinguishing strains among different rhizobia. There are at least two distinct kinds of antigens associated with the rhizobial cell — on the main body of the cell (somatic) and on the flagella. Agglutinations of a suspension of specific *Rhizobium* due to flagellar antigens can be distinguished from those due to somatic ones by the nature of its reaction. By this means, it has been shown that rhizobia are serologically heterogeneous. The combined results of both somatic and flagellar reactions have served to distinguish strains within a cross-inoculation group. Serological methods have helped in collecting information on the distribution of strains in different agroclimatic zones and within a plant or within a nodule. One of the important uses of serological methods is to distinguish nodules formed by inoculum applied to seeds from those formed by strains of *Rhizobium* already present in soil (Dudman and Brockwell, 1968; Vincent, 1970).

The work done at the Microbiology Division of the Indian Agricultural Research Institute on the serology of rhizobia has revealed interesting results. It has been shown that rhizobia from *Cicer arietinum* are antigenetically related to *R. leguminosarum,* whereas *Rhizobium* of *Vigna radiata* (mung) is related to *R. japonicum* (Dadarwal and Sen, 1973). The competitiveness of efficient strains of three different species of *Rhizobium* introduced into a given soil have been shown to decrease in the following order: *R. japonicum, Rhizobium* sp. (cowpea group from *C. arietinum*), and *R. leguminosarum.* Similarly, the competitive ability of a strain of *Rhizobium* from *V. radiata* is dependent on the genotype of the host (Dadarwal and Sen, 1974). It has also been shown that bacteroids from nodules differ in their internal antigenic constitution from the cultured rhizobial cells of the same species (Dadarwal *et al.,* 1973). Dadarwal *et al.* (1974) isolated rhizobia from five wild species of *Arachis (A. duranensis, A. prostrata, A. villosa, A. glaberata,* and *A. marginata).* By immunodiffusion technique, the authors have grouped 44 rhizobial isolates from *Arachis* spp. into 33 different strain serotypes. From serological and nodulation studies, Gaur and Sen (1977) have stated that *Rhizobium* of *C. arietinum* cannot be grouped with any existing cross-inoculation groups and has to be given a special status.

Maintenance

A collection of cultures in any microbiological laboratory may be regarded as its nerve centre. The purity of cultures maintained reflects the reputation of the institution and hence great care has to be exercised in maintaining cultures in any permanent culture collection. An additional essential feature of a good collection of rhizobia is the constant check to be exercised in verifying the nodulation ability of cultures on their respective hosts. Under the auspices of the International Biological Programme, a world catalogue of culture collections of rhizobia has been published (Hamatova *et al.,* 1971) which may be consulted.

Agar culture — Maintaining cultures on YEMA (see Appendix) after periodic sub-culturing at intervals (15–30 days) has been recognized as the time honoured method. It is a very convenient method for retaining cultures used in routine work, provided duplicates are preserved permanently by the lyophilization method. The longevity of the cultures may be enhanced by preserving agar cultures at low temperatures (4°C) after incubating them initially for 3–10 days at 28°C to ensure enough growth of the bacteria without any contamination. In tropical climate, premature desiccation of cultures can be avoided by keeping a glass tray filled with water in the incubator to raise the humidity of the chamber.

Agar culture stored under paraffin oil — After the cultures are grown for 3–10 days and checked for freedom from contamination, sterile medicinal grade liquid paraffin is poured over the agar slope until the bacterial growth is fully covered. To ensure complete sterilization of paraffin, the oil is sterilized in moist tubes. The cultures under paraffin can be stored under low temperature (4°C) when covered aseptically with screw caps.

Porcelain bead method — The following materials are needed for this method: airtight screw cap small bottles, silica gel, and unglazed porcelain beads (electrical equipment). The glass bottles and the screw caps are sterilized in an autoclave separately, dried in a hot-air oven, and cooled before assembling the pieces. Silica gel (3–4 g) is packed in a piece of tough gauze or translucent cloth material. The porcelain beads are washed well and air-dried, and both the gel and the beads are sterilized in a hot-air oven. The silica gel pack is inserted into the bottle before stoppering.

The sterilized beads are dipped in an actively growing bacterial culture broth, the excess of broth drained over sterilized cotton wool, or suitable absorbing material, and the beads inserted into the bottle following the usual aseptic measures. Dry silica gel is blue and turn pink when it absorbs moisture and therefore, as long as the gel is blue, the culture is satisfactory. Cultures can be preserved and transported in this way. As and when required, one bead is transferred to fresh YEMA for reisolation (for further details refer to Norris, 1963).

Lyophilization — For this purpose, small ampoules are used. The tapering side of the ampoule is opened, plugged lightly with cotton wool, and sterilized. A strip of filter paper, on which the code number of the culture is typed, may be introduced into ampoule. A bacterial suspension from an actively growing agar slant is made from scrapings of bacterial growth. The suspending medium is an aqueous solution of 10 per cent sucrose and 5 per cent peptone which is sterilized prior to use. The cotton wool in each ampoule is gently removed, 0.1 ml aliquots of the rhizobial suspension introduced, and the cotton plug replaced. Ampoules are centrifuged in a centrifuge carrier which consists of a glass bell-jar which is sealed to circular base plate by a rubber gasket as shown in Fig 4. Centrifugation increases the surface area by dispersion of bacterial suspension on the walls of the ampoule, which, in turn helps in rapid freezing of the material. Simultaneously, high vacuum is applied in the presence of a desiccant such as phosphorus pentoxide (P_2O_5) to remove all the moisture in the ampoule within a few hours. The cotton plug is now pushed half way into the ampoule and the stem of the ampoule constricted to facilitate sealing at a later stage. Drying is continued by maintaining the vacuum for an additional 12 hours with simultaneous exposure to P_2O_5. A minimum of 10 g of loosely packed P_2O_5 powder is required for every ml of water to be absorbed and therefore, the tray should be heaped with the powder and replaced as and when necessary. Great care has

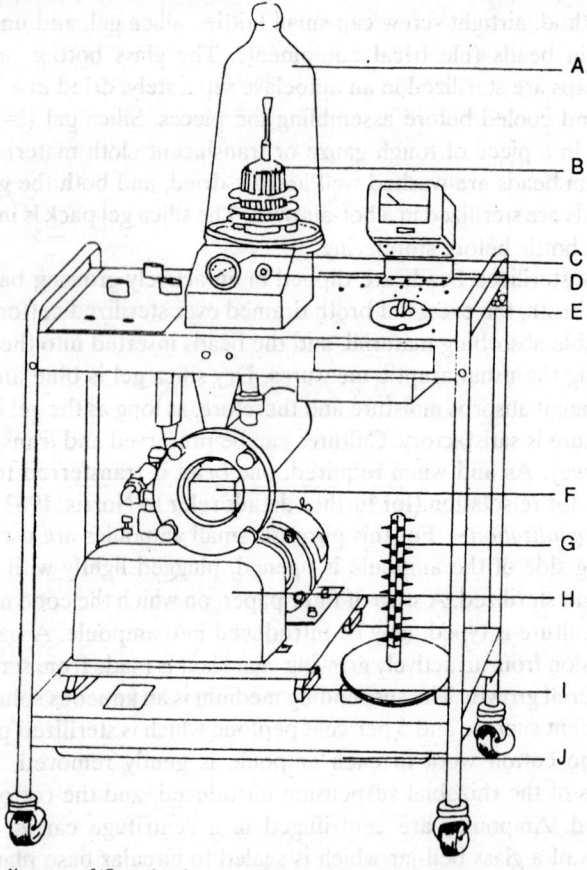

Fig. 4. A diagram of 'Speedvac' model SPS centrifuge freeze dryer (not to scale) — (A) bell-jar, (B) ampoule carrier, (C) vacuum dial gauge, (D) air admittance valve, (E) selector switch, (F) moisture trap (P_2O_5), (G) sealing header, (H) rotary vacuum pump, (I) anti-vibration mounts, and (J) storage tray.

to be exercised in handling P_2O_5. The ampoule is now sealed with the help of a burner, care being taken not to burn the cotton inside. Intact ampoules are stored in room temperature. Initially 10–50 per cent of the original population will survive the lyophilization process and loss of viability is 10-fold after two years' storage (Vincent, 1970).

Sterilization Procedures

In the preparation of inoculants, sterilization of apparatus and materials is generally done by applying heat in the form of saturated steam under pressure. The laboratory apparatus designed to use steam under regulated pressures is known as an autoclave. It is a double-jacketed steam chamber with provisions for inlet and outlet for steam, measuring gauges, and safety valve. It is the high temperature in the autoclave which kills microorganisms and to achieve the desired temperature, steam pressure is increased from 0 lb/sq. inch (100°C) to 15 lb/sq. inch (121°C) or 20 lb/sq. inch (126.6°C) and held at that pressure for varying periods depending on the nature and volume of the materials to be sterilized.

Certain items of laboratory glassware, oils, powders, and similar substances can be sterilized by dry heat or hot air in electric or gas ovens, exposed to temperature of 160°C. Dry sterilization is most suitable for petri dishes and pipettes which are commonly used in microbiological work.

Sterilization of liquids without denaturing the solutes is done by filtering them in bacteriological filters made of asbestos pad (Seitz filter), diatomaceous earth (Berkefield filter), porcelain (Chamberlain filter), and sintered glass filters. Membrane or molecular filters are being increasingly used for identification or enumeration of microorganisms.

Dust-free and bacteriologically pure surroundings are needed for microbiological work to ensure freedom from contaminants. This has been achieved by means of high efficiency particulate air filters. This type of filter with 'laminar air flow' system is now being increasingly used for dust-free environment in modern microbiological laboratories.

Inoculation rooms are equipped with ultraviolet lamps with wavelengths around 2650 Å which have maximum bactericidal effect. These are used to sterilize the surface of transfer hoods or rooms prior to handling selected microorganisms. The action of ultraviolet rays is primarily on nucleic acids (the formation of pyrimidine dimer) thereby preventing DNA replication.

Gamma radiations are capable of penetrating microorganisms and destroying them. In some countries, gamma rays are used in the sterilization of peat, which is a carrier for *Rhizobium* inoculant.

For further details on control of microorganisms by physical and chemical agents, the reader is referred to textbooks on fundamentals of microbiology (Pelczar *et al.*, 1977).

Rhizobium in Soil

Rhizobium is known to survive in soil and in the rhizospheres of legumes as well as non-legumes. There is evidence that the bacterium thrives on root excretions, although no single component in the root exudates has any special role in stimulating its growth. *Rhizobium* secretes extracellular polysaccharides (slime) which may help in binding soil particles together.

Continuous use of nitrogenous fertilizers does not seem to influence the effectiveness of rhizobia. *Rhizobium* can survive at low temperatures and tolerate temperatures up to 50°C for more than a few hours. It is sensitive to plant protectants, antibiotics, and other agricultural chemicals (Nutman, 1965). The bacterium can survive in soil for several years under dry storage conditions, although the mechanism of its survival is unknown (Sen and Sen, 1958). Several soil microorganisms (Chhonkar and Subba Rao, 1966; Sethi and Subba Rao, 1968; Bhalla and Sen, 1973) and bacteriophages are known to inhibit the growth of rhizobia although, in nature, nodulation is rarely inhibited by the activity of these antagonistic microorganisms. Soil amoebae are known to be predators of rhizobia (Alexander, 1977). *Rhizobium* is more tolerant towards salt than its host legume and therefore survives in saline soils (Subba Rao *et al.*, 1972, 1974).

Selective methods are unsuitable for counting rhizobia in soil. Serological methods or methods involving labelling with flourescent antibody (Schmidt *et al.*, 1968) are not only accurate but also useful in distinguishing strains within a rhizobial species. The only recommended method to count rhizobia in soil is to conduct nodulation tests using soil dilutions and specific hosts. This method is an indirect one and is known as 'plant infection count method' (Brockwell, 1963; Vincent, 1970). It indicates the most probable number of rhizobia in a given soil sample.

The plant infection count method is better applicable to small-seeded legumes (clovers, lucerne, etc.) grown in test tubes on agar slopes or stubs. However, for large-seeded legumes many other methods of growing plants can be used. To count *Rhizobium* sp. (cowpea) nodulating large-seeded legumes in the tropics, small-seeded siratro (*Macroptilium atropurpureum*) could be used as a test plant. Soil dilutions are made in the way adopted for plate counts. Aliquots of dilutions (0.2 to 1.0 ml depending on the method) are added to duplicate or quadruplicate tubes containing aseptically grown seedlings. Appropriate control tubes with or without in-oculation with standard strains or with nitrate (0.05 per cent KNO_3) have to be maintained for comparison. The plants are expected to nodulate in about 2–3 weeks when nodulation in each tube is scored as present ($+$) or absent ($-$). From the number of plants nodulated in different dilutions in an experiment, the most probable number (MPN) of rhizobia per gram of soil sample can be calculated by two methods: the density estimate and the maximum likelihood method.

Based on the density estimates of Fisher and Yates (1963), Vincent (1970) provides several tables for calculating the MPN of rhizobia, one of which is reproduced in Table 7. It applies to dilution series in which duplicate aliquots (0.2 ml) are examined for the presence of rhizobia at each dilution ranging from 10^1 to 10^8. When plants are scored for nodulation at the end of 2–3 weeks and assuming that the data gathered as follows:

Dilution	10^1	10^2	10^3	10^4	10^5	10^6	10^7	10^8
Plus tubes	2	2	2	1	1	0	0	0

The total number of plus tubes is 8. Going back to the table, it can be seen that for a reading of 2 replicates and 8 plus tubes, the likely number is 1.7 and the multiplier is 10^3 equalling 1700 rhizobia at the original tube (10^1).

The number of rhizobia per gram of soil is then calculated as follows:

$$\text{rhizobial count} = \frac{m \times d}{v \times w} = \frac{1700 \times 10}{0.2 \times 1.5} = 57,000/\text{gram of soil}$$

Where m is likely count at the original tube in dilution series

  d is dilution of sample at tube 1 in series

  v is aliquot of volume

  w is weight of sample

At the bottom of Table 7 fiducial limits are shown for duplicate and quadruplicate tubes and by applying this factor the confidence intervals can be determined. For tests made with duplicate tubes, the

Table 7: Number (M) of rhizobia[•] estimated by the plant infection count:
C. Ten-fold dilutions (A = 10)

Positive tubes		Dilution steps (s)			
$n = 4$	$n = 2$	$s = 10$	$s = 8$	$s = 6$	$s = 4$
40	20	7×10^8			
39					
38	19	6.9			
37		3.4			
36	18	1.8			
35		1.0			
34	17	5.9×10^7			
33		3.1	$s = 8$		
32	16	1.7	7×10^6		
31		1.0			
30	15	5.8×10^6	6.9		
29		3.1	3.4		
28	14	1.7	1.8		
27		1.0	1.0		
26	13	5.8×10^5	5.9×10^5		
25		3.1	3.1	$s = 6$	
24	12	1.7	1.7	7×10^4	
23		1.0	1.0		
22	11	5.8×10^4	5.8×10^4	6.9	
21		3.1	3.1	3.4	
20	10	1.7	1.7	1.8	
19		1.0	1.0	1.0	
18	9	5.8×10^3	5.8×10^3	5.9×10^3	
17		3.1	3.1	3.1	$s = 4$
16	8	1.7	1.7	1.7	7×10^2
15		1.0	1.0	1.0	
14	7	5.8×10^2	5.8×10^2	5.8×10^2	6.9
13		3.1	3.1	3.1	3.4
12	6	1.7	1.7	1.7	1.8
11		1.0	1.0	1.0	1.0
10	5	5.8×10^1	5.8×10^1	5.8×10^1	5.9×10^1
9		3.1	3.1	3.1	3.1
8	4	1.7	1.7	1.7	1.7
7		1.0	1.0	1.0	1.0
6	3	5.8×1	5.8×1	5.8×1	5.8×1
5		3.1	3.1	3.1	3.1

Contd.

Table 7 continued

Positive tubes		Dilution steps (s)			
4	2	1.7	1.7	1.7	1.7
	3	1.0	1.0	1.0	1.0
2	1	0.6	0.6	0.6	0.6
	1	0.6	0.6	0.6	0.6
0	0				

Source: Vincent, 1970.

Approx. range Factor, 95%	10^9	10^7	10^5	10^3
Fiducial limits	n = 2	6.6		
(X, ÷):	n = 4	3.8		

*Calculated from Table VIII of Fisher and Yates (1963), Cochran (1970).

multiplier is 6.6. The true count lies in the range of 57,000 x 6.6 to 57,000 ÷ 6.6 or 380,000 to 8600 rhizobia/g. The accuracy can be improved by increasing the number of replicated tubes, although for practical purposes duplicate tubes will do (Vincent, 1970). A simplified version (Table 8) for arriving at MPN of rhizobia has been described by Dye (1979).

Brockwell (1963) provides tables for the maximum likelihood method. One of the calculations for MPN meant for five-fold dilutions of the original sample from tests with quadruplicate seedling tubes is reproduced from Vincent (1970) in Table 9. In this procedure, 1 ml of the initial suspension is diluted with 4 ml of a diluting medium. One ml each of the resulting suspension is distributed in four test tubes containing seedlings on agar slopes and the remaining 1 ml is diluted again with fresh 4 ml of the diluting medium and the process is repeated until six successive dilution levels are obtained. At the end of 2–3 weeks, the quadruplicate tubes in each dilution are scored for presence or absence of root nodules. An example of a typical scoring is as follows (Vincent, 1970):

Dilution	1	5	25	125	625	3125
Plus tubes	4	4	2	1	0	0

This would mean that the characteristic is 442,100 and on matching this figure with Table 8, the number of rhizobia will be 108 and the total number will be 108×10^2/g. The fiducial limit at 95 per cent level is expressed by a factor of 2.6, when the range of MPN would be $108 \times 10^2 \times 2.6$ to $108 \times 10^2 \div 2.6 = 28,000$ to 4000/g of rhizobia.

Table 8: Most probable number: (MPN) of *Rhizobium* by the plant dilution method[1]

Number of nodulated plants in four dilutions when tested in			MPN is the aliquot of the lowest dilution[2]
Duplicate	*Triplicate*	*Quadruplicate*	
8	12	16	> 2300
		15	> 1300
	11		> 1080
7		14	690
	10		420
		13	340
6	9	12	180
		11	100
	8		87
5		10	59
	7		37
		9	31
4	6	8	17
		7	10
	5		8.5
3		6	5.8
	4		3.7
		5	3.1
2	3	4	1.7
		3	1.0
	2		0.85
1		2	0.58
	1		< 0.37
		1	< 0.31
0	0	0	No detectable rhizobia

Source: Dye, 1979.

[1] Modified from Date and Vincent (1962) and calculated from Fisher and Yates (1953).
[2] Factors for 95 per cent fiducial limits are 6.6 for duplicates, 4.7 for triplicates, and 3.8 for quadruplicates (Cochran, 1970).

Example: A 30 g sample of soil was suspended in 270 ml of water (to give a 10^{-1} dilution) and 10 fold dilutions made to 10^{-10}. Duplicate plants were inoculated with 1 ml of the 10^{-7}, 10^{-8}, 10^{-9}, and 10^{-10} dilutions. After growth the number of nodulated plants was found to be 5.

From Table 8 the MPN in 1 ml of the 10^{-7} dilution is 59. Hence, the number of rhizobia in the original soil was 59×10^{-7}/g. The 95 per cent fiducial limits are $59 \times 10^{7} \overset{x}{+} 6.6$ i.e $8.9 \times 10^{7} - 39 \times 10^{8}$.

Table 9: Most probable number[1] according to distribution of tubes with nodulated plants five-fold dilutions in quadruplicate

Characteristic[2]	Estimate	Characteristic	Estimate	Characteristic	Estimate	Characteristic	Estimate
100000	1.1	401000	10.8	440200	71	444030	450
2−	2.6	411−	15.1	−12−	98	−13	630
3−	4.6	421−	21.5	−22−	141	−23	910
4−	8.0	431−	32.8	−32−	218	−33	1410
010000	1.0	402000	14.1	440300	91	444410	1430
11−	2.3	412−	19.6	−13−	126	−20	2030
21−	4.0	422−	28.3	−23−	182	−30	3020
31−	6.5	432−	43.6	−33−	282	−40	5050
020000	2.1	403000	18.1	444100	290	444401	1350
12−	3.5	413−	25.2	−2−	410	−11	1880
22−	5.5	423−	36.4	−3−	600	−21	2690
32−	8.7	433−	56.5	−4−	1010	−31	4100
030000	3.0	441000	57	444010	270	444402	1770
13−	4.9	−2−	81	−11−	380	−12	2450
23−	7.2	−3−	121	−21−	540	−22	3530
33−	11.3	−4−	202	−31−	820	−32	5440
410000	11.4	440100	54	444020	350	444403	2260
42−	16.2	−11−	75	−12−	490	−13	3140
43−	24.2	−21−	108	−22−	710	−23	4550
44−	40.4	−31−	164	−32−	1090	−33	7060
						444441	7100
						−2	10100
						−3	15100
						−4	25200

Source: After Brockwell, 1963; reproduced from Vincent, 1970.

[1] Number of rhizobia/ml of suspension from which the first five-fold dilution is made.

[2] Number of positive tubes in successive five-fold dilutions: 1–3125; common digits not repeated within groups.

Approximate range = 25,000.

Factor for 95 per cent fiducial limits, $(X, \div)$ approx. $2.6 x \geq 9$; 2.7–$7.7, x \leq 8$.

Plant dilution counting methods for rhizobia have been used to estimate cell number in soil, carrier-based inoculants, liquid cultures, and seed washings from inoculated seeds. Practical experience has shown that 'skip tubes' or non-nodulated plants may arise in the middle of nodulated ones in a series of dilutions. Such tubes are regarded as plus tubes for calculation. If microbial antagonism is the cause for skip tubes, adding mycostatin to agar tubes (Robinson, 1968) may obviate non-nodulated plants. The reader is advised to consult original references on plant dilution methods for counting rhizobia for detailed information (Brockwell, 1963; Vincent, 1970).

Fluorescent antibody procedure has been used to study rhizobia in soil (Schmidt, 1974). When soil suspensions are stained with a fluorescent antibody and examined by incident light fluorescent microscopy, rhizobia fluoresce yellow-green, whereas other bacteria fluoresce differently. This method has enabled the detection of *R. japonicum* strains in soil. There is, however, one limitation of non-specific fluorescence exhibited by plant tissue remains and other microorganisms in soil which may interfere with the result obtained.

Antibiotic-resistant markers are useful in monitoring rhizobia in soil (Pugashetti and Wagner, 1980). Streptomycin-resistant strains of *R. trifolii* and *R. japonicum* have been introduced into soil and their survival in soil followed by periodic plating on streptomycin-containing YEMA medium (Danso and Alexander, 1974).

Rhizobium in Root Nodules

Rhizobia enter the roots of legumes either through root hairs (as in clovers and lucerne) or directly at the point of emergence of lateral roots (as in groundnut). Many legumes have not been examined for the mode of entry of *Rhizobium* into their roots. Thread-like structures carrying rod-shaped bacteria known as 'infection thread' have been seen in *Rhizobium*-infected clovers and lucerne although the precise mechanism of entry of rhizobia into root hairs is not clear. Two modes of entry of rhizobia into the root hairs have been suggested: entry of small coccoid swarmers through the gaps in cellulose microfibrils and direct invagination of the root hair cell (Nutman, 1965; Subba Rao, 1967; Fahraeus and Ljunggren, 1968; Dart, 1974). Quite recently, investigations on the preferential attachment of *Rhizobium* to its host legume have revealed the possibility that lectins (phytohaemagglutinins) in clover roots function as molecular bridges between the common antigens on the bacterial cell and root surfaces. For instance, a protein celled 'trifoliin' in roots of clover binds to a polysaccharide on the surface of *R. trifolii* but not the polysaccharide on the surface of *R. japonicum*. In other words, the recognition of a *Rhizobium* species by its homologous host seems to be mediated by a lectin (Bauer, 1977).

A transverse section of a nodule reveals a central 'bacteroid zone' which is enveloped in a nodule cortex. The bacteroid zone is made up of host cells containing 'bacteroids' encased in membranous envelopes which are of host origin. Bacteroids are non-motile stages in the life cycle of Rhizobium. In nature, bacteroids are only present in nodules and possess certain distinct characteristics. A fully developed bacteroid has no flagella and is surrounded by three membranes. The nuclear region of bacteroids appears fragmented and is associated with granular cytoplasm.

There is no simple physiological or biochemical test to distinguish between effective and ineffective strains of Rhizobium. Several attempts have been made in this direction. A positive and significant correlation between the amount of asparagine nitrogen utilized and the effectiveness of rhizobial isolates of pea (Pisum sativum) and fenugreek (Trigonella foenum-graecum) has been observed. Different strains of rhizobia also showed a tendency to consume glucose to different degrees, a characteristic which could be used to distinguish strains (Gupta and Sen, 1963). The respiratory activity (μl O_2 consumed/hr/mg dry cells) of efficient strains of R. trifolii and R. leguminosarum on a glucose substrate is stimulated significantly in the presence of glycine whereas the respiratory activity of ineffecient strains under similar conditions remains static. This may provide a clue to explore the possibility of distinguishing strains (Magu and Sen, 1969). A significant and inverse correlation between symbiotic efficiency of R. meliloti strains and their nitrate utilization has been observed by Sarma et al. (1973). In spite of these attempts, the only reliable method to distinguish between efficient and inefficient strains of Rhizobium is the response of plants to rhizobial inoculation.

Ineffective strains of rhizobia form ineffective nodules which are generally small and contain poorly developed bacteroid tissue showing accumulation of starch in host cells which do not contain Rhizobium and of dextran in host cells infected by Rhizobium. The bacteroids of an ineffective nodule contain glycogen. On the contrary, effective nodules formed by effective strains of rhizobia are well developed, they possess pink colour due to the presence of a pigment 'leghaemoglobin' (akin to the haemoglobin of human blood), and the bacteroid tissue is well organized with plenty of bacteroids (Bergersen and Briggs, 1958; Jordan, 1962; Dart and Mercer, 1963).

Function of the Nodule

The nodule is merely a protective structure since it is now well established that bacteroids are the seats of nitrogen fixation. Nitrogenase is the enzyme which mediates the reduction of N_2 to NH_3.

Nitrogenase can be obtained by the disintegration of bacteroids by mechanical processes. This enzyme is made up of two components — one with both iron (Fe) and molybdenum (Mo) having a molecular weight of about 200,000 and the second with Fe and without Mo having a molecular weight of about 65,000 (Quispel, 1974).

Nitrogen fixation is essentially an anaerobic process and hence the nodule must have a mechanism to exclude oxygen from the bacteroid which is the site of fixation. This is accomplished by the presence of leghaemoglobin around bacteroids enclosed by membranous envelopes of host origin. In recent years, the exact location of leghaemoglobin has become a debatable point, since fresh evidence has been obtained to demonstrate that the pigment is distributed in the cytoplasm of the host cell. This pigment limits oxygen supply and helps in providing low oxygen conditions near the bacteroids with the result that not only is the oxygen-sensitive nitrogenase prevented from damage but also enough oxygen is available at the site for ATP generation. The amount of leghaemoglobin and the extent of bacteroid tissue in nodules have a direct bearing on the amount of nitrogen fixed be legumes (Bergersen and Briggs, 1958; Chopra and Subba Rao, 1967; Verma and Bal, 1976).

The nitrogenase-catalysed reaction requires a source of ATP and reductant. Products of photosynthesis are translocated from leaves to nodules which provide the necessary ATP and reductant for nitrogen fixation. Most measurements indicate a requirement of 12 molecules of ATP per molecule of N_2 fixed. The Fe of nitrogenase is believed to be involved in the binding of nitrogenase to nitrogen while Mo is responsible for the decrease in the strength of nitrogen bonds($N \equiv N$) to an optimum extent to facilitate reduction. The enzyme nitrogenase couples ATP hydrolysis to ADP with electron transfer from a reduced electron donor, probably a ferredoxin or a flavodoxin, to reduce N_2 to $2NH_3$. The first stable intermediate in nitrogen fixation is ammonia. Between N_2 and NH_3, hydrazine, hydroxylamine, diimide, and carbamyl phosphate have been variously proposed as intermediates without convincing evidences. The ammonium ion (NH_4^+) produced during nitrogen fixation is assimilated through GS-GOGAT (glutamine synthetase-glutamate synthase) pathway which is present in most higher plants (Postgate, 1971; Quispel, 1974; Nutman, 1976). Many aspects of the biochemistry of symbiotic nitrogen fixation are still to be understood. Nevertheless, an overall picture can be built up (Fig. 5) from results available from experiments with nodule homogenates

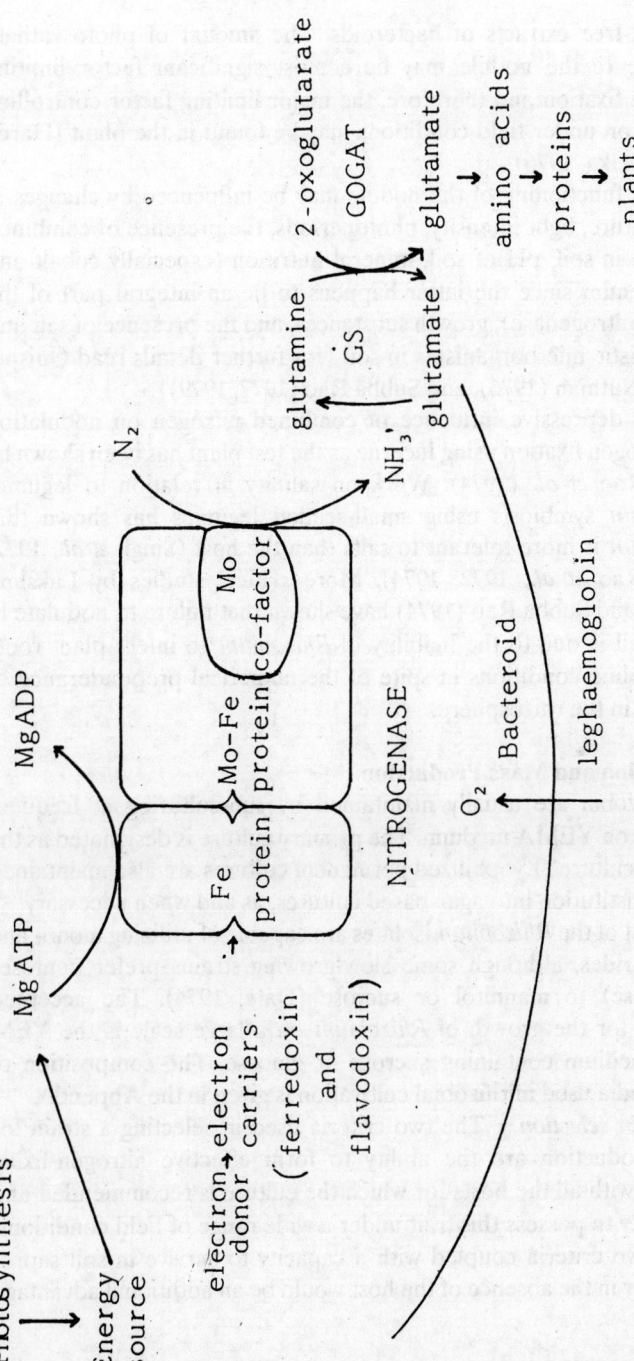

Fig 5: An overall scheme for biological nitrogen fixation in a root nodule.

and cell-free extracts of bacteroids. The amount of photosynthate available to the nodule may be a most significant factor limiting nitrogen fixation and therefore, the major limiting factor controlling N_2 fixation under field conditions may be found in the plant (Hardy and Havelka, 1976).

The functioning of the nodule may be influenced by changes in temperature, light intensity, photoperiods, the presence of combined nitrogen in soil, pH of soil, mineral nutrition (especially cobalt and molybdenum since the latter happens to be an integral part of the enzyme nitrogenase), growth substances, and the presence of salt and antagonistic microorganisms in soil {for further details read Quispel (1974), Nutman (1976), and Subba Rao (1977, 1979)}.

The depressive influence of combined nitrogen on nodulation and nitrogen fixation using lucerne as the test plant has been shown by Subba Rao et al. (1974). Work on salinity in relation to legume-Rhizobium symbiosis using small-seeded legumes has shown that Rhizobium is more tolerant to salts than the host (Singh et al., 1972; Subba Rao et al., 1972, 1974). More critical studies by Lakshmi Kumari and Subba Rao (1974) have shown that failure to nodulate in saline soil is due to the inability of Rhizobium to infect plant roots under saline conditions in spite of the numerical preponderance of rhizobia in the rhizosphere.

Cultivation and Mass Production

Rhizobia are usually maintained by sub-culturing at frequent intervals on YEMA medium. The primary culture is designated as the 'mother culture'. Lyophilized permanent cultures are also maintained for reconstitution into agar-based cultures, as and when necessary.

Most of the Rhizobium isolates are capable of utilizing mono- and disaccharides, although some slow-growing strains prefer pentoses (arabinose) to mannitol or sucrose (Date, 1974). The accepted medium for the growth of Rhizobium on a large scale is the YEM liquid medium containing sucrose or glucose. The composition of some media used in rhizobial cultivation is given in the Appendix.

Strain selection — The two criteria used in selecting a strain for mass production are the ability to form effective nitrogen-fixing nodules with all the hosts for which the culture is recommended and the ability to possess this trait under a wide range of field conditions. These two criteria coupled with a capacity to survive in soil sapro-phytically in the absence of the host would be an additional advantage

(Date, 1974). The ability of an introduced rhizobial strain to out-perform the native strains in soil is perhaps a foremost consideration in selecting a suitable strain and is a criterion which can be arrived at by careful laboratory work, field testing, and serological studies. Other considerations have been proposed which include prompt nodulation over a range of root temperatures, greater survival in carriers and on seed, and tolerance to pesticides, fertilizers, and other agricultural chemicals (Date, 1976; Roughley, 1976).

One of the basic questions which remains to be fully answered is whether inoculants should be designed for individual leguminous species or for a group of legumes based on the system of cross-inoculation groups. The use of 'multi-strain' inoculants for different hosts or for a single host in an inoculation group, according to Date (1974), cannot be recommended since one strain is likely to domi-nate over other strains. The practice of using wide-spectrum strains of the cowpea miscellany is generally based on results obtained in greenhouse trials where effective cross-infections within a range of legumes have been demonstrated. However, no serious field investigations on the validity of using wide-spectrum strains for all cowpea type of legumes have been undertaken with tropical grain legumes. Therefore, for individual cowpea type of legumes, single-strain inoculants are usually used in India. The use of multi-strain inoculants may be considered if effective strains for a limited number of host species have been identified by field testing host responses to inoculants containing different strains. An additional precaution to be borne in mind is that when mixed inocula are added to the carrier (say peat or a suitable substitute), the added strains must possess equal growth rates in the carrier devoid of any mutual competition. Burton (1967) has stated that the composite cultures of meticulously screened wide- spectrum strains of rhizobia are far more practical and desirable than those which can be used on only one species or variety of the host plant. In his experiments, three of the nine strains tested were moderately effective on cowpea, mung bean, groundnut, guar, and lespedeza. Based on this experience, an inoculant con-taining these three multiple strains should be effective for all the crops mentioned provided no ineffective strain is included in the inoculant, because it has been pointed out by several investigators that ineffective strains of rhizobia may hinder nodulation by effective strains.

Preparation of broth — The selected strain of *Rhizobium* is grown on YEMA slants for 3–9 days depending on the rate of growth (fast or slow). After the culture is checked for purity and proper growth, the culture is transferred from tubes to large flasks containing sterile solid or liquid midium for 4–9 days. This is known as the 'starter culture'. Later, the starter culture is transferred to a seed tank fermentor and incubated for 4–9 days. At this stage large quantity of the liquid medium (broth) is formulated in large production fermentors and sterilized after adjusting the pH to 6.5 to 7.0, with KOH or H_2SO_4. When the production fermentor with the sterilized medium is cooled to 30°C and is ready for use, inoculum from the seed tank fermentor is transferred aseptically to the production fermentor at the rate of 1 per cent by volume. In Nitragin Co., USA, cultures are aerated by forcing sterile air through porous carborundum or stainless steel spargers in the bottom of the production fermentor. An oxygen partial pressure of 0.15 atmosphere is optimum and rhizobia grow best in the range of 30° to 32°C (Burton, 1967). According to Burton (1967), rhizobial count of 5×10^9 can be attained in 96 hours with a lag phase of 48 hours for *R. japonicum* and 24 hours for *R. meliloti* when the initial inoculum in the fermentor is 5 per cent of the volume of the medium. By increasing the inoculum level, the lag phase can be considerably reduced.

The underlying objective in the preparation of the primary inoculum for seeding into fermentors is to attain high populations of rhizobia within a short time ranging from 3 to 9 days depending on the species or *Rhizobium* (fast or slow growing). The size of the fermentors and the method of aeration differ and personal preferences and experiences of individual institutions in different countries have to be taken into account in this regard. Thus, the factors influencing the output of cells are aeration, volume, initial inoculum level, bacterial strain, temperature, and incubation time. The prime objective is to attain high populations in minimum time and Vincent (1970) mentions that viable counts up to 2000×10^6 or 4000×10^6 could be attained by regulating these factors.

In the United States, large fermentors (Burton, 1967) with complicated devices for steam sterilization, media formulation, foam control, and monitoring growth are used, whereas in Australia a container such as a drum up to 100 l capacity with up to 50 l of broth with an air inlet, an air outlet, an inoculation point, and a sampling tap has proved statisfactory (Date, 1974). An air filter is attached to the air inlet port and the whole unit (Fig. 6) is autoclaved with the medium leaving one of the inlets open to accommodate pressure changes. After cooling, filtered air at about 0.7 kg/sq.cm pressure is supplied. The Australian experience has been that autoclavable fermentation units work more satisfactorily than self-operating, complicated fermentors requiring steam sterilization.

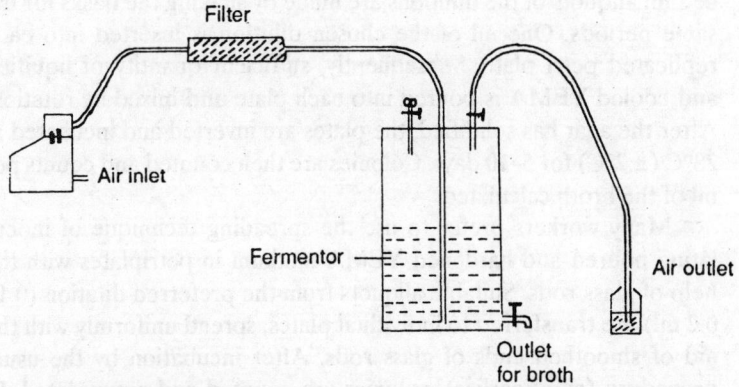

Fig. 6. Diagrammatic representation of a simple Australian fermentor for *Rhizobium*, according of Date (1974).

Checking the broth — At the end of fermentation, the broth is checked for freedom from contaminants by the following methods (Vincent, 1970): (1) pH test — if above 8 or below 6, the broth is suspected to be contaminated; (2) agglutination test (if facilities are available) against 1/100 antiserum specific for the strain used; (3) a Gram smear test from diluted broth culture (see Appendix for details) for detection of Gram-positive contaminants, spore formers, and other extraneous forms. Vincent (1970) indicates that the occasional occurrence of a few Gram-positive cells in a microscopic field is permissible; (4) inoculation of the broth on peptone agar medium (see Appendix for details) — if abundant growth takes place within 2 days, suspect contamination of the broth; and (5) streaking the broth on YEMA for verification of the pattern of growth of *Rhizobium*.

Counts of cells in the broth — This is done by the normal plate count method to determine the viable count at 28°C (± 2°C) incubation. When counted in this manner, broths having viable cells higher than 10^9/ml cells may be used. In this method, standard microbiological procedures for counting rhizobia by the serial dilution and plating methods have to be strictly followed (Vincent, 1970).

Serial dilutions of the broth are prepared so as to provide a dilution at which 30–300 viable bacteria (Vincent, 1970) appear on petri plates. This is best done with a series of flasks having 99 ml aliquots of sterilized water, using 1 ml of the broth in the first aliquot. After shaking the flask uniformly for a constant period, serial transfers of 1 ml aliquots of the dilutions are made by shaking the flasks for the same periods. One ml of the chosen dilution is inserted into each replicated petri plate. Subsequently, sufficient quantity of liquified and cooled YEMA is poured into each plate and mixed by rotation. After the agar has solidified, the plates are inverted and incubated at 28°C (±2°C) for 5–10 days. Colonies are then counted and counts per ml of the broth calculated.

Many workers prefer to use the spreading technique of inoculating poured and hardened YEMA medium in petriplates with the help of glass rods. Suitable aliquots from the preferred dilution (0.1–0.2 ml) are transferred to individual plates, spread uniformly with the aid of smoothed ends of glass rods. After incubation by the usual procedure (cited earlier), colonies are counted and enumerated. In this case, best results are obtained if plates contain 75 to 150 colonies at the desired dilution.

Counting viable number of rhizobia by the plate count gives a reliable estimate of numbers in a broth to be used for preparation of inoculants. However, using a phase contrast microscope, the number can be determined from fresh broths after suitable dilutions in a bacterial counting chamber or haemocytometer. Vicent (1970) indicates that numbers more than twice those of viable rhizobia determined by the plate count method may be taken as a guide to accept broths for preparation of inoculants when the microscopoic method of counting is followed.

Storage of broth — It is not advisable to store the broth after fermentation for periods longer than 24 hours even at 4°C since counts of viable rhizobia begin to decrease. Hence, the broth has to be incorporated and dispersed evenly into a carrier. However, in Northrup King and Co., USA, the mature broth is centrifuged and the cells collected in the form of a paste (1×10^{11} cells/g wet paste). The paste is immediately frozen ($-28°C$) in suitable containers, care being taken not to thaw the paste. When required, the paste is diluted to a count of about 1×10^9/ml and could be stored in the diluted state for several weeks at 4°C (quoted from a bulletin and subject to verification).

Agar and Broth Inoculants

Agar-based inoculants have become outdated except for small-scale experiments. Broth cultures are in vogue in European countries and in the United States. When broth is directly used for inoculation, large quantities of fresh broth are necessary to obtain good nodulation comparable to that obtained by peat-based inoculants. Secondly, the experience of both Australian and US scientists has been that both agar and broth cultures are inferior to peat-based inoculants because peat provides the natural protection to rhizobia and thus enhances it survival on seeds.

Carrier-based Inoculants

In the United States, sedge peat is ground to fine powder capable of passing through 100 mesh sieve and heat-treated followed by neutralization with $CaCO_3$ to raise the pH of the peat carrier to 6.8. Diluted broth having rhizobial cell population in excess of 10^9 cells/ml is blended with the peat carrier so as to bring the final moisture content of peat to 35–40 per cent on wet basis. The resulting product shall have at least 300 million (3×10^8) rhizobia per g of peat (Burton, 1967). In the process of mixing, the broth is sprayed to powdered peat and left in tubs, in trays, or on a floor covered with polythene sheets for 2 to 10 days at 22 to 24°C for curing when the heat generated is driven off. The product is again milled and packed in polyethylene bags where rhizobia increase in numbers. For instance, *R. japonicum* reaches a maximum population of more than 25×10^9 cells/g in 4 weeks while *R. meliloti* reaches the same level in 2 weeks (Burton, 1967). At higher temperatures (25–35°C), the number of rhizobia falls below optimum when carrier-based inoculants are stored beyond 2–3 months, whereas storage at 4°C prolongs the shelf life of cultures up to 12 months.

Gas exchange in polythene has been stressed by US manufacturers (pinholes on bags are advocated), whereas Date (1974) states that the Australian experience has been that such pinholes on bags are unnecessary.

In Australia milled dry peat (15 per cent moisture) is packed in sealed polythene bags (0.089 mm gauge of medium density and 0.038–0.051 mm of the high density sheets) and sterilized by gamma radiation. The broth is introduced into polythene bags by means of a hollow needle to bring the moisture level of peat to 50 per cent and incubated for 5–10 days, depending on the strain used. In this way, cell count from 10^9 to 10^{10}/g peat can be reached at the time of manufacture (Date, 1974).

In India, peat-like material available in the Nilgiri valley to an estimated extent of 5.5 million tons has been found to be a good carrier (Iswaran *et al.*, 1969) Lignite is another carrier which is widely used (Kandasamy and Prasad, 1971) and an estimated quantity of 3 million tons is available annually from Neyveli Lignite mines in South India.

Rhizobial broth is grown on YEM medium in large flasks on a shaker for small requirements or in fermentors for large requirements. The powdered carrier (passing through 100 mesh sieve) is neutralized with $CaCO_3$ and autoclaved at 15 lbs pressure for 4 hours. After cooling, a high count broth is mixed so as to attain a 40 per cent moisture-holding capacity of the carrier. The carrier and the broth are mixed either manually or by means of a mechanical mixer, cured in trays for 2–5 days, and packed in polythene bags. The entire procedure is schematically represented in Fig. 7.

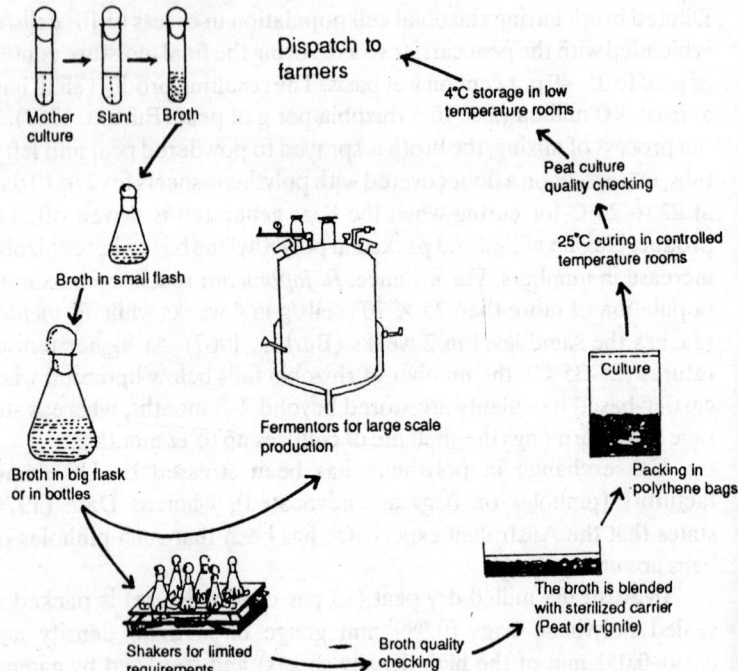

Fig. 7. Schematic representation of procedures in mass culturing of rhizobia.

Several indigenously available carriers have been compared with American peat for their ability to support the growth of *R. japonicum* (Tilak and Subba Rao, 1978). Among the different carriers, combinations of Indian peat soil, farmyard manure, compost, or pressmud with charcoal (1:1) which were capable of passing through 200 mesh sieve gave higher rhizobial count than individual carriers. At the end of one month the population of rhizobia started declining when incubated at 30°C but charcoal, farmyard manure, and pressmud helped to retain the viability of rhizobia up to 3 months in peat soil which could be extended to 12 months when stored at 4°C (Fig. 8a, b). The physical properties of the carrier (Table 10) were improved by the addition of charcoal which indirectly helped in the survival of *R. japonicum*.

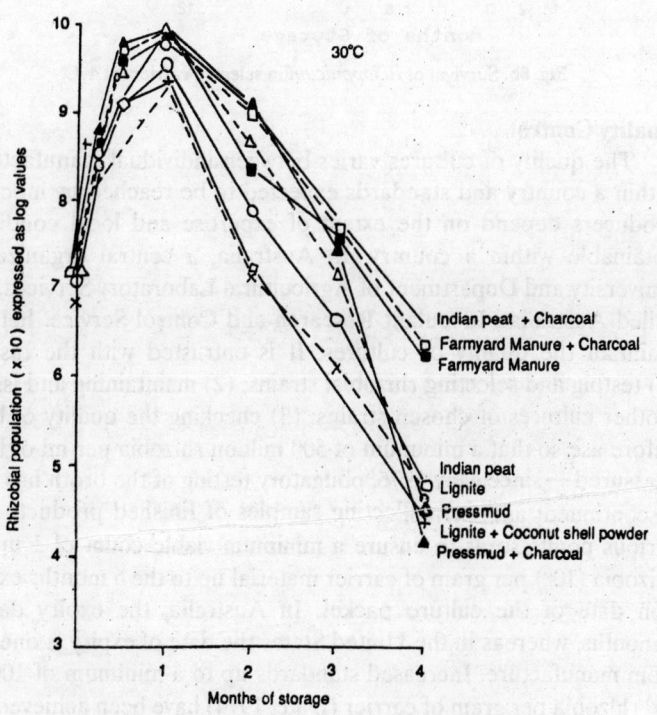

Fig. 8a. Survival of *R. japonicum* in selected carriers at 30°C.

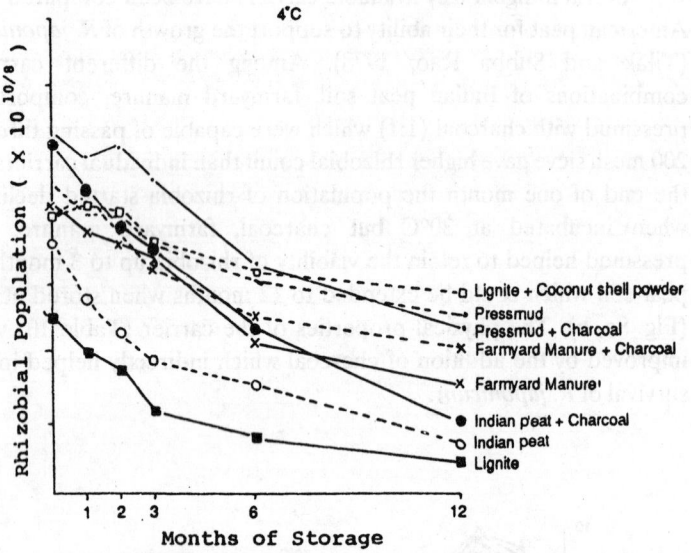

Fig. 8b. Survival of *R. japonicum* in selected carriers at 4°C.

Quality Control

The quality of cultures varies between individual manufacturers within a country and standards expected to be reached by inoculant producers depend on the extent of expertise and local conditions obtainable within a country. In Australia, a central organization, University and Department of Agricultural Laboratory Services, now called Australian Inoculant Research and Control Service, helps to maintain the quality of cultures. It is entrusted with the task of: (1) testing and selecting rhizobial strains; (2) maintaining and issuing mother cultures of chosen strains; (3) checking the quality of broth before use so that a minimum of 500 million rhizobia per ml of broth is assured — since May 1976, obilgatory testing of the broth has been discontinued; and (4) collecting samples of finished products from various points so as to ensure a minimum viable count of 1 million rhizobia (10^6) per gram of carrier material up to the 6 months expiration date of the culture packet. In Australia, the expiry date is 6 months, whereas in the United States the date of expiry is one year from manufacture. Increased standards up to a minimum of 1000 × 10^6 rhizobia per gram of carrier (Date, 1974) have been achieved.

In the United States, the Australian approach has been described as disadvantageous since it tends to diminish competition and free

Table 10: Some physical and chemical characteristics of different carriers mean of four replicates

Carriers	Organic matter (per cent)	Total nitrogen (per cent)	Bulk density (g/cm³)	Particle density (g/cm³)	Porosity (per cent)	Water holding capacity (per cent)	Total surface area (sq.m/g)
American peat	76.15	0.95	0.82	1.48	44.58	208.5	1063.3
Indian peat-soil	41.65	0.69	1.02	2.18	53.16	149.3	646.6
Indian peat-soil + charcoal (1:1)	34.91	0.66	0.87	1.88	53.73	182.4	766.8
Farmyard manure	79.05	0.93	0.79	1.77	55.39	153.4	911.1
Farmyard manure + charcoal (1:1)	58.19	0.78	0.64	1.72	62.70	169.4	885.8
Pressmud	76.50	0.83	0.75	1.70	56.12	155.4	889.0
Pressmud + charcoal (1:1)	55.25	0.85	0.72	1.80	65.50	165.4	870.1
Compost	55.00	0.55	0.75	1.82	58.84	171.3	940.8
Compost + charcoal (1:1)	42.71	0.57	0.61	1.77	65.52	177.2	888.5
Clay (vermiculite)	1.07	0.01	0.98	2.66	63.24	152.4	109.3
Teak leaf meal	65.19	1.14	0.46	1.65	71.96	219.9	821.1
Clay + teak leaf meal (1:1)	40.00	0.55	0.81	1.95	58.91	196.7	563.6
Lignite	75.46	0.31	1.08	1.66	34.79	198.9	556.4
Coconut shell powder	72.16	0.78	1.02	1.57	30.25	185.8	540.1
Lignite + coconut shell powder (1:1)	75.25	0.72	0.75	1.49	50.75	225.3	840.9
Lignite + teak leaf meal (1:1)	70.46	0.71	0.72	1.55	53.03	212.2	810.9
Soil	3.37	0.25	1.33	2.59	48.69	59.8	70.2
Charcoal	21.60	0.01	0.43	1.62	73.39	200.0	870.9
C.D. at 5 per cent	6.45	0.03	0.12	0.09	2.44	19.19	65.42

Source: Tilak and Subba Rao, 1978.

enterprise (Burton, 1967). Hence, individual manufacturers control their own quality. In India, the Indian Standards Institution has evolved methods to check the quality of inoculants and issue ISI marks to qualified producers (see ISI bulletin No. IS: 8268-1976). This bulletin can be had on payment from Director-General, Indian Standards Institution, Manak Bhavan, Bahadur Shah Zafar Marg, New Delhi 110002. The following are the relevant clauses from the ISI specifications for rhizobial cultures:

1) The inoculant shall be a carrier-based one.

2) The inoculant shall contain a minimum of 10^8 viable cells of *Rhizobium* per gram of the carrier on dry-mass basis within 15 days of manufacture and 10^7 within 15 days before the expiry date marked on the packet when the inoculant is stored at 25°–30°C.

3) The inoculant shall have a maximum shelf life of 6 months from the date of its manufacture.

4) The inoculant shall not have any contamination by other microorganisms.

5) The pH of the inoculant shall be between 6.0 and 7.5.

6) The inoculant shall show effective nodulation on all those species/cultivars listed on the packet before the expiry date. If good effective pink nodulation is obtainable in the inoculated species together with the total absence or sometimes presence of stray nodules in the controls, it should be concluded that the inoculant contains effective rhizobia. The total dry mass of inoculated plants shall be significantly higher than that of the uninoculated controls and at least 50 per cent more than the controls.

7) The carrier material shall be in the form of powder (capable of passing through 75–106 μ sieve) that is, peat, lignite, peat-soil, humus, or similar material neutralized with calcium carbonate and sterilized.

8) The manufacturers shall control the quality of broth and maintain records of tests. They shall also maintian: (a) records of isolation and identification of *Rhizobium* cultures together with records of nodulating ability of pure cultures, and (b) data on effectiveness of pure cultures for every season and crop.

9) The inoculant shall be packed in 50–75 μ low density polyethylene packets or any other suitable container.

10) Each packet shall be marked legibly to give the following information:

    a) name of the product, specifically as *Rhizobium* inoculant,

    b) leguminous crop for which intended,

c) name and address of manufacturer,
d) type of carrier,
e) batch or code number,
f) date of manufacture,
g) date of expiry,
h) net quantity meant for 0.4 ha, and
i) storage instructions worded as follows:

'STORE IN COOL PLACE AWAY FROM DIRECT
SUN AND HEAT'

11) The above items should be printed on a coloured ink background.

12) Each packet may also be marked with the ISI certification mark.

13) The inoculant shall be stored by the manufacturer in a cool place away from direct heat preferably at a temperature of 15°C and not exceeding 30°C ± 2°C. It shall also be the duty of the manufacturer to instruct the retailers and, in turn, the users about the precautions required during storage.

14) Tests shall be carried out from time to time by the methods prescribed in items 2 to 6.

According to Date (1974), Czechoslovakian cultures have a minimum of 300 × 10^6 rhizobia per gram of sterilized soil-peat mixtures and cultures from Holland possess 4000 × 10^6 to 25000 × 10^6 per gram of sterilized loam-peat-lucerne meal mixture.

Quality control measures in Uruguay described here are based on notes supplied by Margarita Sicardi de Mallorca, Laboratory for Soil Microbiology and Inoculant Control, Plant Agropecuario, Ministerio de Ganaderia y Agricultural Uruguay. The programme of inoculant control initiated in 1963 includes (1) strain selection in lighted room, glass house, and field, (2) qualitative and quantitative broth checks, and (3) plant infection counts of peat cultures before storage and distribution by the use of *Macroptilium atropurpureum* (Siratro) which is infected by many species of rhizobia.

The standard in New Zealand is 100 million rhizobia (10^8) per gram of peat, whereas in Russia, the standard ranges from 50 to 100 million rhizobia per gram of the carrier (Burton, 1967).

Methods of Inoculation

Agar-based cultures are scraped by means of a needle or scalpel and suspended in water and applied to seed by sprinkling and mixing.

The use of 10 per cent sugar or 40 per cent gum arabic in the suspending fluid enhances the survival of rhizobia on seed.

Carrier-based cultures are mixed with minimum amount of water to form a slurry (sugar or gum arabic, as stated above, may be added) and seeds are added to the slurry so as to uniformly coat the seeds with the inoculant. The seeds are dried in shade and sown immediately (Fig. 9).

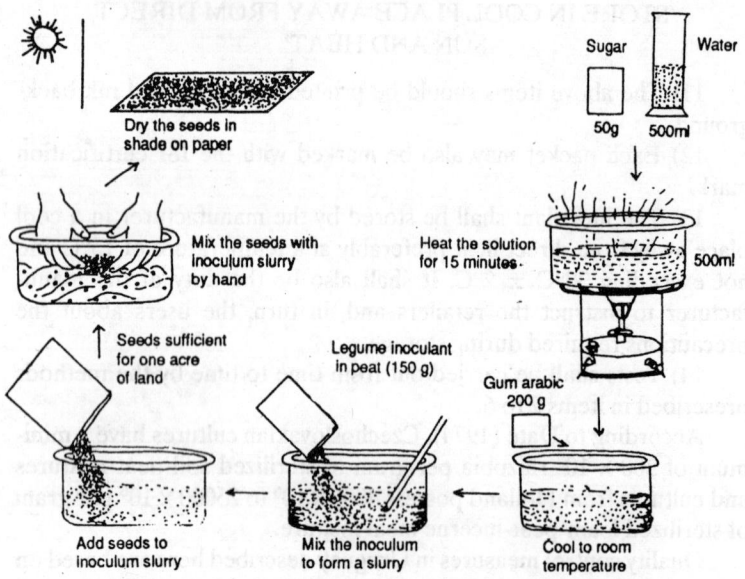

Fig. 9. The procedure for inoculating seeds with *Rhizobium*.

The following special methods of inoculation are recommended to meet adverse situations of soil conditions or special requirements. Many of the methods are quoted by Burton (1979) and some are US patented. These methods have been summarized from Burton (1979) as follows:

Pelleted seed.—A pelleted seed protects the rhizobial inoculum on seed from the toxic effects due to acidity of soil or due to hazards of fertilizer and pesticide applications. The usual method of pelleting involves additions of 40 per cent gum arabic or 5 per cent carboxy methyl cellulose to the inoculant slurry before application to seeds. Finely ground calcium carbonate capable of passing through 300 mesh sieve is added to freshly inoculated wet seeds in a container and mixed rapidly for 2 minutes until seeds are evenly coated. The lime-coated seeds appear as white tablets and they are allowed to harden for an hour by spreading on a clean surface. A good lime-pelleted seed should have an even surface and no black markings of inoculum should be visible outside. In New Zealand and Australia, cement mixers are used to achieve uniform lime pelleting when large quantities of pelleted seed are necessary for use in acidic soils. The seed should be sown immediately but if absolutely necessary can be stored up to 2 weeks at low temperatures (4°C) in a refrigerator.

Besides lime, other forms of pelleting agents such as dolomite, gypsum, bentonite, rock phosphate, superphosphate, talc, charcoal, and basic slag have been used and methods of application described in detail (Brockwell, 1977).

Pre-inoculated seed — Some manufacturers in the United States sell pre-inoculated seed, which is practical only in areas where the seeds are inoculated in winter for sowing in spring. The number of viable rhizobia tend to diminish in pre-inoculated seeds stored indefinitely.

Liquids and frozen concentrates — This type of inoculant is suitable for direct soil application and requires refrigeration and air shipment.

Granular soil inoculant — In this process, marble or calcite grains or cores are wetted by peat-based cultures using adhesives. Granular inoculants are designed for broadcasting by aeroplane or with the aid of suitable farm machinery. They have short shelf life.

Porous gypsum granule — Granules of calcium sulphate paste are prepared by extruding calcium sulphate paste through small circular openings and segmenting with a knife. They are designed for mixing with legume seeds and distribution through a seed hopper. Such granules of porous gypsum are sprayed with a broth culture of appropriate rhizobia mixed with 12.5 per cent milk powder and an equal volume of saturated sucrose solution. Viability of cells on granules is repeatedly poor and declines rapidly in storage.

Natural peat granule — This is Nitragin's 'Soil Implant' inoculum. It consists of natural peat granule in which rhizobia are cultured. The granules are designed to provide inoculum in a furrow in soil along with seed using mechanical farm machinery. Populations of 10^8 to 10^9/g can be expected in the granules. Soybean and groundnut have shown good response to this type of inoculant in the United States.

Agronomic Importance

Both inoculation successes and failures at field levels have been well documented in literature from time to time (Taha *et al.*, 1967a, 1967b; Subba Rao and Balasundaram, 1971; Ham *et al.*, 1976; Hamdi, 1976; Hera, 1976; Subba Rao, 1976, 1979; Vojinovic, 1976; Balasundaram and Subba Rao, 1977; Subba Rao and Tilak, 1977). Failure to obtain the desired response may be due to: (1) the presence of native ineffective strains, which could not be displaced by the

Table 11: Effect of *Rhizobium* inoculation on the yield of different pulses at different locations — results of all-India coordinated experiments under ICAR Pulse Project

Location	Yield q/ha [*]			
	Control	Inoculated	Increase	% Increase
Chick-pea or gram (*Cicer arietinum*)				
Delhi	19.56	22.28	2.72	13 [**]
Kanpur	10.86	14.99	4.13	38 [**]
Hissar	13.42	16.46	3.04	22 [**]
Varanasi	19.51	26.62	7.11	36 [**]
Dholi	26.74	32.31	5.47	20 [**]
Jabalpur	20.27	22.12	1.85	9 [**]
Sardar Krishi Nagar	13.56	23.93	10.37	76 [**]
Durgapura	11.23	13.10	1.87	16
Ludhiana	7.27	8.26	0.99	13
Pigeon pea or arhar (*Cajanus cajan*)				
Jabalpur	4.82	6.93	2.11	44 [**]
Ludhiana	6.21	7.49	1.28	20 [**]
Hissar	19.85	21.87	2.02	10
Coimbatore	3.58	4.16	0.58	16
Hyderabad	11.30	16.52	5.22	46
Baroda	14.76	17.89	3.13	21
Mungbean or mung (*Vigna mungo*)				
Dholi	4.48	6.78	2.30	51 [**]
Ludhiana	7.97	10.02	2.05	26 [**]
Delhi	4.89	7.58	2.69	55 [**]
Hissar	11.83	12.83	1.00	9
Madurai	11.47	15.12	3.65	32 [**]
Hyderabad	3.73	4.56	0.83	22 [**]

Source: Dr. R.B. Rewari and associates.
[*] 1 quintal = 100 kg
[**] Significant.

introduced effective strains, (2) the presence of antagonists of rhizobia which minimize the number of rhizobia in the rhizosphere, (3) the availability of soil conditions which limit symbiosis caused by acidity, alkalinity, other factors relating to soil structure, application of pesticides and high nitrate to soil, and (4) the presence of effective native rhizobial strains in large numbers.

Responses to *Rhizobium* inoculation (Plate 1) have been demonstrated with principal grain legumes such as arhar (*Cajanus cajan*), gram (*Cicer arietinum*), mung bean (*Vigna mungo*), and broad bean (Tables 11, 12).

Table 12: Significant increase in yield of broad bean and lentil due to rhizobial inoculation in the presence of superphosphate

Superphosphate (kg/ha)	Mean yield (kg/ha)			
	Broad bean		Lentil	
	Uninoculated	Inoculated	Uninoculated	Inoculated
0	1310	1550	1376	1638
117	1572	1716	1638	1733
233	1716	1856	1615	1873
350	1786	1856	1638	1873
466	1642	1893	1756	1972

Source: Taha *et al.,* 1967a, 1967b.

Legumes are known to leave behind some residual nitrogen in soil. In some experiments, the residual effect was judged by the yield of a subsequent crop of wheat or rice (Table 13) which was always more in *Rhizobium* inoculated series than in uninoculated ones (Subba Rao and Tilak, 1977). Maximum residual effect was seen in soybean which increased the yield of the subsequent crop of wheat by 65.9 per cent over corresponding uninoculated controls.

Pay-off to the farmers by the use of Rhizobium inoculant — The use of rhizobial cultures in the establishment of legumes has been widely recognized, especially in areas where indigenous nodulation has been found to be inadequate. A rough calculation on the benefits derived by the use of *Rhizobium* inoculants (Table 14) shows that quite a good deal of money can be saved by the marginal farmers of India provided they use quality tested inoculants on the farm. In this connection, small- or large-scale industries suitable for each agro-climatic region must be encouraged and backed by guidance and know-how from centrally sponsored government agencies for achieving proper quality control standards. The approximate cost involved in setting up such industries in India is given in Table 15.

Table 13: Effect of legume inoculation with *Rhizobium* on the yield of subsequent crops (soil pH 7.3)

Previous crop	Yield of wheat (Triticum aestivum) var. Kalyansona (kg/ha)	Previous crop	Yield of rice (Oryza sativa) var. IR-8 (kg/ha)
Arhar (Cajanus cajan) (uninoculated)	2075	Gram (Cicer arietinum) (uninoculated)	2515
Arhar (inoculated)	2415 (16.4)	Gram (inoculated)	2715 (7.9)
Urid (Vigna mungo) (uninoculated)	2075	Lentil (Lens culinaris) (uninoculated)	2257
Urid (inoculated)	2125 (2.4)	Lentil (inoculated)	2555 (13.2)
Soybean (Glycine max) (uninoculated)	1350		
Soybean (inoculated)	2240 (65.9)		

Source: Subba Rao and Tilak, 1977.
The figures in parenthesis indicate the per cent increase in yield due to *Rhizobium* inoculation over uninoculated control.

Table 14: Possible pay off to the farming community in India by the application of good quality *Rhizobium* inoculant in the cultivation of three grain legumes, (Calculations are based on extensive field trials at several locations during successive years; the cost of inoculant per ha is taken as Rs. 20–30. Rs. 30 = 1 U.S. dollar)

Grain legume	Mean yield increase (kg/ha)	Monetary benefit by inoculation (Rs/ha)	Total acreage in the country (million ha)	Total increase in yield possible by inoculation (million t)	Possible monetary gain to the country (million rupees)
Bengal gram, chick-pea (Cicer arietinum)	500	5000	8.25	4.125	41250.0
Masur or lentil (Lens culinaris)	175	1225	0.85	0.149	1041.25
Soybean (Glycine max)	1002	8016	0.04	0.040	320.64

*If the prevailing retail selling price is taken as follows: Bengal gram Rs 10/kg; Lentil Rs. 7/kg; Soybean Rs. 8/kg. Even if one assumes that 1/10th of above responses actually occur in farmers fields, the benefit to the farmer is noteworthy considering the nominal amount of Rs. 20–30 as the price of the inoculant per ha.

Table 15: Cost involved in setting up plants for *Rhizobium*, *Azotobacter* and *Azospirillum* inoculant production (add appropriate sum to account for any possible increase in price)

	Cost in Rupees[*]
I. Small-scale industry (20,000 ha)	
Requirements	
Autoclave (1)	250,000
Shakers (2)	250,000
Incubator (1)	20,000
Oven (1)	20,000
Refrigerator (1)	30,000
Air-conditioners (2)	100,000
Sealers (2)	10,000
Metallic trays (60)	10,000
Ultraviolet lamps (4)	10,000
Glassware	175,000
Chemicals	175,000
pH meter	10,000
Space for production (building costs)	
a. Cold storage room	
b. Inoculation room	
c. Mixing and packing room	Variable
d. Shaker room	
e. Quality control laboratory	
Raw materials for production	200,000
Total cost or say Rs. 1.26 million excluding building costs	1,260,000
II. Large-scale industry (above 40,000 ha)	
Requirements same as above	1,260,000
Fermentor (25 to 150 cap.)	800,000
Mixer	100,000
Sealers, automatic (3)	50,000
Extra chemicals and glasswares	200,000
Extra raw material for production	200,000
Total cost (excluding building costs)	261,0000
or say Rs. 2.61 million excluding building costs	

[*]Approximately Rs. 30 = 1 U.S. dollar.

REFERENCES

Alexander, M. (1977). *Introduction to Soil Microbiology,* John Wiley & Sons, New York.

Balasundaram, V.R., and Subba Rao, N.S. (1977). A review of development of rhizobial inoculants for soybeans in India. *Fertilizer News,* **22,** 42–46.

Barrios, S., Raggio, N., and Raggio, M. (1963). Effect of temperature on infection of isolated bean roots by rhizobia. *Plant Physiol.,* **38,** 171–174.

Bauer, W.D. (1977). Lectins as determinants of specificity in legume-*Rhizobium* symbiosis. In *Genetic Engineering for Nitrogen Fixation,* Ed. A. Hollaender, Plenum Press, New York. pp. 283–297.

Bell, F., and Nutman, P.S. (1971). Experiments on nitrogen fixation by nodulated lucerne. *Biological Nitrogen Fixation in Natural and Agricultural Habitants.* Plant and Soil, Special volume, Martinus Nijhoff, The Hague, The Netherlands. pp. 231–264.

Bergersen, F.J., and Briggs, M.J. (1958). Studies on the bacterial component of soybean root nodules. Cytology and organization in the host tissue. *J. Gen. Microbiol.,* **19,** 482–490.

Bhalla, H., and Sen, A.N. (1973). Effect of rhizosphere bacteria of gram (*Cicer artetinum*) of different morphological, nutritional and physiological groups on *Rhizobium* nodulating the same host. *Sci. and Cult.,* **39,** 191–193.

Brockwell, J. (1963). Accuracy of a plant infection technique for counting populations of *Rhizobium trifolii. Appl. Microbiol.,* **11,** 377–383.

Brockwell, J. (1977). Application of legume seed inoculants. In *A treatise on Dinitrogen Fixation.* Eds. R.W.F. Hardy and A.H. Gibson. Section IV, *Agronomy and Ecology.* John Wiley and Sons, New York. pp. 277–310.

Bunting, A.H., and Horrocks, J. (1964). An improvement in the Raggio technique for obtaining nodules on excised roots on *Phaseolus vulgaris,* in culture. *Ann. Bot.,* **28,** 229–237.

Burris, R.H. (1974). Methodology. In *The Biology of Nitrogen Fixation.* Ed. A. Quispel. North Holland Publishing Co., Amsterdam. pp. 9–33.

Burris, R.H., Eppling, F.J., Wahlin, H.B., and Wilson, P.W. (1943). Detection of nitrogen fixation with isotopic nitrogen. *J. Biol. Chem.* **148,** 349–357.

Burton, J.C. (1967). *Rhizobium* culture and use. In *Microbial Technology.* Ed. J. Peppler. Reinhold Publishing Corporation, New York. pp. 1–33.

Burton, J.C. (1979). New developments in inoculating legumes. In *Recent Advances on Biological Nitrogen Fixation.* Ed. N.S. Subba Rao. Oxford & IBH Publishing Co., New Delhi. pp. 380–405.

Chhonkar, P.K., and Subba Rao, N.S. (1966). Fungi associated with legumes root nodules and their effect on rhizobia. *Canad. J. Microbiol.,* **12,** 1253–1261.

Chopra, C.L., and Subba Rao, N.S. (1967). Mutual relationship among bacteroids, leghaemoglobin and nitrogen content of Egyptian clover (*Trifolium alexandrinum*) and gram (*Cicer arietinum*). *Arch fur Mikrobiol.,* **58,** 71–76.

Cochran, W.G. (1970). Estimation of bacterial densities by means of 'most probable number'. *Biometrics,* **6,** 105–116.

Dadarwal, K.R., and Sen, A.N. (1973). Serological studies with strains of *Rhizobium* isolated from some pulse crops of India. *Indian J. Microbiol.,* **13,** 7–12.

Dadarwal, K.R., and Sen, A.N. (1974). Varietal specificity of rhizobial serotypes in relation to nodulation and crop yield. *Proc. INSA (B),* **40,** 548–553.

Dadarwal, K.R., Sen, A.N., and Subba Rao, N.S. (1973). Comparison of antibiotic properties of rhizobia cultured *in vitro* and their bacteriod form from root nodules. *Curr. Sci.*, **42**, 686–687.

Dadarwal, K.R., Singh, C.S., and Subba Rao, N.S. (1974). Nodulation and serological studies of rhizobia from six species of *Arachis. Plant and Soil*, **40**, 535–544.

Danso, S.K.A., and Alexander, M. (1974). Survival of two strains of *Rhizobium* in soil. *Soil Sci. Soc. Amer. Proc.*, **38**, 86–89.

Dart, P.J. (1974). The infection process, pp. 381–429. In *The Biology of Nitrogen Fixation*. Ed. A. Quispel. North Holland Publishing Co., Amsterdam.

Dart, P.J., and Mercer, F.V. (1963). Development of bacteroid in the root nodule of barrel medic (*Medicago tribuliodes* Desr) and subterraneum clover (*Trifolium subterraneum* L.). *Arch. fur Mikrobiol.*, **46**, 382–401.

Date, R.A. (1974). Legume inoculant production. *Proc. INSA (B)*, **40**, 667–686.

Date, R.A. (1976). Principles in *Rhizobium* strain selection. In *Symbiotic Nitrogen Fixation in Plants*. Ed. P.S. Nutman. Cambridge University Press, Cambridge, pp. 137–150.

Date, R.A., and Vincent, J.M. (1962). Determination of the number of root nodule bacteria in the presence of other organisms. *Aust. J. Exp. Agric. Anim. Husb.*, **2**, 5–7.

De Ley, J., and Russel, A. (1965). DNA base composition, flagellation and taxonomy of the genus *Rhizobium. J. Gen. Microbiol.*, **31**, 85–91.

Dilworth, M.J. (1966). Acetylene reduction by nitrogen fixing preparations from *clostridium pasteurianum. Biochem. Biophys. Acta*, **127**, 285–294.

Dudman, F.W., and Brockwell, J. (1968). Ecological studies of root nodule bacteria introduced to field environments. I. A survey of field performance of clover inoculants by gel immune-diffusion serology. *Aust. J. Agric. Res.*, **19**, 739–740.

Dye, M. (1979). Functions and maintenance of a *Rhizobium* collection. In *Recent Advances in Biological Nitrogen Fixation*. Ed. N.S. Subba Rao. Oxford & IBH Publishing Co., New Delhi. pp. 435–471.

Elkan, G.H. (1984). Taxonomy and metabolism of *Rhizobium* and its genetic relationship. In *Biological Nitrogen Fixation*, Ed. M. Alexander. Plenum Press, New York. pp. 1–38

Fahraeus, G., and Ljunggren, H. (1968). Pre-infection phases of legume symbiosis. In *The Ecology of Soil Bacteria*. Eds. T.R.G. Gray and D. Parkinson. Liverpool University Press, Liverpool. pp. 396–421.

Fielder, R., and Proksch, G. (1975). The determination of nitrogen-15 by emission and mass spectrometry in biochemical analysis. A review. *Anal. Chim. Acta.*, **78**, 1–62.

Fisher, R.A., and Yates, F. (1953). *Statistical Tables for Biological Agricultural and Medical Research*, 4th ed. Oliver and Boyd, London.

Fisher, R.A., and Yates, F. (1963). *Statistical Tables*, 6th ed. Oliver and Boyd, London.

Fred, E.B., Baldwin, I.L., and McCoy, E. (1932). *Root Nodule Bacteria and Leguminous Plants*. Univ. Wisconsin, Madison, Wisc.

Fried, M., and Broeshart, H. (1967). *The Soil Plant System in Relation to Inorganic Nutrition*, Academic Press, New York.

Fried, M., and Broeshart, H. (1975). An independent measurement of the amount of nitrogen fixed by a legume crop. *Plant and Soil*, **43**, 707–711.

Gaur, Y.D., and Sen, A.N. (1977). Taxonomical position of *Cicer* rhizobia, Abstr. In *Limitation and Potentials for Biological Nitrogen Fixation in the Tropics*. Plenum Press, New York. pp. 362–363.

Gibson, A.H. (1963). Physical environment and symbiotic nitrogen fixation. I. The effect of root temperature on recently nodulated *Trifolium subterraneum* L. plants. *Austral. J. Biol. Sci.,* 16, 28–42.

Graham, P.H. (1964). An application of computer techniques to the taxonomy of the root nodule bacteria of legumes. *J. Gen. Microbiol.,* 35, 511–517.

Gupta, K.C., and Sen, A. (1963). Utilization of combined nitrogen by *Rhizobium* spp. from some common cultivated legumes in relation to their effeciencies. *Indian J. Agric. Sci.,* 33, 240–243.

Ham, G.E., Lawn, R.J., and Brun, W.A. (1976). Influence of inoculation, nitrogen fertilizer and photosynthetic sources — Sink manipulations of field grown soybeans. In *Symbiotic Nitrogen Fixation in Plants.* Ed. P.S. Nutman. Cambridge University Press, Cambridge. pp. 239–253.

Hamdi, V.D. (1976). Field and green house experiments on the response of legumes in Egypt to inoculation and fertilizers. In *Symbiotic Nitrogen Fixation in Plants.* Ed. P.S. Nutman. Cambridge Univ. Press, Cambridge. pp. 289–298.

Hamatova, E. (1971). World catalogue of rhizobia collections, IBP Subcommittee on N2 Fixation.

Hardy, R.W.F., and Havelka, U.D. (1976) Photosynthate as a major factor limiting nitrogen fixation by field grown legumes with emphasis on soybeans. In *Symbiotic Nitrogen Fixation in Plants.* Ed. P.S. Nutman. Cambridge University Press, London. pp. 421–439.

Hera, C. (1976). Effect of inoculation and fertilizer application on the growth of soybean in Rumania. In *Symbiotic Nitrogen Fixation in Plants.* Ed. P.S. Nutman. Cambridge Univ. Press, Cambridge. pp. 269–279.

Holsten, R.D., Burns, R.C., Hardy, R.W.F., and Hebert, R. (1971). Establishment of symbiosis between *Rhizobium* and plant cells *in vitro, Nature,* Lond., 232, 173–176.

Iswaran, V., Sundara Rao, W.V.B., Magu, S.P., and Jauhri, K.S. (1969). Indian peat as a carrier of *Rhizobium. Curr. Sci.,* 38, 468–469.

Jensen, H.L. (1942). Nitrogen fixation in leguminous plants II. Is symbiotic nitrogen fixation influenced by *Azotobacter? Proc. Linn. Soc. N.S.W.,* 57, 205–212.

Jordan, D.C. (1962). The bacteroids of the genus *Rhizobium. Bact. Rev.,* 26, 119–141.

Kandaswamy, R., and Prasad, N.N. (1971). Lignite as a carrier of rhizobia. *Curr. Sci.,* 40, 496.

Koch, B., and Evans, H.J. (1966). Reduction of acetylene to ethylene by soybean root nodules. *Plant Physiology,* 41, 1748–1750.

Lakshmi Kumari, M., and Subba Rao, N.S. (1974). Effect of salinity and alkalinity on early phases of infection in lucerne (*Medicago sativa*). *Plant and Soil,* 40, 261–268.

Legg, J.O., and Sloger, C. (1975). A tracer method for determining symbiotic nitrogen fixation in field studies. In *Proc. International Conference on Stable Isotopes.* Eds. E.R. Klein and P.D. Klein. Oak Brook, Illinois. pp. 661–666.

Leonard, L.T. (1944). Method of testing bacterial cultures and results of tests of commercial inoculants, USDA Circ. No. 703, Washington, DC.

Magu, S.P., and Sen, A.N. (1969). Studies on the respiration of efficient and inefficient strains of *Rhizobium. Arch. Microbiol.,* 68, 355–361.

Mosse, B. (1964). Electron microscope studies of nodule development in some clover species. *J. Gen. Microbiol.,* 36, 49–66.

Norris, D.C. (1963). A porcelain bead method for storing *Rhizobium. J. Exp. Agric.,* 31, 255–258.

Nutman, P.S. (1965). The relation between nodule bacteria and the legume host in the rhizosphere and the process of infection. In *Ecology of Soil-borne Plant Pathogens*. Eds. K.F. Baker and W.C. Snyder. Univ. California Press, Berkeley and Los Angeles. pp. 231–246.

Nutman, P.S. (Ed.) (1976). *Symbiotic Nitrogen Fixation in Plants*. Cambridge University Press, Cambridge.

Pelczar, M.J., Reid, R.D., and Chan, E.C.S. (1977). *Microbiology*, Fourth Edition. McGraw-Hill Book Co., New York.

Postgate, J.R. (Ed.) (1971). *The Chemistry and Biochemistry on Nitrogen Fixation*. Plenum Press, London.

Pugasheti, B.K., and Wagner, G.H. (1980). Survival and multiplication of *Rhizobium japonicum* strains in Slit loam. *Plant and Soil*, **56**, 217–227.

Quispel, A. (Ed.) (1974). *The Biology of Nitrogen Fixation*. North Holland Publishing Co., Amsterdam.

Raggio, M., Raggio, N., and Torrey, J.G. (1957). The nodulation of inoculated leguminous roots. *Amer. J. Bot.*, **44**, 325–334.

Ranga Rao, V., Sopory, S., and Subba Rao, N.S. (1973). Establishment of symbiosis *in vitro* between *Rhizobium* and pea (*Pisum sativum*) root callus. *Curr. Sci.*, **43**, 503–505.

Robinson, A.C. (1968). The effect of anti-fungal antibiotics on the nodulation of *Trifolium subterraneum* and the estimation of *Rhizobium trifolii* populations. *Aust. J. Exp. Agric. Anim. Husb.*, **8**, 327–331.

Roughley, R.J. (1976). The production of high quality inoculants and their contribution to legume yield. In *Symbiotic Nitrogen Fixation*. Ed. P.S. Nutman. Cambridge Univ. Press, Cambridge. pp. 125–136.

Sarma, K.S.B., Lakshmi Kumari, M., Apte, R., and Subba Rao, N.S. (1973). Some physiological characteristics of *Rhizobium melioti* and *R. trifolii* in relation to efficiency of symbiosis with lucerne and Egyptian clover. *Plant and Soil*, **28**, 299–305.

Schmidt, E.L. (1974). Quantitative and ecological study of microorganisms in soil by immunofluorescence. *Soil Sci.*, **118**, 141–149.

Schmidt, E.L., Bankola, B.B., and Bohlool, R.O. (1968). Fluorescent antibody approach to study of rhizobia in soil. *J.Bact.*, **95**, 1987–1992.

Schollhorn, R. and Burris, R.H. (1967). Acetylene as a competitive inhibitor of N_2 fixation. *Proc. Natl. Acad. Sci. USA*, **38**, 213–216.

Sen, A.N., and Sen, A. (1958). Survival of *Rhizobium* in stored air dry soil. *J. Indian Soc. Soil Sci.*, **4**, 215.

Sethi, R.P., and Subba Rao, N.S. (1968). Inhibitory or stimulatory effect of soil fungi on rhizobia. *J. Gen. Appl. Microbiol.*, **14**, 325–327.

Singh, C.S., Lakshmi Kumari, M., Biswas, A., and Subba Rao, N.S. (1972). Nodulation of lucerne (*Medicago sativa* L.) under the influence of chlorides of magnesium and potassium. *Proc. Indian Acad. Sci.*, **76(8)**, 90–96.

Subba Rao, N.S. (1967). Mechanism of infection of legume roots by *Rhizobium*. *J. Sci. Ind. Res.*, **26**, 24–37.

Subba Rao, N.S. (1976). Field response of legumes in India to inoculation and fertilizer application. In *Symbiotic Nitrogen Fixation in Plants*. Ed. P.S. Nutman. Cambridge Univ. Press, Cambridge. pp. 255–268.

Subba Rao, N.S. (1977). *Soil Microorganisms and Plant Growth*, Oxford & IBH Publishing Co., New Delhi.

Subba Rao, N.S. (Ed.) (1979). *Recent Advance in Biological Nitrogen Fixation.* Oxford and IBH Publishing Co., New Delhi.

Subba Rao, N.S., and Balasundaram, V.R. (1971). *Rhizobium* inoculants for soybean. *Indian Farming,* **21**, 22–23.

Subba Rao, N.S., Lakshmi Kumari, M., Singh, C.S., and Magu, S.P. (1972). Nodulation of lucerne (*Medicago sativa* L.) under the influence of sodium chloride. *Indian J. Agric. Res.,* **42**, 386–388.

Subba Rao, N.S., Lakshmi Kumari, M., Singh, C.S., and Biswas, A. (1974). Salinity and alkalinity in relation to legume- *Rhizobium* symbiosis. *Proc. INSA,* **40**, 544–547.

Subba Rao, N.S., Pahwa, M.R., and Lakshmi Kumari, M. (1974). Effect of combined nitrogen in legume root nodulation. *Acta Botanica Indica,* **1**, 54–63.

Subba Rao, N.S., and Tilak, K.V.B.R. (1977). Rhizobial cultures —Their role in pulse production. *Souvenir Bulletin,* Directorate of Pulses Development, Government of India, Lucknow. pp. 31–34.

Taha, S.M., Mahmoud, S.Z., and Salem, S.H. (1976a). Effect of inoculation with rhizobia on some leguminous plants in UAR. I. Phosphorus manuring. *J. Microbiol. United Arab Republic*, **2**, 17–29.

Taha, S.M.., Mahmoud, S.Z., and Salem, S.H. (1967b). Effect of inoculation with rhizobia on some leguminous plants in UAR. II. Nitrogen Fertilization. *J. Microbiol. United Arab Repubilc,* **2**, 31–41.

Thornton, H.G. (1930). The early development of root nodules of lucerne (*Medicago sativa L.*). *Ann. Bot.* **44**, 385–392.

Tilak, K.V.B.R., and Subba Rao, N.S. (1978). Carriers for legume (*Rhizobium*) inoculants. *Fertilizer News,* **23(2)**, 25–28.

t Mannetje, L. (1967). A reexamination of the taxonomy of the genus *Rhizobium* and related genera using numerical analysis. *Antonie van Leeuwenhoek,* **33**, 477–491.

Verma, D.P.S., and Bal, A.K. (1976). Intracellular site of synthesis and localization of leghaemoglobin in root nodules. *Proc. Natl. Acad. Sci. USA,* **73**, 3843–3847.

Vincent, J.M. (1970). *A Manual for the Practical Study of the Root Nodule Bacteria,* IBP Hand Book No. 15, Blackwell Scientific Publications, Oxford.

Vojinovic, Z.D. (1976). Some studies on the necessity of legume inoculation in Serbia (Yougoslavia). In *Symbiotic Nitrogen Fixation in Plants.* Ed. P.S. Nutman. Cambridge Univ. Press, Cambridge, pp. 191–199.

3

Azotobacter Inoculant

The fixation of atmospheric nitrogen by free-living microorganisms as distinguished by fixation in association with another host plant system is known as non-symbiotic nitrogen fixation. Non-symbiotic nitrogen fixation is restricted to certain microorganisms, mostly bacteria and blue-green algae.

Free-living nitrogen-fixing bacteria are classified into aerobic, anaerobic, and facultative anaerobic types depending on the growth and survival of the organisms in the presence or absence of oxygen. The aerobic bacteria capable of fixing nitrogen belong to entirely different families and have been isolated from different habitats — soil, freshwater, marine, animal, and others. In some instances, claims of fixation of nitrogen have been confirmed, whereas in others they remain unconfirmed. The species of aerobic bacteria which have the ability to fix molecular nitrogen come under the genera *Azotobacter, Azomonas, Beijerinckia, Derxia, Mycobacterium,* and *Azospirillum* (micro-aerophilic). The species which fix nitrogen and are facultative anaerobes come under the genera *Bacillus, Enterobacter, Escherichia, Klebsiella, Rhodopseudomonas,* and *Rhodospirillum.* The strict anaerobic species which fix nitrogen come under the genera *Clostridium, Desulfovibrio, Chlorobium,* and *Chromatium.*

Among these bacteria, many are heterotrophic (e.g. *Azotobacter*) and depend on the energy derived from the degradation of plant residues. Photoautotrophic nitrogen fixation mediated by energy derived from photosynthesis is restricted to few bacteria (e.g. *Rhodopseudomonas*). In *Desulfovibrio,* nitrogen fixation is accompanied by reduction of sulphates (Mishustin and Shilnikova, 1971; Dobereiner, 1974; Mulder and Brontonegoro, 1974; Knowles, 1978).

Beijerinck was the first to isolate and describe *Azotobacter*—*A. chroococcum* and *A. agilis*. The former species was described as a soil-inhabiting species and the latter as a water-borne organism. During subsequent years, several other species have been described—*A. vinelandii, A. beijerinckii, A. insignis, A. macrocytogenes,* and *A. paspali*. Related to *Azotobacter* are other species known as *Beijerinckia indica* and *Derxia gummosa* (Mulder and Brontonegoro, 1974).

Isolation

Azotobacter spp. can be isolated by the soil dilution plating method. A weighed sample of soil (10 g) is suspended in 90 ml of sterilized water and serial dilutions of the suspension prepared (refer to method for isolation of *Rhizobium*) by further dilutions. Petri plates and pipettes are sterilized in the manner described for the isolation of *Rhizobium*. Any one of the nitrogen-free agar media for *Azotobacter* described in the Appendix is prepared and poured into petri plates. One ml aliquots of appropriate dilutions are evenly spread over cooled and set agar medium in petri plates. The plates are incubated at 28°C (± 2°C) in an incubator. After 3 days' incubation, flat, soft, milky, and mucoid colonies of *Azotobacter* develop on agar plates.

Azotobacter chroococcum is the dominant species in arable soils. Direct isolation of *Azotobacter* from soil has been practised by Russian workers (cited by Mishustin and Shilnikova, 1969, 1971). Lumps of soil are spread out on a nitrogen-free nutrient medium. After incubation of 3 days, *Azotobacter* colonies develop on the agar medium. Another method is to prepare a paste of soil in nitrogen-free liquid nutrient medium. This paste is incorporated in a layer of washed charcoal placed in a petri plate. The soil is aerated by burying a glass tube in it. After incubation of the plates at 28°C for 3–4 days, small *Azotobacter* colonies, if present, will develop on the soil surface. The method is known as the 'soil plate' method and has been widely used in Russian soil ecological studies.

Identification

In general, *Azotobacter* cells are polymorphic, the size of young rod-shaped cells varying from 2.0 to 70 × 1.0 to 2.5 μ; occasionally an adult cell may measure 10–12 μ. The morphology of cells, however, is dependent upon the composition of the medium. Young cells have peritrichous flagella which serve as locomotory organs (Mishustin and Shilnikova, 1969). Cells of *A. paspali* possess a tendency to form filaments (1.2 × 4–10 μ). After few days of cultivation, very long filaments (60 μ) are formed. *Azotobacter chroococcum, A vinelandi,* and *A. beijerinckii* are related species and their cells are generally rod-shaped with variable cell size. On the other hand, in *A. agilis* and *A. insignis,* the size of the cell and its oval to coccoid shape undergo little change due to ageing or nutritional conditions. *Azotobacter macrocytogenes* characterized by slime and capsules has coccoid cells which often associate into tetrads or groups under the influence of slime (Mulder and Brontonegoro, 1974).

Azotobacter chroococcum, A vinelandii, A. beijerinckii, and *A. paspali* are known to form cysts to withstand adverse conditions. Each cyst has a living cell with two coats. The cysts accumulate poly B-hydroxybutyric acid (PHB). With the onset of favourable conditions, the cysts give rise to vegetative cells.

Polysaccharide or gum production is another characteristic feature of A. chroococcum, A. beijerinckii, and *A. vinelandii,* although the related *Beijerinckia indica* and *Derxia gummosa* also produce abundant gum. On the other hand, *A. agilis* produces very little gum and *A. insignis* none at all (Mulder and Brontonegoro, 1974).

Azotobacter chroococcum produces characteristic black pigment, melanin, especially in older cultures. This pigmentation is due to the oxidation of tyrosine by tyrosinase, an enzyme which has copper. The formation of yellow pigment is characteristic of *A. beijerinckii. Azotobacter vinelandii* produces green-yellow water-soluble fluorescent pigment, while older cultures of *A. insignis* are yellow-brown. The related *Derxia* which fix nitrogen are yellow to mahogany brown, whereas *B. indica* is rust brown (Mulder and Brontonegoro, 1974; Mishustin and Shilnikova, 1971).

Classification

Most of the workers (Tchan, Jensen, Rubenchik, Norris, Mishustin) approve the grouping *Azotobacter* spp. under Azotobacteraceae, while others (Krasilnikov) group them under Bacteriaceae. In Azotobacteraceae, three genera — *Azotobacter, Beijerinckia,* and *Derxia* — have been recognized. However, De Ley and Park (1966) and De Ley (1968) did DNA analyses and DNA hybridization tests of different species of *Azotobacter, Beijerinckia,* and *Derxia.* Based on the differences in percentage (G + C) composition between species, they concluded that the genera *Beijerinckia* and *Derxia* are genetically distinct from the genus *Azotobacter.* In addition, within *Azotobacter,* they recognized three groups: (1) *A. chroococcum, A. beijerinckii,* and *A. vinelandii* group; (2) *A. insignis* and *A. macrocytogenes* group; and

(3) the *agilis* group. Accordingly, group 1 was retained as genus *Azoto-bacter,* group 2 was named *Azotomonas,* and group 3 *Azotococcus.* Mulder and Brontonegoro (1974) recognize the following species of *Azotobacter—A. chroococcum* (soil inhabitant, cyst and moderate slime producer with brown-black pigmentation), *A. vinelandii* (soil and water inhabitant, cyst and moderate slime producer with green fluorescent pigmentation). *A. beijerinckii* (soil inhabitant, cyst and moderate slime producer with yellow-light-brown pigmentation), *A. paspali* (soil inhabitant, cyst and moderate slime producer with green fluorescent pigmentation), *A. macrocytogenes* (soil inhabitant, cyst-less, abundant slime producer with pink pigmentation), *A. insignis* (water inhabitant, cystless, gumless with greyish-blue pigmentation), and *A. agilis* (cystless, little gum producer with green fluorescent pigmentation).

In the taxonomy of *Azotobacter,* the main criteria used are flagell-lation, pigmentation, and cyst formation and recently, as cited above, DNA analysis has also been taken into consideration.

Azotobacter in Soil

The numbers of *A. chroococcum* in Indian soils rarely exceed 10^4 to 10^5/g soil. There are two factors which have major influence on the population of *Azotobacter* in soil. They are the associative and antagonistic action of soil microflora and organic matter content of soil. Many microorganisms are known to accelerate the growth of *Azotobacter* and its nitrogen fixation. Similarly, other microorganisms inhibit the growth of *Azotobacter* and consequently its ability to fix nitrogen. Cellulolytic microorganisms which degrade plant residues in soil are known to encourage the proliferation of *Azotobacter* in soil. For earlier literature from the USSR on this subject, consult Mishustin and Shilnikova (1969, 1971). *Cephalosporium* spp., a common soil inhabitant, is known to inhibit the growth of *Azotobacter* and its nitrogen fixation (Iswaran and Subba Rao, 1966). These effects have been shown in pure cultures under laboratory conditions and have less relevance to field conditions. *Azotobacter* is also known to produce an ether-soluble fungistatic substance which inhibits the growth of fungi like *Alternaria, Helminthosporium,* and *Fusarium* when tested under laboratory conditions on agar media (Lakshmi Kumari *et al.,* 1972; Singh, 1977).

The lack of organic matter in soil is a limiting factor in the proliferation of *Azotobacter* in soil. The beneficial effects of small amounts of humus on the growth of *Azotobacter* and its nitrogen fixation are known (Jensen, 1951; Iswaran, 1958; Gaur and Mathur, 1966; Bhardwaj and Gaur, 1970). Table 16 illustrates this point.

Table 16: Effect of sodium humate and fulvic acid on the growth of *Azotobacter chroococcum* and its nitrogen fixation

Sodium humate or fulvic acid added (ppm)	Sodium humate 2		Fulvic acid	
	Growth (cell number × 10⁶/ml)	N fixed (mg)/g sugar oxidized	Growth (cell cumber × 10⁶/ml)	N fixed (mg)/g sugar oxidized
0	2.4	11.5	2.4	12.0
20	4.3	12.0	6.1	14.0
100	8.3	13.0	12.0	15.0
200	20.0	15.5	25.0	16.0
300	36.0	16.0	37.0	17.0
500	40.0	18.6	38.0	19.6
700	35.0	18.3	38.0	19.9
1000	25.0	15.9	28.0	17.5
Sig at 5% level	CD 0.464	CD 0.893	CD 0.745	CD 0.954

Source: Bhardwaj and Gaur, 1970.

The distribution of *Azotobacter* in different soils of the USSR has been extensively studied by the soil plate method. It has been shown that a considerable number of colonies of *Azotobacter* develop on soil plates from cultivated and manured soil samples of the USSR in contrast to virgin meadow and forest soils where the numbers are low or negligible. Studies on the occurrence of *Azotobacter* in some soil types of India have been done by Rangaswami and Sadasivam (1964). Inorganic fertilization of soil influences *Azotobacter* numbers. While addition of nitrogenous fertilizers to soil inhibits the growth of *Azotobacter,* addition of phosphatic fertilizers improves bacterial growth and proliferation (for earlier literature from Russia refer to Mishustin and Shilnikova, 1969, 1971).

Azotobacter cells are not usually present on the rhizoplane (root surface) but are abundant in the rhizosphere (the soil immediately surrounding roots). The dominance of *Azotobacter* in the rhizosphere of plants has been consistently shown by several investigators although some plants like wheat are known to harbour more anaerobic clostridia type of bacteria in their rhizosphere than aerobic *Azotobacter* types (Kavimandan et al., 1978). Root exudates or excretions which contain amino acids, sugars, vitamins, and organic acids together with the decaying portions of root system serve as energy sources for *Azotobacter* multiplication. Readers are advised to consult Vancura and Macura (1961) and Rovira (1965) for relevant literature on this subject.

Physiology and Function

The ability to fix elemental nitrogen is a vital physiological characteristic of *Azotobacter* spp. Different strains of *A. chroococcum* are known to vary in this regard. The range of fixation is 2–15 mg N fixed/g of carbon source utilized, although higher values have been often reported.

Azotobacter can utilize a variety of carbon sources (mono-, di-, and certain polysaccharides), organic acids of the fatty and aromatic series, ethyl alcohol, glycerol, mannitol vapours of acetone, and other volatile organic acids (see Mishustin and Shilnikova, 1969, 1971). The essentiality of calcium at optimum levels for better growth of *Azotobacter* and its nitrogen fixation has been pointed out (Iswaran and Sen, 1960). Similarly, the presence of combined nitrogen, trace elements, and sodium chloride in the medium can influence nitrogen fixation by *Azotobacter* (Iswaran, 1960b; Iswaran and Sundara Rao, 1960; Iswaran *et al.*, 1966).

The ability of *A. chroococcum* to synthesize and secrete thaimine, riboflavin, pyridoxin, cyanocobalamine, nicotinic and pantothenic acid, indole acetic acid, and gibberellins or gibberellin-like substances has been well documented by Russian workers. As indicated earlier, *A. chroococcum* also produces antifungal antibiotics which inhibit a variety of soil fungi. In fact, these twin attributes of *Azotobacter* can explain the beneficial effects of the bacteria on the germination of seeds (Shende *et al.*, 1977).

Primarily, the function of *Azotobacter* is to fix molecular nitrogen but as mentioned earlier, the ability of *A. chroococcum* to synthesize auxins, vitamins, growth substances, and antifungal antibiotics confers on it additional advantages. Most of these physiological attributes have been measured *in vitro* and no quantitative estimates of metabolites produced by *Azotobacter in vivo* in soil are available.

The overall reaction in the enzymic reduction of atmospheric nitrogen to ammonia could be stated as follows:

$$N_2 \xrightarrow[2e]{2H^+} NH=NH \xrightarrow[2e]{2H^+} H_2N-NH_2 \xrightarrow[2e]{2H^+} 2NH_3$$

(Dinitrogen)   (Diimide)   (Hydrazine)   (Ammonia)

Six electrons are needed to reduce N_2 to NH_3. It has been calculated that 12 moles of ATP are needed for reducing 1 mole of N_2 to 2 moles of ammonia. The electrons are derived from various carbon-containing compounds. The compound pyruvate provides electrons as well as ATP. These electrons flow to ferredoxins which are naturally occurring iron-sulphur (Fe-S) electron carrier proteins capable of undergoing reversible oxidation and reduction. Recently, iron-containing flavodoxins have been shown to be electron carriers in some nitrogen-fixing bacteria. Subsequently, the electrons pass through nitrogenase and reduce N_2 to NH_3. These sequences can be summarized as follows (Fottrell, 1968; Postgate, 1971, 1974):

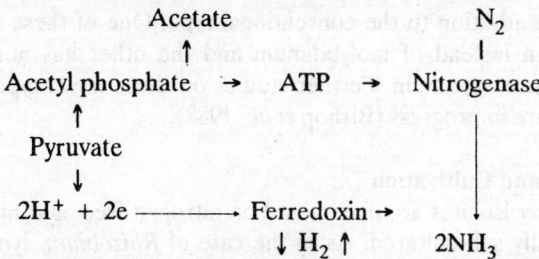

Azotobacter is an aerobic organism and oxygen is required for ATP formation, but nitrogen fixation is an anaerobic process. Obviously, oxygen must be excluded from the site of nitrogen fixation. Various proposals have been offered from time to time to explain the oxygen protection mechanism — the presence of membranes around nitrogenase to prevent oxygen damage, conformational protection of nitrogenase by rearrangement of the physical structure of nitrogenase so as to afford moderate resistance to oxygen, and the presence of large amounts of slime around bacterial cells which minimize oxygen entry. However, many workers believe that increased respiration by *Azotobacter* excludes oxygen from nitrogenase which may serve as a natural tool to scavenge oxygen from the site of nitrogen fixation (Postgate, 1971, 1974).

The MoFe protein is known as 'dinitrogenase', since N_2 binds to this moiety, whereas the Fe protein which serves the specific function of reducing the MoFe protein is referred to as 'dinitrogen reductase'. During the catalytic activity of nitrogenase, protons and N_2 compete for electrons. Therefore, in an environment consisting of N_2, H_2 production takes place simultaneously when N_2 is reduced to NH_3. The hydrogen evolution costs 25–30 per cent of the energy (reductants) available to the entire nitrogenase reaction, which is regarded as wasteful. The overall nitrogenase reaction can also be summarized as follows:

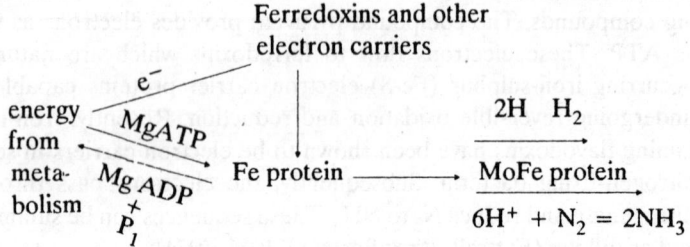

In mutants of *A. vinelandii*, two more nitrogenases have been recognized, in addition to the conventional type. One of these contains vanadium instead of molybdenum and the other has neither molybdenum nor vanadium. Further studies on these novel types of nitrogenases are in progress (Bishop *et al.*, 1988).

Maintenance and Cultivation

Azotobacter isolates are maintained on nitrogen-free agar media and periodically sub-cultured. As in the case of *Rhizobium*, lyophilization of cultures helps in permanently preserving different strains and species.

Large-scale cultivation of *A. chroococcum* for preparing inoculants in India is done by growing the cultures either in large flasks on a rotary shaker or in batch fermentors depending on the quantity needed. All precautions and sterilization procedures followed in the case of *Rhizobium* are also observed in the mass cultivation of *Azotobacter*. The media used in *Azotobacter* cultivation are given in the Appendix.

Agar- and carrier-based inoculant — In Russia the importance of *Azotobacter* as a seed inoculant was first recognized and used on a large scale to measure the benefits on crop growth. Agar-based cultures were used and the surface growth of bacteria on agar in large bottles was scraped, suspended in water, and the suspension used for inoculating seeds. In the case of transplanted crops (rice, cauliflower, etc.), the seedlings from nursery beds were dipped in the suspension of bacterial cells before planting.

Agar-based cultures were used in India for inoculation until 1973 but with the advent of carrier-based inoculants of *Rhizobium*, materials such as powdered peat soil, lignite, or powdered farmyard manure are also being increasingly used by manufacturers to produce

Azotobacter inoculants. The carrier-based cultures of *Azotobacter* are prepared in the same way as *Rhizobium* cultures.

The powdered carrier is neutralized with $CaCO_3$, autoclaved, and mixed with a broth culture of *Azotobacter*. The mixture is cured in trays for 2–5 days and then packed in polythene bags. All the mixing procedures followed for *Rhizobium* culture are also followed for *Azotobacter* culture preparation.

A slurry of the carrier-based culture is made with a minimum amount of water and the seeds are inoculated by mixing seeds with the slurry. The seeds are dried in shade and sown. For transplanted crops, the seedlings are dipped in the slurry for a certain period (10 to 30 minutes) and planted immediately. Individual manufacturers advertise their own methods of application including the doses of inoculum to be used. For sugarcane and millets, many packets are recommended at intervals for secondary inoculation in the early stages of plant growth. The second and subsequent inoculations are done by pouring the slurry near the root zone. The inoculant is also mixed in farmyard manure and broadcast near the root zone.

Crop Response

In Russia, between 1958 and 1960, 23 field experiments were done to measure the response of crops to *Azotobacter* inoculation. Out of them, significant increase in yield was obtained in eight experiments. Mishustin and Shilnikova (1969) summarized the innumerable field experiments in Russia (Table 17). The results show that there is a positive benefit of at least 7 to 12 per cent increase in yield due to inoculation.

Table 17: Effect of Azotobakterin on yield of field crops

Crop	Average yield in control (metric Cwt/ha)	Increase from Azotobacter (%)
Spring wheat	15.8	8.2
Winter wheat	21.3	9.8
Oats	17.1	12.0
Barley	21.0	9.0
Maize	36.2	8.0
Sugarbeet	283.1	7.0
Potato	178.0	8.0
Average		8.86

Source: Mishustin and Shilnikova, 1969.

Table 18: Summary of published results on field response of crops to *Azotobacter chroococcum* in India

Crop	Basal dressing	Increase (% over corresponding uninoculated control; * indicates significant increase)	Method of inoculation	Authors
Onion	0 kg N/ha, 40 cart loads of manure/ha, 50 kg P$_2$O$_5$ ha, 100 kg K$_2$O/ha	22	Roots dipped in a slurry of lignite-based inoculant at transplanting	Joi and Shinde (1976)
Onion	100 kg N/ha, 40 cart loads of manure/ha, 50 kg P$_2$O$_5$/ha, 100 kg P$_2$O$_5$/ha	18	"	"
Wheat Sonora 64	At varying levels of NPK	2 to 8	Seed inoculation with suspension of cells	Mehrotra and Lehri (1971)
Rice	" " "	1 to 22	"	"
Rice	At 120 kg N/ha 60 kg P$_2$O$_5$/ha 60 kg K$_2$O/ha	23*	"	"

Crop	Fertilizer level	Increase (range)	Method of inoculation	Reference
Brinjal	At varying levels of NPK and manure	1 to 42	Roots dipped in a slurry of lignite-based inoculant at transplanting	Mehrotra and Lehri (1971)
Tomato	"	2 to 29	"	"
Cabbage	"	26 to 45	"	"
Brinjal	"	15 to 62	"	Lehri and Mehrotra (1972)
Cabbage	"	25 to 50	"	"
Wheat	12,000 kg/ha manure	10 to 20	Seed inoculation with cell suspension	Lehri and Mehrotra (1968)
Wheat	Nil	10 to 30	"	"
Sorghum	Nil	9.3 to 38.1	"	Sundara Rao et al., (1963)
Maize	Nil	36.5 to 71.7	"	"
Cotton	Nil	6.7 to 26.6	"	Shende and Apte (1982)

Field experiments have also been done in India on *Azotobacter* inoculation of seed or seedlings of wheat (*Triticum aestivum*), rice (*Oryza sativa*), Onion (*Allium cepa*), brinjal (*Solanum melangena*), tomato (*Lycopersicum esculentum*), and cabbage (*Brassica oleracea*) under different agroclimatic conditions (Sundara Rao *et al.*, 1963; Lehri and Mehrotra, 1968, 1972; Mehrotra and Lehri, 1971; Joi and Shinde, 1976). The results, summarized in Table 18, show that significant increases in yield are seen in rice, cabbage, and brinjal, whereas in others there is only evidence of a positive increase in yield.

Shende *et al.*, (1977) have observed enhanced seed germination by *Azotobacter* inoculation. This effect is variable depending on the strains of *Azotobacter* used (Table 19). This is partly due to the ability of *Azotobacter* to produce growth substances and anti-fungal antibiotics (Brown, 1962; Mishustin and Shilnikova, 1969, 1971; Lakshmi Kumari *et al.*, 1975). The observed beneficial response of crop plants to inoculation with *Azotobacter* can be attributed to growth substances produced by the organism in addition to the fixed nitrogen made available to plants (Plate 2).

Table 19: Effect of *Azotobacter* strains on the germination of cotton seeds

Strains of A. chroococcum	Germination % (mean of 60 seeds)	Strains of A. chroococcum	Germination % (mean of 60 seeds)
Control (without Azotobacter)	43.3	P₁	30.0
Bar 1	45.0	P₂	38.3
B₁	33.3	P₄	46.6
B₂	60.0	W₁	33.3
M₂	76.6	W₂	43.3
M₄	60.0	W₃	35.0
M₅	41.6	W₄	43.3
M₆	66.6	W₅	45.0
M₇	50.0	mp₃	26.6
M*f*	55.0		
F value			Significant
C.D. at 5%			10.2

Source: Shende *et al.*, 1977.

REFERENCES

Bhardwaj, K.K.R., and Gaur, A.C. (1970). The effect of humic and fulvic acids on the growth and efficiency of nitrogen fixation of *Azotobacter chroococcum. Folia Microbiol.,* 15, 364–367.

Bishop, P.E., Premkumar, R., Joerger, R.D., Jacobson, M.R., Dalton, D.A., Chisnell, J.R., and Wolfinger, E.D. (1988). Alternative nitrogen fixation systems in *Azotobacter vinelandii.* In *Nitrogen Fixation: Hundred Years After.* Eds. H. Bothe, F.J. de Bruijn and W.E. Newton. Gustav Fischer, Stuttgart. pp. 71–79.

Brown, M. (1962). Population of *Azotobacter* in the rhizosphere and effect of artificial inoculation. *Plant and Soil,* 17(3), 15.

De Ley, J. (1968). DNA base composition and classification of some more free-living nitrogen fixing bacteria. *Antonie van Leeuwenhoek,* 34, 66–70.

De Ley, J., and Park, I.W. (1966). Molecular biological taxonomy of some free-living nitrogen fixing bacteria. *Antonie van Leeuwenhoek,* 32, 6–16.

Dobereiner, J. (1974). Nitrogen fixing bacteria in the rhizosphere. In *The Biology of Nitrogen Fixation.* Ed. A. Quispel. North Holland, Amsterdam. pp. 86–120.

Fottrell, R.F. (1968). Recent advances in biological nitrogen fixation, *Sci. Prog.,* Lond., 56, 541–555.

Gaur, A.C., and Mathur, R.S. (1966). Stimulating influence of humic substances on nitrogen fixation by *Azotobacter. Sci. Cult.,* 32, 319.

Iswaran, V. (1958). Effect of humus of legume and non-legume origin on the nitrogen fixation in *Azotobacter chroococcum. Curr. Sci.,* 27, 489–490.

Iswaran, V. (1960a). Effect of humified matter on nitrogen fixation by *Azotobacter. J. Indian Soc. Soil Sci.,* 8, 107.

Iswaran, V. (1960b). Influence of combined nitrogen on fixation of nitrogen by *Azotobacter. Proc. Indian Acad. Sci.,* 51(8), 103–115.

Iswaran, V., and Sen, A. (1960). Effect of calcium salts on nitrogen fixation by *Azotobacter* sp. *Ann. Biochem. Exp. Med.,* 20(8), 197–204.

Iswaran, V., and Subba Rao, N.S. (1966). A study of interaction between *Cephalosporium* sp. and *Azotobacter chroococcum. Indian Phytopath.,* 19, 87–91.

Iswaran, V., and Subba Rao, N.S., and Sundara Rao, W.V.B. (1966). Sodium chloride tolerance by *Azotobacter chroococcum. Curr. Sci.,* 35, 126–127.

Iswaran, V., and Sundara Rao, W.V.B. (1960). The effect of trace elements on nitrogen fixation by *Azotobacter. Proc. Indian Acad. Sci.,* 51(8), 103–115.

Jensen, H.L., (1951). Notes on the biology of *Azotobacter. Proc. Soc. Appl. Bacterial.,* 74(1), 89–94.

Joi, M.B., and Shinde, P.A. (1976). Response of onion crop to Azotobacterization. *J. Maharashtra Agric. Universtities.,* 1 (2–6), 161–162.

Kavimandan, S.K., Lakshmi Kumari, M., and Subba Rao, N.S. (1978). Non-symbiotic nitrogen fixing bacteria in the rhizosphere of wheat, maize and sorghum. *Proc. Indian Acad. Sci.,* 878, 299–302.

Knowles, R. (1978). Free-living bacteria. In *Limitations and Potentials for Biological Nitrogen Fixation in the Tropics.* Eds. J. Dobereiner, R.H. Burris and A. Hollaender. Plenum Press, New York. pp. 25–40.

Lakshmi Kumari, M., Vijayalakshmi, K., and Subba Rao, N.S. (1972). Interaction between *Azotobacter* sp. and fungi. 1. *In vitro* studies with *Fusarium moniliforme* Sheld. *Phytopath. Z.,* 75, 27–30.

Lehri, L.K., and Mehrotra, C.L. (1968). Use of bacterial fertilizers in crop production in UP. *Curr. Sci.,* 37, 494–495.

Lehri, L.K., and Mehrotra, C.L. (1972). Effect of *Azotobacter* inoculation on the yield of vegetable crops. *Indian J. Agric. Res.*, 9(3), 201–204.

Mehrotra, C.L., and Lehri, C.K. (1971). Effect of *Azotobacter* inoculation or crop yields. *J. Indian Soc. Soil Sci.*, 19(3), 243–248.

Mishustin, E.N., and Shilnikova, V.K. (1969). Free-living nitrogen-fixing bacteria of the genus *Azotobacter*. In *Soil Biology, Reviews of Research*, UNESCO Publication. pp. 72–124.

Mishustin, E.N., and Shilnikova, V.K. (1971). *Biological Fixation of Atmospheric Nitrogen*. MacMillan, London.

Mulder, E.G., and Brontonegoro (1974). Free-living heterotrophic nitrogen-fixing bacteria. In *Biology of Nitrogen Fixation*, Ed. A. Quispel. North Holland, Amsterdam. pp. 37–85.

Postgate, J.R. (Ed.) (1971). *The Chemistry and Biochemistry of Nitrogen Fixation*, Plenum Press, London, New York.

Postgate, J.R. (1974). Prerequisites for biological nitrogen fixation in free-living heterotrophic bacteria, In *Biology of Nitrogen Fixation*. Ed. A. Quispel. North Holland Publishing Co., Amsterdam. pp. 663–686.

Rangaswami, G., and Sadasivam, K.V. (1964). Studies on the occurrence of *Azotobacter* in some soil types, *J. Indian Soc. Soil Sci.*, 1, 12(1), 43–49.

Rovira, A.D. (1965). Effect of *Azotobacter, Bacillus* and *Clostridium* on the growth of wheat, *Plant Microbes Relationship*. Prague, Czechosl. Acad. Sci., 193–200.

Shende, S.T., and Apte, R. (1982). *Azospirillum* inoculation — A highly remunerative input for agriculture, In *Biological Nitrogen Fixation, Proc. National Symp.*, IARI, New Delhi. pp. 532–543.

Shende, S.T., Apte, R.G., and Singh, T. (1977). Influence of *Azotobacter* on germination of rice and cotton seeds, *Curr. Sci.*, 46, 675.

Singh, T. (1977). Studies on interaction between *Azotobacter chroococcum* and some plant pathogens, IARI Ph.D. thesis, New Delhi.

Sundara Rao, W.V.B., Mann, H.S., Pal, N.B., and Mathur, R.S. (1963). Bacterial inoculation experiments with special reference to *Azotobacter Indian J. Agric. Sci.*, 33, 279–290.

Vancura, J., and Macura, J. (1961). The effect of root excretion on *Azotobacter, Folia Microbiol.*, 6(4), 250–259.

4

Azospirillum Inoculant

In 1925, Beijerinck described a nitrogen-fixing bacterium under the name *Spirillum lipoferum*. Since fixation of nitrogen in pure cultures of this organism could not be confirmed at that time, the bacterium was deleted from the list of nitrogen fixers. However, Becking (1963) isolated a strain of *Vibrio* or *Spirillum* from African soils which resembled Beijerinck's *S. lipoferum* and fixed nitrogen as revealed by $^{15}N_2$ incorporation studies. Later, Bulow and Dobereiner (1975) ascribed the nitrogen-fixation potential of some tropical forage grasses such as *Digitaria, Panicum, Brachiaria,* maize, sorghum, wheat, and rye to the activity of *S. lipoferum* in their roots (Dobereiner and Day, 1975a). A survey in various countries revealed that the N_2-fixing *S. lipoferum* is a very common root- and soil-inhabiting nitrogen-fixing bacterium in the tropics (Dobereiner *et al.,* 1976). The distribution of the bacterium in India, the mode of bacterial colonization in plant roots, and the response of grasses and crops to inoculation with Indian isolates have also been reported (Lakshmi Kumari *et al.,* 1976; Lakshmi *et al.,* 1977; Kavimandan *et al.,* 1978; Subba Rao *et al.,* 1979a, 1979b). The nomenclature of this organism was revised and designated as *Azospirillum* (Tarrand *et al.,* 1978). In the pages to follow, the name *Azospirillum* will therefore be used. It must also be noted that in earlier papers, the organism was referred to as *Spirillum* until the revised nomenclature was proposed.

Isolation

Conventional methods of isolation of aerobic and anaerobic bacteria are not applicable to the isolation of *Azospirillum*. The bacterium is widespread in soil and occurs outside as well as inside the roots. Enrichment procedures are necessary to obtain cultures of the organism from plant roots as well as soil samples. Cultures can be isolated from surface-sterilized as well as unsterilized washed roots.

Small pieces of washed roots (0.5 cm pieces) or small samples of soil (few μg) are placed on a semi-solid agar medium containing sodium malate or calcium malate as the carbon source (see Appendix for composition). After incubation at 28°–30°C for 2 days, pellicles of *Azospirillum* can be seen 1–2 mm below the upper surface of the medium. Usually, small screw-cap bottles are used for isolation of the organism by the enrichment method (Bulow and Dobereiner, 1975; Lakshmi Kumari *et al.*, 1976; Burris *et al.*, 1977).

The semi-solid medium allows the organism to develop at low partial pressure of oxygen, which is favourable for the organism in its nitrogen-fixing state. If ammonia is supplied to the medium, *Azospirillum* grows as an aerobe on agar slopes or in liquid medium but is incapable of fixing nitrogen. On ammonia-containing medium, the doubling time is 1 hour, whereas on a malate containing semi-solid medium, the doubling time is 5.5 to 7 hours (Okon *et al.*, 1977). The advantage of growing *Azospirillum* on ammonia-containing medium is that a rich harvest of cells could be obtained for inoculation purposes.

In India, *Azospirillum* has been isolated from the roots of several plants (Lakshmi *et al.*, 1977) and their nitrogen-fixing potential varies (Table 20). The organism has also been isolated from the stems of several varieties of wheat (Kavimandan *et al.*, 1978) and found to occur in xylem vessels of *Cicer arietinum* (Lakshmi *et al.*, 1977).

Table 20: Occurrence of *Azospirillum lipoferum* bacteria in the roots of several plants and the amount of N_2 fixed by them

Plant	Variety	mg N_2 fixed/g of substrate
Oryza sativa	var. Madhu	28
	var. Mashuri	20
Sorghum bicolor	var. CSH2	20
	var. CSV5	16
Zea mays	var. not known	24
Panicum sp.		28
Cynodon dactylon		36
Setaria sp.		12
Amaranthus spinosa		16

Source: Lakshmi *et al.*, 1977.

Enumeration

Enumeration can be done by MPN method for counting *Azospirillum* from soils and roots. Adequate dilutions (up to 10 fold) are made in mineral salt solution without malate. Aliquots (0.1 ml) of each dilution are placed in the centre of screw-capped vials with semi-solid nitrogen-free bromothymol blue (NFB) medium in which 0.5 per cent malate is replaced with 0.025 per cent malate and 0.025 per cent cane sugar. The presence of *Azospirillum* and other diazotrophs in the serial dilution is determined by C_2H_2 reduction tests. The formation of a dense pellicle is a good evidence for *Azospirillum* growth but this should be checked microscopically from the highest dilution which can reduce C_2H_2. The C_2H_2 reduction test must be carried out at two-day intervals in all the vials having apparent growth since aged cultures fail to reduce C_2H_2 (Dobereiner, personal communication). The MPN counts can be calculated as per tables provided by Cochran (1950) and reproduced by Alexander (1965).

Identification and Classification

On the semi-solid malate medium, the development of white, dense, and undulating fine pellicles is very characteristic of *Azospirillum*. Microscopic examination reveals polymorphism but the dominant forms on a sodium malate medium are characteristic curved rods of varying sizes with prominent refractive fat droplets. The organism is Gram-negative and contains PHB granules. The cells have a one half spiral turn and show spirillar movement (Dobereiner *et al.,* 1976). Thin pellicles are less contaminated with other microorganisms than thick pellicles and show high nitrogenase activity. The contaminants in thick pellicles are *Azotobacter*, pro-actinomycetes, and protozoa (Lakshmi Kumari *et al.,* 1976). Stale cultures show a high level of protozoa with no *Azospirillum*. Serial transfers of *Azospirillum* from thin pellicles into fresh semi-solid medium are necessary to obtain pure cultures. The size of cells is variable even among isolates from the same roots. Electron micrographs of strains Sp 7 and Br 17 of *Azospirillum* show lateral flagella in addition to single polar flagellum (Krieg and Tarrand, 1978).

Based on the vibrioid and helical shape of cells and their affinity to salts of organic acids (malate, succinate, etc.) as the carbon source, *Spirillum lipoferum* was initially assigned to the genus *Spirillum* Ehrenberg by Beijerinck in 1925. However, ever since Dobereiner and associates described the organism in greater detail, certain strains of *Spirillum* were found to require low levels of yeast extract for growth on mineral media (Dobereiner *et al.,* 1976; Okon *et al.,* 1976). Yeast extract requiring strains (at low levels) exhibited growth with glucose as the source of carbon, whereas strains that did not require yeast extract failed to grow on glucose. Therefore, Krieg and Tarrand (1978) and others suspected the existence of more than one group among the *S. lipoferum* strains. The taxonomy of the genus was thus confusing and necessitated further inquiry.

Tarrand *et al.,* (1978) examined 61 strains of root-associated nitrogen-fixing *S. lipoferum* strains from various sources for substrate utilization, flagellation, and DNA base composition. They concluded that the existing strains described hitherto under *S. lipoferum* can be assembled in two groups (I and II) and assigned to a new genus *Azospirillum* (azote means nitrogen and spira means spiral) with the following characteristics: cells generally vibrioid but may be S-shaped or helical in semi-solid nitrogen-free medium containing 0.005 per cent yeast extract; cell diameter about 1 μ; single polar flagellum in liquid medium and numerous lateral flagella on solid medium; prominent PHB granules in cell; no formation of slime; has mainly respiratory type of metabolism but some fermentative character may be seen; under O_2 deficiency, nitrate is dissimilated to nitrate, nitrous oxide, or nitrogen gas; molecular nitrogen is fixed; grows well on salts of organic acids — malate, succinate, pyruvate, or lactate; certain carbohydrates may also serve as carbon sources; the mol percentage G + C of the DNA is about 70 by thermal denaturation methods. Type species is *A. lipoferum*.

Two species of *Azospirillum* had earlier been proposed — *A. lipoferum* (Beijerinck) comb. nov. and *A. brasilense* sp. nov.

The characteristics of *A. lipoferum* which fall under group II of Tarrand *et al.,* (1978) are as follows: lipus means fat and fero means to carry; capable of using glucose as a sole source of carbon for growth on a nitrogen-free semisolid medium containing biotin; biotin required for growth; when grown on peptone-containing glucose medium under aerobic conditions growth takes place with the production of acid but scant growth and acidification may also take place in glucose- and fructose-containing media under anaerobic conditions. Similarly, acid production takes place in media containing ribose, mannitol, or sorbitol; cell size is 1.4–1.7 μ in semisolid nitrogen-free malate medium containing 0.005 per cent yeast extract but cells tend to become wider, longer, S-shaped or helical, and non-motile. The original strain of *S. lipoferum* isolated by Beijerinck probably belongs to *A. lipoferum*. The characteristics of *A. brasilense* which fall under group I of Tarrand *et al.,* (1978) are as follows: incapable of utilizing glucose as a sole carbon source for growth on nitrogen-free semisolid medium; weak acidification may occur on media without peptone buffered with phosphate but no acidification of peptone-containing glucose medium or media with ribose mannitol or sorbitol takes place; sugars not fermented; no need for vitamins in semisolid nitrogen-free malate medium containing 0.005 per cent yeast extract; cell size 1.0 μ, short, vibrioid, motile, but S-shaped cells may occur in aged cultures.

The cultures isolated from Delhi, which were earlier descirbed under *S. lipoferum,* were reexamined on the criteria proposed by Tarrand *et al.,* (1978). The results show that all the strains so far isolated could be clubbed under group I of Tarrand *et al.,* (1978) and hence belong to *A. brasilense* (Sathyanarayana Rao, 1977).

One of the characteristics of *Azospirillum* is its ability to reduce nitrate and denitrify (Krieg, 1977). Both *A. lipoferum* and *A. brasilense* may comprise strains which can actively or weakly denitrify or reduce nitrate to nitrite and therefore, for inoculation studies, it would be necessary to select strains which do not possess these characteristics.

New N$_2$-fixing Bacteria Associated with Cereals and Sugarcane

Several new N$_2$-fixing bacteria have been isolated and characterized by Brazilian microbiologists (Dobereiber and others) from root systems of several plants. Two new species of *Azospirillum* have been isolated from sugarcane, rice, sorghum, and maize. They are *A. amazonense* (Magalhaes *et al.,* 1983) and *A. halopraeferans* (Reinhold *et al.,* 1987). *Azospirillum amazonense* is acid tolerant, uses sucrose, and has been frequently isolated from sugarcane and sweet sorghum roots. It has also been isolated from palm trees of the Amazon region (Magalhaes *et al.,* 1983). *Azospirillum halopraeferans* is common on the root surface of Kallar grass (*Diplanchne fusca* (Linn) Beauv) in Pakistan's salt-affected soils but it is not found in the cell interior of roots (Reinhold *et al.,* 1987). The bacterium has adapted to the harsh ecological surroundings with an optimum requirement of 41°C temperature and 0.25 per cent salt requirements. A new genus different from azospirilla has been erected based on isolation of N$_2$-fixing bacteria from washed and surface-sterilized roots of maize, rice, and sorghum in Rio de Janeiro. The bacterium has bipolar flagella and N_2 fixation is more O_2- and pH-tolerant than those of azospirilla. It has been named *Herbaspirillum seropedicae* (Baldani *et al.*, 1986). The microbiologists at the International Rice Research Institute (IRRI) in the Philippines (Watanabe and others) have isolated *Pseudomonas diazotrophicus* from the roots of rice and weeds growing in wetlands but the species was not found in plants growing in dry soils (Watanabe *et al.*, 1987). A nitrogen-fixing bacterium very sensitive to oxygen was earlier isolated from a water weed (*Spartina alterniflora*) and identified as a new species of *Campylobacter* (McClung and Patriquin, 1980). *Bacillus azotofixans*, an efficient nitrogen fixer, was isolated from surface-sterilized roots of grasses, wheat, and sugarcane (Seldin *et al.*, 1984) and this isolate is capable of fixing nitrogen in the presence of nitrate and is in fact nitrate-dependent for growth. This characteristic is also shared by *Azotobacter paspali*, which was originally described by Dobereiner (1966).

Acetobacter nitrocaptans (syn. *Saccharobacter nitrocaptans*) has been isolated from many sugarcane cultivars in many parts of Brazil. It exists in rhizosphere soil, washed roots, surface-sterilized soils and cane trash in the range of 10^3 to 10^7/g wet weight basis. Sugarcane-free soil or soil in the vicinity of other weeds associated with sugarcane cultivation do not harbour this bacterium, which reflects that the residual sugar in the sugarcane biomass encourages the growth of this N_2- fixing organism. The isolation and enumeration medium consists of 10 per cent cane sugar and 1 per cent cane juice, acidified with acetic acid to pH 4.5. The bacterium is a small Gram-negative aerobic rod showing pellicle formation and exhibiting acetylene-reducing activity in nitrogen-free semisolid medium without sugarcane juice. The growth is maximum when sugar content is 10 per cent and after 5 days forms a thick pellicle leading to a fall in pH to 3.0 or below, at which hydrogen ion concentration, N_2 fixation continues for several days (more than 100 n moles/hr/ml). The bacterium uses ethyl alcohol for growth, oxidizing it to CO_2 and H_2O. On potato agar with 10 per cent sugar the bacterium forms dark brown colonies, whereas on nitrogen-limited medium having 0.005 per cent yeast extract, mineral medium with 10 per cent sugar, and bromothymol blue, the bacterium exhibits orange colonies (Cavalcante and Dobereiner, 1988; Dobereiner *et al.*, 1988).

Azospirillum in Soil and in Roots

In a survey conducted by Dobereiner *et al.,* (1976) it was found that *Azospirillum* is a common soil inhabitant of tropics (four African countries and Brazil). As mentioned earlier, the occurrence of *Azospirillum* in Indian soils has already been reported (Lakshmi *et al.,* 1977). Differences between plant species in relation to *Azospirillum* occurrence and its nitrogenase activity have been observed. The occurrence of the bacterium in soil is dependent on pH. Soil pH between 5.6 and 7.2 registers nitrogenase activity while pH below 5.6 does not encourage nitrogenase activity of soil around roots of *Panicum maximum*. Maximum nitrogenase activity of soil inoculum was observed at pH of soil between 6.7 and 7.0. The nitrogenase activity of *P. maximum* roots could be detected even in acid pH up to 5.2 probably due to the proliferation of *Azospirillum* within roots. Nitrogenase activity of roots was highest at pH 6.7 (Dobereiner *et al.,* 1976). *Azospirillum* is known to get established in callus cultures as well as cultured cells of plants (Lakshmi *et al.,* 1977; Vasil *et al.,* 1977).

Table 21: Isolation of *Spirillum lipoferum* from air-dried and stored soil samples

Time of storage (years)	Nature of soil	Organic matter (%)	pH	Present (+) or absent (−)
1	Silt loam	2.75	7.2	+
2	Silty clay loam	2.85	7.0	+
3	Sandy loam	0.47	8.0	+
4	Sandy loam	0.3	6.2	+
5	Sandy loam	0.4	4.8	−
6	Loamy sand	0.5	5.8	+
5	Sandy	0.2	5.7	−
6	Sandy	0.41	4.8	−
7	Sandy clay	0.3	5.8	+
7	Silty loam	3.2	7.1	+
10	Sandy	0.3	6.9	+
10	Sandy	0.4	4.8	−
10	Silty clay loam	1.5	7.8	+
12	Sandy	0.2	5.5	−
15	Silty clay loam	3.5	7.2	+
15	Sandy	0.25	5.2	−
15	Clayey loam	1.2	6.2	+

Source: Lakshmi *et al.,* 1977.

Work done in India (Lakshmi *et al.,* 1977) has revealed that soil samples of all ages even up to 15 years and of varying texture and organic matter content had *Azospirillum* but soils below pH 5.7 were free of this bacterium. Sandy soils devoid of organic matter were generally not favourable for *Azospirillum*, whereas soils rich in organic matter were (Table 21). At the Central Rice Research Institute, Cuttack, it has been shown that the occurrence of N_2-fixing *A. lipoferum* is widespread in roots of several cultivars of rice and weeds associated with rice plants (Nayak and Rao, 1977).

Light microscopic observations and staining agents such as 2, 3, 5-triphenyl-tetrazolium dichloride (TTC) have served to describe the colonization of roots by diazotrophic bacteria. Because TTC reduction may be due to respiratory electron transport by a variety of fermentative bacteria, the question of actual location of diazotrophs within roots still remains unanswered. By the use of the protein A gold technique coupled with silver amplification and light microscopy to render diazotrophs visible in semi-thin section of roots, it has been shown that diazotrophic rods predominate as large aggregates in the endorhizosphere of Kallar grass (*Diplanchne fusca*). However, in aseptically grown and inoculated seedlings, even though such large aggregates were not seen, the bacteria had the potentiality to colonize the aerenchyma of roots. Penetration of the bacteria may occur at the epidermal cell junctions where lateral roots emerge (Reinhold and Hurek, 1989).

Earlier studies have also revealed that *Beijerinckia* cells colonized aseptically grown rice (Diem *et al.*, 1978). Electron micrographs have also shown *Campylobacter* bacteria in the aerenchyma of field-grown *Spartina alterniflora* (McClung *et al.*, 1983). Similarly, the occurrence of *Azospirillum* has been demonstrated in the cortex of field-grown *Cyanodon dactylon* roots (Schank *et al.*, 1979).

Physiology and Function

Azospirillum grows very well on malate, succinate, lactate, or pyruvate, moderately on galactose or acetate, but poorly on glucose or citrate. The ability to fix nitrogen has been verified by reduction tests with acetylene and uptake of $^{15}N_2$. *Azospirillum* fixes nitrogen best under micro-aerophilic conditions and shaking of cultures inactivates nitrogenase activity temporarily. Reduction of acetylene gets diminished rapidly in cultures whose pH is adjusted to levels beyond 7.8. The organism is highly aerobic in the presence of ammonia in the medium. It does not fix nitrogen under total anaerobic conditions. The amount of agar in the semisolid medium influences the growth and activity of this organism. It grows very well, reduces acetylene efficiently, and forms typical pellicle 2 mm below the surface when the agar concentration is 0.05 to 0.17 per cent. The sensitivity of the bacterium to agar concentrations reflects its characteristic low optimum requirements for oxygen (Dobereiner and Day, 1975b; Day and Dobereiner, 1976; Okon *et al.*, 1976).

Nitrogenase has been recovered from cell-free suspensions of *Azospirillum*. The nitrogenase proteins of *Azospirillum* can cross-react and form active nitrogenase with separated components from several other nitrogen-fixing micro organisms (Burris *et al.*, 1977).

Maintenance and Cultivation

Maintenance of *Azospirillum* cultures can be done on ammonium chloride containing agar medium formulated by Okon *et al.* (1976, 1977). On this medium the bacterium does not fix nitrogen but proliferates profusely under aerobic conditions. The number of cells in the broth can be counted by plating dilutions on agar medium which contains ammonium chloride. Otherwise, the cultures can also be maintained on semisolid malate medium in screw-cap tubes.

For large-scale cultivation, bottles or flasks with liquid medium that contains ammonium chloride (Okon *et al.*, 1976, 1977) could be used and incubated on a rotary shaker. The cells can be harvested for inoculation after 3 days' incubation at 35°C on a rotary shaker. Later, the contents of the flask are incorporated into a carrier. The composition of the media used in *Azospirillum* cultivation is given in the Appendix.

Carrier-based Inoculant

Several indigenously available carriers have been examined for the survival of *Azospirillum* (Lakshmi *et al.*, 1977; Tilak *et al.*, 1979). Of all the carriers tested, powdered and sterilized farmyard manure + soil, manure alone, or manure + charcoal supported the survival of the organism up to 31 weeks (Table 22).

The survival of *Azospirillum* in many other carriers was studied by Tilak *et al.* (1979), who confirmed the fact that soil and farmyard manure gave higher counts of *Azospirillum* than other carriers. The viability of the organism in carriers could be monitored by plating dilutions of the carrier on agar medium that contains ammonium chloride (Okon *et al.*, 1977). On this solid medium it is possible to count the number of *Azospirillum* cells at a given time. Individual colonies are picked up from agar plates and examined for characteristic features of *Azospirillum* under a microscope. The survival of *Azospirillum* in different carriers is shown in Fig. 10.

Table 22: Survival of *A. lipoferum* in different carriers

Carrier	Survival (weeks)
Soil	1
Farmyard manure	31 **
Soil + manure (1:1)	31 **
Soil + manure* (9:1)	15
Soil + sucrose (9:1)	1
Soil + sucrose (9:4)*	1
Soil + sodium malate (9:1)	1
Soil + sodium malate* (9:1)	1
Charcoal	1
Manure + charcoal (1:1)	31 **
Manure + charcoal* (1:1)	15
Indian peat	2

Source: Lakshmi *et al.*, 1977.
*Supplemented with 100 mg K_2HPO_4.
**The reisolated culture fixed N_2.

Crop Response

The response of a few economic species of graminaceous plants to inoculation (Plate 2) with a carrier-based inoculant containing two strains of *A. brasilense* (strain Madhu isolated from roots of rice and a strain from roots of *Cynodon dactylon,* a weed grass) was tested in pots containing unsterilized soil (Subba Rao *et al.*, 1979a). The bacteria were grown on a semisolid sodium malate medium for 72 hours, mixed with a sterilized carrier (soil + farmyard manure powder, 1:1), and incubated at room temperature (28°–32°C) for a week. This inoculant was used to treat seeds. Seed inoculation was done with two grasses (*Cenchrus ciliaris* and *Chrysopogon fulvus*), wheat (*Triticum aestivum*) var. HD 2122, barely (*Hordeum vulgare*) var. S 32, rice (*Oryza sativa*) var. Pusa 2–21, and oats (*Avena sativa*) var. Kent. A sticker (6 g carboxy methyl cellulose in 500 ml water) was sprinkled on seeds. The seeds were spread on a polythene sheet and the carrier-based inoculant powder was sprinkled on seeds and mixed uniformly.

Seed inoculation increased the dry weight of both the grasses but significantly so in *C. ciliaris*. The yield increase was equivalent to that obtainable with 20 kg N/ha of urea. Inoculation with 20 kg N/ha significantly increased the yield of grasses (Table 23).

In grain crops, inoculation significantly increased the yields of straw and grain of barley at 0, 40, and 60 kg N/ha of urea. The trend was also similar with rice in so far as grain yields are concerned. In

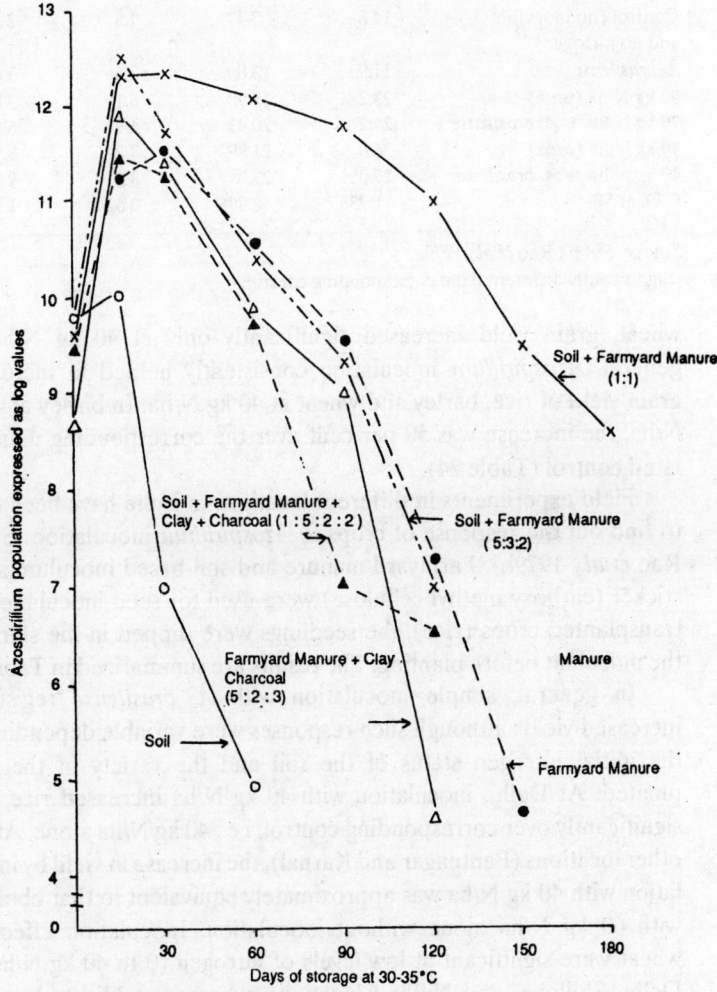

Fig. 10. Survival of *A. brasilense* in different carriers (Tilak *et al.*, 1979).

Table 23: The effect of seed inoculation of two grasses with *A. brasilense*
(Mean of three replicate pots, each having 22 plants)

Treatments	C. ciliaris		C. fulvus	
	Shoot length (cm)	Dry weight of shoot (g)	Shoot length (cm)	Dry weight of shoot (g)
Control (no inoculum and no nitrogen)	14.8	3.47	1.8	2.53
A. brasilense	21.9*	13.06*	3.6*	3.68
20 kg N/ha (urea)	23.2	13.98	6.1	3.89
20 kg N/ha + A. brasilense	24.2	20.43*	6.9*	6.16*
40 kg N/ha (urea)	26.0	21.89	7.7	8.75
40 kg N/ha + A. brasilense	27.0	23.3	8.6*	9.09
C.D. at 5%	1.738	2.896	0.624	1.225

Source: Subba Rao *et al.,* 1979a.
*Significantly different from corresponding control.

wheat, grain yield increased significantly only at 40 kg N/ha. In general, *Azospirillum* inoculation consistently helped in increasing grain yield of rice, barley and wheat at 40 kg N/ha. In barley at 40 kg N/ha, the increase was 50 per cent over the corresponding uninoculated control (Table 24).

Field experiments in different locations in India have been done to find out the response of crops to *Azospirillum* inoculation (Subba Rao *et al.,* 1979b). Farmyard manure and soil-based inoculum and a sticker (carboxy methyl cellulose) were used for seed inoculation. In transplanted crops (rice), the seedlings were dipped in the slurry of the inoculant before planting. The results are summarized in Table 25.

In general, simple inoculation with *A. brasilense* registered increased yields although such responses were variable depending on the initial nitrogen status of the soil and the variety of the crop planted. At Delhi, inoculation with 40 kg N/ha increased rice yield significantly over corresponding control, i.e., 40 kg N/ha alone. At two other locations (Pantnagar and Karnal), the increase in yield by inoculation with 40 kg N/ha was approximately equivalent to that obtained with 60 kg N/ha alone without inoculation. Inoculation effects in wheat were significant at low levels of nitrogen (0 to 40 kg N/ha) at Delhi, Shillong, and Niphad locations, whereas at Hissar location,

Table 24: The effect of seed inoculation of rice (Oryza sativa), barley (Hordeum vulgare), wheat (Triticum aestivum) and fodder oats (Avena sativa), with A. brasilense in India (mean of 5 pots)**

Treatments	Rice var. Pusa-2-21		Barley var. S-32		Wheat var. HD 2122		Fodder oats var. Kent
	Straw yield (g)	Grain yield (g)	Straw yield (g)	Grain yield (g)	Straw yield (g)	Grain yield (g)	Dry matter of shoots at 75 days (g)
Control (uninoculated and no nitrogen)	155.9	15.8	22.5	24.5	7.6	11.5	44.5
A. brasilense	200.1	20.9*	44.4*	37.8	21.6*	15.0	51.4
27 kg N/ha (urea)	—	—	—	—	—	—	48.9
27 kg N/ha + A. brasilense	—	—	—	—	—	—	54.0
40 kg N/ha (urea)	327.9	33.9	22.9	25.2	21.9	19.2*	49.9
40 kg N/ha + A. brasilense	386.1*	41.8*	59.8*	61.0*	32.2	33.3*	56.9
60 kg N/ha (urea)	436.7	48.1	31.1	29.8	21.9	31.1	—
60 kg N/ha + A. brasilense	472.2	54.4*	93.2*	69.1*	35.0*	33.5	—
80 kg N/ha (urea)	—	—	—	—	—	—	70.1
80 kg N/ha + A. brasilense	—	—	—	—	—	—	71.1
120 kg N/ha (urea)	572.8	68.9	33.2	32.9	27.2	27.6	—
120 kg N/ha + A. brasilense	645.1*	70.0	46.5	40.2	23.9	27.5	—
C.D. at 5%	54.48	4.41	18.31	12.15	11.84	12.02	7.24

Source: Subba Rao et al, 1979a.

*Significant over corresponding control.

**Each pot had 10 plants in barley and wheat, 15 plants in oats, and 4 plants in rice.

— Not tried.

Table 25: Summary of results on field response of crops to *A. brasilense* in India (1977–1978).

Crop	Location (variety of crop in parenthesis)	Initial N level (kg N/ha)	Grain yield (q**/ha)		Per cent increase in yield over corresponding control
			Uninoculated	Inoculated	
1	2	3	4	5	6
Rice	Delhi	0	37.33	45.33	21.4
	(Basmati)	40	56.89	66.37	16.7*
	Karnal	0	36.33	41.67	14.7
	(Pusa-2-21)	40	41.33	42.67	3.2
		60	41.33	44.33	7.3
		120	40.00	50.67	5.6
	Pantnagar	0	23.75	41.95	76.7
	(Jaya)	40	53.75	63.06	17.3
		60	60.42	63.19	4.6
	Hyderabad	0	31.33	31.67	1.1
	(IET 1444)	25	39.33	40.00	1.7
		50	43.33	45.00	3.9
	Manuthy	0	23.62	24.69	4.6
	(Threveni)	35	26.86	29.17	8.6
		70	25.77	27.32	6.0
Wheat	Delhi	0	27.63	29.21	5.7*
	(HD 2122)	40	39.19	41.90	6.9*
	Karnal	0	17.24	17.93	4.0
	(HD 2122)	40	29.30	31.33	6.0
		80	35.25	35.94	2.0
	Hissar	0	37.78	38.96	3.1
	(HD 2009)	40	45.39	45.76	0.8
		80	49.38	57.53	16.5
		120	49.47	62.88	27.1*
	Hyderabad	0	14.40	12.23	0.0
	(HD 2189)	40	14.95	16.30	9.0
		80	18.12	19.66	8.5
	Solan	0	30.34	37.14	22.4
	(HD 2009)	40	33.56	35.70	6.6
	Shillong	0	13.79	14.59	5.0
	(HP 1287)	30	16.50	22.20	33.9*
		60	17.53	19.00	8.4
	Niphad	0	7.57	9.22	21.8*
	(Sonalika)				

Contd.

Table 25 continued

1	2	3	4[**]	5[**]	6
Barley	Delhi	0	29.55	35.00	18.4
	(Ratna)	40	32.00	38.50	16.9
	Dehradun	0	29.42	37.25	26.6[*]
	(Ratna)				
Sorghum	Delhi	0	16.50	20.20	23.4
	(CSH 5)	40	20.50	26.00	26.8[*]
	Pantnagar	0	11.70	17.80	63.6
	(CSH 5)	40	15.60	28.10	81.3[*]
	Coimbatore	0	31.30	37.00	15.2
	(CSH 5)	40	49.00	51.40	3.2
	Dharwar	0	23.60	31.60	33.9[*]
	(CSH 5)	40	29.10	36.70	26.1[*]
	Udaipur	0	30.1	39.3	35.6[*]
	(CSH 5)	40	51.4	53.3	3.7[*]
	Hyderabad	0	30.3	41.7	37.6
	(CSH 5)	40	45.6	43.1	—
Fodder	Jhansi	0	26.22	35.66	36.0
oats	(Kent)	40	70.81	79.55	12.2
		60	87.03	93.91	7.9
		120	71.73	103.17	43.8[*]
	Karnal	0	16.51	25.22	54.6
	(Kent)	40	45.41	49.48	9.0
		60	66.64	71.04	6.6
		120	88.41	95.13	7.6
Pearl millet	Durgapura	0	6.40	10.64	66.25[*]
or bajra,	(BJ 104)				
(1979–1980)	Jodhpur	0	3.57	5.56	55.74[*]
	(BJ 104)				
	Aurangabad	0	14.30	17.89	25.10[*]
	(BJ 104)				
	Gwalior	0	12.17	12.67	4.10
	(BJ 104)				
	Kanpur	0	13.25	17.20	29.81[*]
	(BJ 104)				
	Raijinder nagar	0	12.67	10.97	—
	(BJ 104)				
	Hissar	0	22.21	22.79	2.61
	(BJ 104)				
	Jamnagar	0	10.65	11.64	9.29[*]
	(BJ 104)				

Source: Subba Rao *et al.*, 1979b.

[*] Significant increase over corresponding control.

[**] 1 q. (quintal) = 100 kg.

significant yield increase was seen only at a high level of nitrogen (120 kg N/ha). Such significant response at high level of nitrogen was also noticeable in fodder oats at Jhansi location, while at another location, simple inoculation without addition of nitrogen helped to increase yields to a large extent. Simple inoculation without any nitrogen input also brought about significant increase in yield of barley at Dehradun location and of fodder sorghum at Karnal location. At Delhi location, however, significant increase in the yield of sorghum was observable at 40 kg N/ha.

Field response of sorghum (*Sorghum vulgare*) var. CSH 5 to inoculation with *A. brasilense* was tested at six centres. Simple seed inoculation generally increased grain yield from 15.2 to 63.6 per cent over uninoculated (no nitrogen) control, which was significant at Udaipur and Dharwar centres. The response of seed inoculation with *A. brasilense* without nitrogen was equivalent to the application of 40 kg N/ha alone at Delhi, Pantnagar, and Dharwar centres (Table 25).

The results obtained from field experiments in 1979–1980 with regard to pearl millet or bajra (*Pennisetum americanum*) inoculated with *A. brasilense* were highly encouraging. Increases in grain yield due to inoculation were significant in five out of eight centres where field trials were conducted. The increased yields of pearl millet

Table 26: Root biomass and shoot weight of different millets as influenced by seed inoculation with *A. brasilense* at 30 days of plant growth in potted conditions (Mean of 4 replicated pots)[*]

Millet	Treatment	Root weight (g)	Shoot weight (g)
Finger miller	Control	8.5	42.5
(*Eleusine coracana*)	*A. brasilense* (strain Fm 4)	15.5[**]	69.8[**]
	A. brasilense (strain Fm 2)	12.5	55.4
Kodo millet	Control	6.5	35.5
(*Paspalum*	*A. brasilense*		
scrobiculatum*)	(strain Km 1)	10.5	50.2[**]
	A. brasilense (strain Km 2)	12.5[**]	60.5[**]
Italian millet	Control	9.7	67.5
(*Setaria italica*)	*A. brasilense* (strain Im 2)	14.7[**]	80.5
	A. brasilense (strain Im 3)	15.2[**]	86.2[**]
CD at 5%		4.53	13.5

[*] Each pot had 10 plants.
[**] Significant increase over uninoculated control.

obtained by *Azospirillum* inoculation may be attributeed to indoleacetic acid, gibberellins, and cytokinin-like substance produced by the bacterium and their effect on pearl millet (Tien *et al.*, 1979). The effect of inoculation on the biomass of plants is reflected in the results of an experiment in pots with three different millets (Table 26). It can be interpreted that increased root biomass in inoculated plants helped in greater absorption of native nutrients in soil resulting in higher yield.

Based on the results so far obtained the possible pay-off to the farming community has been roughly estimated (Table 27), which is indeed worthwhile for a developing country where fertilizer nitrogen is hardly used in sorghum and millet cultivation.

Table 27: Possible pay-off to the Farming Community in India by the application of *Azospirillum* inoculant in the cultivation of sorghum and pearl millet without using any fertilizer nitrogen; Calculations based on extensive field trials in different locations. The cost of inoculant is approximately Rs. 20/ha. 30 Rs. = 1 U.S. dollar

Crop	Mean yield increase (Kg/ha)	Monetary benefit by inoculation (Rs./ha)*	Total acreage in the country (million ha)	Total possible increase due to inoculation (million t)	Possible gain for India (million Rs.)
Sorghum (*Sorghum bicolor*)	735	5880	16.27	11.958	95667.60
Pearl millet (bajra) (*Pennisetum americanum*)	251	1004	16.00	4.016	16064.0

*If the selling retail price prevailing now is taken as follows: Sorghum — Rs. 8/kg; bajra — Rs. 4/kg. Even if one assumes that V10th of the above responses actually occur in farmers fields, the benefit to the farmer is noteworthy considering the nominal amount of Rs. 20/- as the price of the inoculant per ha.

REFERENCES

Alexander, M. (1965). Most probable number method for microbial populations. In *Methods of Soil Analysis*, Part II. Eds. C.A. Black. American Soc. Agronomy, Malison, wis pp. 1467–1472.

Baldani, J.I., Baldani, V.L.D., Seldin, L., and Dobereiner, J. (1986). Characterization of *Herbaspirillum seropedicae* gen. nov. sp. nov.: A root-associated nitrogen-fixing bacterium. *Int. J. Syst. Bacteriol.*, **36**, 86–93.

Becking, J.H. (1963). Fixation of molecular nitrogen by an aerobic *Vibrio* or *Spirillum* sp. *Antonie van Leeuwenhoek J. Microbio. Serol.*, **29**, 326.

Bulow, J.F.W. Von, and Dobereiner, J. (1975). Potential for nitrogen fixation in maize genotypes in Brazil, *Proc. Natl. Acad. Sci., USA*, **72**, 2389–2393.

Burris, R.H., Okon, Y., and Albrecht, S.L. (1977). Physiological studies of *Spirillum lipoferum*. In *Genetic Engineering for Nitrogen Fixation*. Ed. A. Hollaender. Plenum Press, New York. pp. 445–450.

Cavalcante, V., and Donereiner, J. (1988). A new acid tolerant nitrogen-fixing bacterium associated with sugarcane. *Plant and Soil*, 108, 23–31.

Cochran, W.G. (1950). Estimation of bacterial densities by means of 'most probable number'. *Biometrics*, 6, 105–116.

Day, J.M., and Dobereiner, J. (1976). Physiological aspects of N_2-fixation by a *Spirillum* from *Digitaria* roots. *Soil Biol. Biochem.*, 8, 45–50.

Diem, H.G., Schmidt, E.L., and Dommergues, Y.R. (1978). The use of the fluorescent-antibody technique to study the behaviour of *Beijerinekia* isolate in the rhizosphere and spermatosphere of rice. *Ecol. Bull.* Stockholm, 26, 312–318.

Dobereiner, J. (1966). *Azotobacter paspali* sp n. una bacteria fixadora de nitrogenio na rizosfera de *Paspalum*. *Pesq. Agropec. Bras.*, 1, 357–365.

Dobereiner, J., and Day, J.M. (1975a). Nitrogen fixation in the rhizosphere of tropical grasses, In *Nitrogen Fixation by Free Living Microorganisms*. Ed. W.D.P. Stewart, Cambridge Univ. Press, Cambridge. pp. 39–56.

Doberciner, J., and Day, J.M. (1975b). Associative symbiosis in tropical grasses; characterization of microorganisms and dinitrogen fixing sites. International Symposium on N_2 fixation — interdisciplinary discussions 3–7 June, 1974. Washington State University, Washington State University Press, Pullman.

Dobereiner, J., Marriel, J.E., and Nery, M. (1976). Ecological distribution of *Spirillum Beijerinck. Can. J. Microbiol.*, 22, 1464–1473.

Dobereiner, J., Reis, V.M., and Lazarini, A.C. (1988). New N_2 fixing bacteria in association with cereals and sugarcane, In *Nitrogen Fixation: Hundred Years After*. Eds. H. Bothe, F.J. de Bruin and W.E. Newton. Gustav Fischer, Stuttgart, New York. pp. 717–722.

Kavimandan, S.K., Subba Rao, N.S., and Mohrir, A.V. (1978). Isolation of *Spirillum lipoferum* from different varieties of wheat and nitrogen fixation in enrichment cultures. *Curr. Sci.*, 47, 96.

Krieg, N.R. (1977). Taxonomic studies of *Spirillum lipoferum*, In *Genetic Engineering for Nitrogen Fixation*. Ed. A Hollaender. Plenum Press, New York. pp. 463–472.

Krieg, N.R., and Tarrand, J.J. (1978). Taxonomy of the root-associated nitrogen-fixing bacterium *Spirillum lipoferum*. In *Limitations and Potentials for Biological Nitrogen Fixation in the Tropics*, Eds. J. Dobereiner, R.H. Burris and A. Hollaender, Plenum Press, New York. pp. 317–333.

Lakshmi Kumari, M., Kavimandan, S.K., and Subba Rao, N.S. (1976). Occurrence of nitrogen fixing *Spirillum* in roots of rice, sorghum, maize and other plants. *Indian J. Exp. Biol.*, 14, 638–639.

Lakshmi, V., Satyanarayana Rao, A., Vijayalakshmi, M., Lakshmi Kumari, M., Tilak, K.V.B.R., and Subba Rao, N.S. (1977). Establishment and survival of *Spirillum lipoferum. Proc. Indian Acad. Sci.*, 86(8), 397–404.

Magalhaes, F.M., Baldani, J.I., Souto, S.M., Kuykendall, J.R., and Dobereiner, J. (1983). A new acid tolerant *Azospirillum* species. *Anal di Academi Brasilien de Cience*, 55, 417–430.

McClung, C.R., and Fatriquin, D.G. (1980). Isolation of a nitrogen-fixing *Campylobacter* species from the roots of *Spartina alterniflora* Liosel. *Can. J. Microbiol.*, 26, 881–886.

Nayak, D.N., and Rao, V.R. (1977). Nitrogen dixation by *Azospirillum* sp. from rice roots, *Arch. fur Microbiol.*, 115, 359.

Okon, Y., Albert, S.L., and Burris, R.H. (1976). Factors affecting growth and nitrogen fixation of *Spirillum lipoferum. J. Bacteriol.*, **127**, 1248–1254.

Okon, Y., Albrecht, S.L., and Burris, R.H. (1977). Methods for growing *Spirillum lipoferum* for counting it in pure cultures and in association with plants. *Appl. Environ. Microbio.*, **33**, 85.

Reinhold, B.,, and Hurek, T. (1989). Location of diazotrophs in the root interior with special attention to the Kallar grass association. In *Nitrogen Fixation with Nonlegumes:* Eds. F.A. Skinner, R.M. Boddey and I. Fendrik. Kluwer Academic Publishers, London. pp. 209–218.

Reinhold, B., Hurek, T., Fendrik, I., Pot, B., Gillis, M., Kersters, K., Thielemans, S., and Deley, J. (1987). *Azospirillum halopraeferans* sp. nov., a nitrogen fixing organism associated with roots of Kallar grass (*Leptochloa fusca* (L.) Kunth.). *Int. J. Syst. Bacteriol.*, **37**, 43–51.

Sathyanarayana Rao, A. (1977). Studies on nitrogen fixing *Spirillum* species, M.Sc. Thesis, P.G. School, IARI, New Delhi.

Seldin, L., Van Elsas, J.D., and Penido, E.G.C. (1984). *Bacillus azotofixans* sp. nov., a nitrogen fixing species from brazilian soils and grass roots. *Int. J. Syst. Bacteriol*, **34**, 451–456.

Schank, S.C., Smith, R.L., Weiser, G.C., Zuberer, D.A., Bouton, J.H., Quesenberry, K.H., Tyler, M.E., Milam, J.R., and Littell, R.C. (1979). Fluorescent antibody technique to identify *Azospirillum brasilense* associated with roots of grasses. *Soil Biol. Biochem.*, **11**, 287–295.

Subba Rao, N.S., Tilak, K.V.B.R., Singh, C.S., and Lakshmi Kumari, M. (1979a). Response of a few economic species of graminaceous plants to inoculation with *Azospirillum brasilense. Curr. Sci.*, **48**, 133–134.

Subba Rao, N.S., Tilak, K.V.B.R., Lakshmi Kumari, M., and Singh, C.S. (1979b). *Azospirillum* — A new bacterial fertilizer for tropical crops, *Sci. Rep.*, CSIR (India), **16(10)**, 690–692.

Tarrand, J.J., Krieg, N.R., and Dobereiner, J. (1978). A taxonomic study of *Spirillum lipoferum* group, with description of a new genus *Azospirillum* gen. nov. and two species. *Azospirillum lipoferum* (Beijerinck) comb. nov. and *Azospirillum brasilense* sp. nov., *Canad. J. Microbiol.*, **24**, 967–980.

Tien, T.M., Gaskin, M.H., and Hubell, D.H. (1979). Plant growth substances produced by *Azospirillum brasilense* and their effect on the growth of pearl millet. *Appl. Environ. Microbiol.*, **37**, 1012–1024.

Tilak, K.V.B.R., Lakshmi Kumari, M., and Nautiyal, C. (1979). Survival of *Azospirillum brasilense* in different carriers. *Curr. Sci.*, **48**, 412–413.

Vasil, I.K. Vasil, V., and Hubbell, D.H. (1977). Engineered plant cell or fungal association with bacteria that fix nitrogen. In *Genetic Engineering for Nitrogen Fixation.* Ed. A. Hollander. Plenum Press, New York. pp. 197–211.

Watanabe, I., So, R., Ladha, J.K., Katayama-Fujimura, Y., and Kuraishi, H. (1987). A new nitrogen-fixing species of pseudomonasi *Pseudomonas diaxotrophicus* sp. nov isolated from the roots of wetland rice. *Can. J. Microbiol.*, **33**, 670–678.

5

Blue-green Algal Inoculant

Rice (*Oryza sativa*) is largely grown in wetland conditions with a layer of standing water. The flooded rice plant ecosystem is extremely complex, physically, chemically, and microbiologically (Fig. 11). One

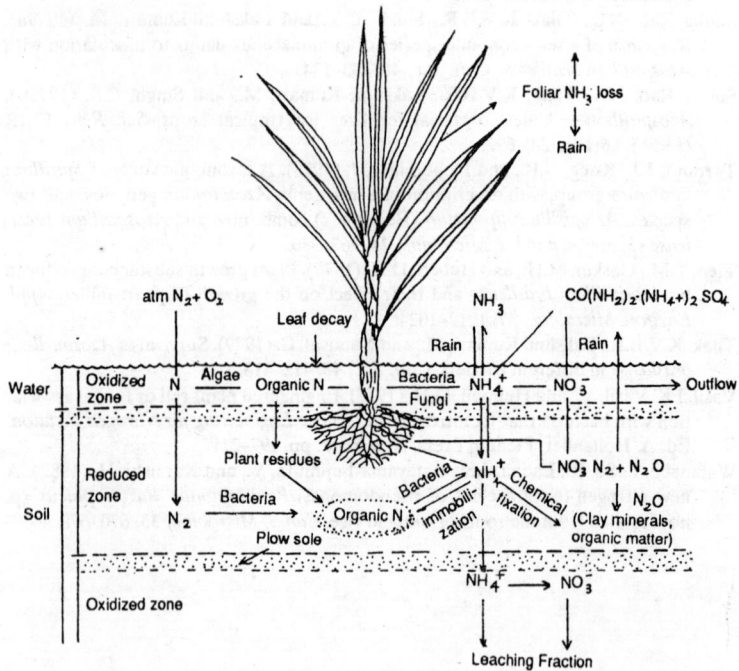

Fig. 11. Schematic representation of nitrogen transformations in a lowland rice ecosystem.

of the effects of flooding in uncropped rice field is a fall in O_2 content. However, in rice-cropped soil, due to aeremyma in the rice plant, O_2 is capable of moving from the leaf blade to the root cortex. This results in the oxidation of soil around the actively growing root system. Flooding of soil results in ammonium accumulation and nitrate instability. Ammoniacal nitrogen, the dominant form of mineral nitrogen in lowland rice soil, is liable to fixation by clay, loss by volatilization, nitrification, denitrification, leaching, runoff, and seepage. About 60–80 per cent of nitrogen absorbed by crops (40–50 kg N/ha) can be attributed to the native nitrogen pool. Approximately 60 per cent of the rice yields (2–4 t/ha) can be obtained without the application of nitrogen fertilizer. The soil nitrogen does not show decreasing trends by rice plantings and harvest, indicating the existence of biological mechanisms to renew the depleted nitrogen from the soil nitrogen pool. Legumes, *Azolla,* nitrogen-fixing bacteria, and blue-green algae take part in biological fixation of nitrogen. The fixed nitrogen is mostly mineralized to NH_4^+, which is the key process of nitrogen nutrition in waterlogged soil which is subjected to environmental stresses (Roger and Watanabe, 1986; De Datta, 1987).

Analysis of the blue-green algal flora from rice fields has revealed the occurrence of species of *Anabaena, Anabaenopsis, Aulosira, Cylindrospermum, Nostoc, Calothrix, Scytonema, Tolypothrix, Fischerella, Hapalosiphon, Mastigocladus, Stigonema, Westiella, Westiellopsis, Campylonema,* and *Microchaete* as dominant nitrogen fixers. Besides fixing nitrogen, these algae excrete vitamin B_{12}, auxins, and ascorbic acid which may also contribute to the growth of rice plants (De, 1939; Fogg, 1939; Singh, 1961; Venkataraman and Neelakantan, 1967; Watanabe, 1967; Stewart, 1970, 1971, 1974).

Heterocysts

Fixation of nitrogen takes place in specialized cells called 'Heterocysts' on the algal filament. However, there are reports that unicellular and filamentous non-heterocystous forms of blue-green algae (*Plectonema, Trichodesmium, Lyngbya,* and *Oscillatoria*) exhibit abilities to fix molecular nitrogen as evidenced by demonstrable nitrogenase activity of cellular preparations of such algae under experimental conditions. Heterocysts are large, thick-walled, apparently empty cells growing in between pigmented cells on the algal filament. The nature, physiology, and function of heterocysts have been extensively investigated and there is little doubt about their positive role in the process of biological nitrogen fixation. Vegetative cells and heterocysts are interdependent when active nitrogen fixation takes place. Heterocysts derive a reductant such as glucose-6 phosphate, pyruvate, or isocitrate from photosynthesizing vegetative cells to reduce atmospheric nitrogen into fixed nitrogen. It is also possible that vegetative cells help in maintaining reducing conditions at the boundary between vegetative cells and heterocyst. The vegetative cells, in turn, depend on heterocysts for nitrogen nutrition in the form of glutamine, glutamate, or other amino acids (Talpasayi, 1967; Stewart, 1970, 1971, 1974; Thomas and David, 1972; Fay, 1979).

The transition or metamorphosis of a vegetative cell of a blue-green alga into a heterocyst is a gradual process from a CO_2-fixing and O_2-evolving cell into an anaerobic cell conducive to active nitrogen fixation. The heterocyst has a multilayered cell wall and is connected by cytoplasmic bridges to neighbouring photosynthetic vegetative cells. These bridges regulate the flow of molecules between the two types of cells and therefore a series of regulated physiological and biochemical changes lead to nitrogen fixation and assimilation (Fig. 12).

Isolation of Blue-green Algae

Blue-green algae are generally covered with mucilage and it is easy to locate them as colonies floating on flooded rice fields. The mucilage contains bacteria and therefore for practical purposes, no attempt is made to isolate bacteria-free algal cultures. It is relatively easy to prepare unialgal cultures as follows: Several conical flasks or bottles containing a nitrogen-free blue-green algal liquid medium are prepared (for composition see Appendix) and autoclaved at 121°C for 20 minutes (Chu, 1942; Allen, 1949; Pringsheim, 1964). Sterile water blanks are prepared (as suggested in earlier chapters) and serial dilutions of soil or of algal sample from a field location are prepared with the help of sterilized pipettes. Aliquots of appropriate dilutions are then inoculated into liquid media in flasks and incubated for several weeks in an illuminated growth room at 28°–32°C. As and when individual colonies arise, they are picked up either for enrichment on fresh aliquots of liquid media or on agar slants for growth, identification, and preservation.

Agroclimatic Variations

There is noticeable variation in nitrogen-fixing ability within a given species. For instance, a strain of Nostoc punctiforme from the soils of Chandigarh fixed 1.3 mg/100 ml/30 days in pure culture

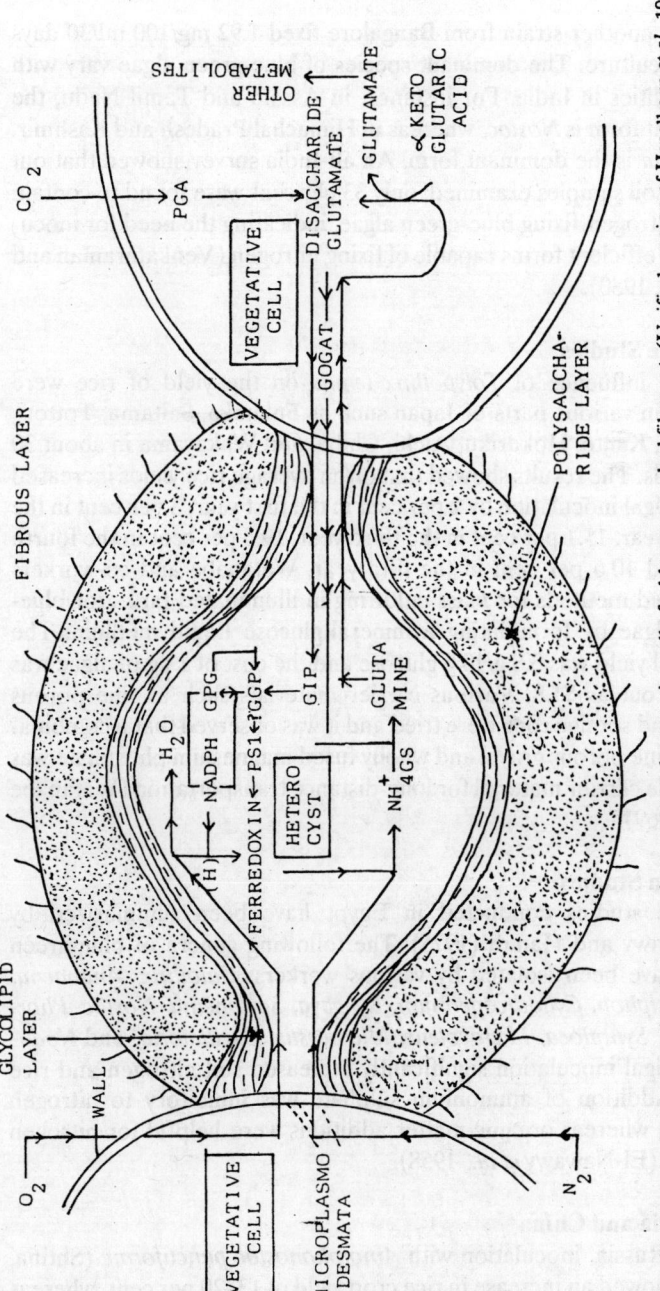

Fig. 12. The principal interactions between a heterocyst and vegetative cell of a blue-green algal filament. (Unified version of Haselkorn et al. 1980 and Wolk, 1980).

GS — glutamine synthetase; GOGAT — glutamine oxoglutarate amidotransferase; NADPH — pyridine nucleotide; G6P — glucose-6-phosphate dehydrogenase; 6PG — 6 phosphogluconate dehydrogenase; PGA — phosphoglyceric acid.

whereas another strain from Bangalore fixed 1.92 mg/100 ml/30 days in pure culture. The dominant species of blue-green algae vary with the localities in India. For instance, in Assam and Tamil Nadu, the dominant form is *Nostoc,* whereas in Himachal Pradesh and Kashmir, *Anabaena* is the dominant form. An all-India survey showed that out of 2213 soil samples examined, only 33 per cent were found to contain useful nitrogen-fixing blue-green algae, indicating the need for inoculation of efficient forms capable of fixing nitrogen (Venkataraman and Kaushik, 1980).

Japanese Studies

The influence of *Tolypothrix tenuis* on the yield of rice were studied in various parts of Japan such as Fukuoka, Saitama, Tottori, Shikoku, Kanto, Hokuriku, Aichi, Chiba, and Wakayama in about 30 rice fields. The results showed that on an average rice yields increased due to algal inoculation by 2 per cent in the first year, 8 per cent in the second year, 15.1 per cent in the third year, 19.5 per cent in the fourth year, and 10.6 per cent in the fifth year. Watanabe and co-workers developed methods for mass culturing in illuminated tanks for blue-green algae by formulating a mineral-glucose liquid medium. The algal cell yield was 3.8 g/10 g glucose and the cost of 1 kg of algae was worked out as $1.8. Various carrier materials such as fine porous gravel and sponge rock were tried and it was observed that a combination of fine porous gravel and wholly fused magnesium phosphate was a suitable carrier material for long-distance transportation (Watanabe *et al.,* 1969).

Egyptian Studies

The studies conducted in Egypt have been summarized by El-Nawawy and Hamdi (1975). The following genera of blue-green algae have been isolated by various workers: *Calothrix, Anabaena, Hapalosiphon, Cylindrospermum, Lyngbya, Scytonema, Nostoc, Phormidium, Symploca, Microcoleus, Microcystis, Oscillatoria,* and *Nodularia.* Algal inoculation significantly increased soil nitrogen and rice yield. Addition of ammonium sulphate was inhibitory to nitrogen fixation, whereas organic matter additions were helpful for nitrogen fixation (El-Nawawy *et al.,* 1958).

In Russia and China

In Russia, inoculation with *Amorphonostoc punctiforme* (Shtina, 1965) showed an increase in rice crop yield of 13–20 per cent, whereas yield increases of 24 per cent under field conditions have been report-ed in China by inoculation of rice with *Anabaena azotica* (Ley, 1959; Kuksa and Orleanskii, 1965).

Algalization Experiments in India

In India, the benefits of blue-green algal inoculation have been demonstrated in pot as well as field trials by a number of workers in different soil conditions using different varieties of rice. Recently, it has also been demonstrated that high-yielding varieties which need high levels of nitrogenous fertilizers also respond to algal inoculation by increasing yields up to 10–15 per cent, which has been attributed to the growth-promoting substances secreted by blue-green algae. The Indian work has shown that in areas where nitrogenous fertilizers are scarcely used, blue green algal inoculation can supply 25–30 kg N/ha of nitrogen needs of the rice crop. It is, however, possible that for various reasons, the introduced algae may not be able to establish where response to algal inoculation may be poor (Singh, 1961; Relwani and Subramanyam, 1963; Subramanyam *et al.*, 1964; Goyal and Venkataraman, 1971; Sankaram, 1971; Aiyar *et al.*, 1972; Venkataraman, 1972).

Preparation of Blue-green Algae in Open-air Shallow Culture

Each farmer can prepare his own algal biofertilizer as follows: It has been recommended that trays (6' × 3' × 9") of galvanized iron sheet or brick and mortar or pits lined with polythene be prepared. A mixture of 10 kg soil and 200 g superphosphate is added to trays and water filled in the trays to a level of 2–6 inch. It is necessary to keep the pH of soil to neutral and liming is recommended for acidic soils. When the soil settles, sawdust is sprinkled and a soil-based starter culture consisting of *Tolypothrix, Nostoc, Anabaena,* and *Plectonema* is sprinkled over the water in the tray. Within a week's time, a thick algal scum is formed on the surface. The water is allowed to dry at this stage, and the dried algal flakes are collected from the trays and stored in polythene bags (Plate 3). It is recommended that such an algal preparation be applied at the rate of 10 kg/ha in the field, one week after rice transplantation (Venkataraman, 1972; IARI, 1978).

Multiplication of Blue-green Algae in the Field and Effect of Inoculation on the Yield of Rice

Srinivasan and Ponnaya (1978) recommend the following proce-dure: About 5 kg of the algal preparation for each cent is spread in the field and the field flooded with water to a level of 2.5 cm followed by broadcasting of 2 kg of superphosphate. The application of phosphate promotes algal multiplication in 2 weeks on clay soils and in 3–4 weeks in sandy soils. Application of pesticides may be necessary to prevent pests like daphnids, snails, and mosquitoes. The average yield of algae ranges from 16 to 35 kg for each cent area of land.

These authors carried out experiments in experimental stations and in farmers' fields. In experimental stations, at all levels of initial nitrogen, algal application increased yields equivalent to that obtainable by the addition of 25 kg N/ha (Table 28). Similar results were also obtained in farmers' fields as revealed by 29 adaptive research trials in Tamil Nadu (Table 29). Field experiments have also been done in other parts of India with encouraging results on the use of algal inoculants in rice cultivation (Venkataraman, 1972).

Table 28: Rice yields, with and without algal application, at different nitrogen levels

N	Treatment		Grain yield kg/ha	
	P	K	Adt. 31	IR-20
	(kg/ha)			
0	50	50	4175	4106
0	50	50 + Algae	4650	4715
25	50	50	4675	4814
25	50	50 + Algae	5025	5518
50	50	50	4900	5611
50	50	50 + Algae	5200	638
75	50	50	5150	6311
75	50	50 + Algae	5550	7091
100	50	50	5575	6948
100	50	50 + Algae	6000	7819
		C.D.	420	232

Source: Srinivasan and Ponnaya, 1978.

Pay-off from Blue-green Algae Inoculant

The cost of the algal material when produced on the farmers' field is negligible although commercially the cost for 10 kg/ha of algae may come to Rs. 30. The saving on fertilizer nitrogen by this input is Rs. 100/ha if 25 kg N/ha is provided for rice cultivation by blue-green algae. An average increase of 300 kg/ha of grain is possible by algal inoculation even under high fertilizer nitrogen applications. This works out to an additional income of Rs. 300 for an investment of Rs. 30 for the algal inoculum (Venkataraman and Kaushik, 1980). In recent years, the cost of materials has increased and the benefits have proportionately calculated.

Table 29: Blue-green algal trials in farmers' fields

Details			Mean yield data (kg/ha)		
N	P	K	Vellore	Trichy	Cuddalore
	(kg/ha)		(11 trials)	(8 trials)	(10 trials)
50	25	25	4235	4557	3789
50	25	25 + Algae	4455	4785	3884
75	37.5	37.5	4400	4485	3953
75	37.5	37.5 + Algae	4565	5117	4156

Source: Srinivasan and Ponnaya, 1978.

REFERENCES

Aiyar, R.S., Salahudeen, S., and Venkataraman, G.S. (1972). On a long term algalization field trial with high yielding rice varieties: Yield and economics, Indian J. Agric. Sci., 42, 380–383.

Allen, D.N. (1949). Experiments in Soil Bacteriology, 1st Edition, Burgers Publishing Co., Minneapolis, Minn.

Chu, S.P. (1942). The influence of the mineral composition of the medium on the growth of planktonic algae. I. Methods and culture media, J. Ecol., 30, 284–325.

De, P.K. (1939). The role of blue-green algae in nitrogen fixation in rice fields, Proc. R. Soc., 127B, 121–139.

DeDatta, S.K. (1987). Nitrogen transformation processes in relation to improved cultural practices for lowland rice. Plant and Soil, 100, 47–69.

El-Nawawy, A.S., and Hamdi, Y. (1975). Research on blue-green algae in Egypt, 1958–1972. In Nitrogen Fixation by Free Living Microorganisms. Ed. W.D.P. Stewart. Cambridge Univ. Press, London. pp. 219–228.

El-Nawawy, A.S., Lotfi, M. and Fahmy, H. (1958). Studies on the ability of some blue-green algae to fix atmospheric nitrogen and their effect on growth and yield of paddy, Agri. Res. Rev. Cairo, 36, 308–319.

Fay, P. (1979). Nitrogen fixation in heterocysts. In Recent Advances in Biological Nitrogen Fixation. Ed. N.S. Subba Rao. Oxford & IBH Publishing Co. Pvt. Ltd., New Delhi. pp. 121–165.

Fogg, G.E. (1939). Nitrogen fixation. In Physiology and Biochemistry of Algae. Ed. R.A. Lewin. Academic Press, New York. pp. 161–170.

Goyal, S.K., and Venkataraman, G.S. (1971). Response of high yielding rice varieties to algalization. II. Interaction of soil types to algal inoculation, Phykos, 10, 32–33.

IARI (1978). Research bulletin No. 9. Algal Technology for Rice. IARI, New Delhi.

Kuksa, I.N., and Orleanskii, V. (1965). Development of scientific research on nitrogen fixing blue-green algae and their practical use in agriculture. Mikrobiologiya, 34, 743–747.

Ley, S.H. (1959). The effect of nitrogen fixing blue-green algae on the yields of rice plant. *Acta Hydrobiol., Sinica,* **4,** 440–444.

Pringsheim, E.G. (1964). *Pure Cultures of Algae: Their Preparation and Maintenance.* Hafner Publishing Co., New York and London.

Relwani, L.L., and Subramanyam, R. (1963). Role of blue-green algae, chemical nutrients and partial sterilization on paddy yield, *Curr. Sci.,* **32,** 441–443.

Roger, P.A., and Watanabe, I. (1986). Technologies for utilizing biological nitrogen fixation in wetland rice: Potentialities, current usage and limiting factors. In *Nitrogen Economy of Flooded Rice Soils.* Eds. S.K. DeDatta and W.H. Patrick Jr. Martinus Nijhoff Publishers, Desseldorf. pp. 39–77.

Sankaram, A. (1971). *Work Done on Blue-green Algae in Relation to Agriculture.* ICAR, New Delhi.

Shtina, E.A. (1965). Fixation of free nitrogen in blue-green algae. In *The Ecology and Physiology of Blue-green Algae.* Ed. V.D. Federov and M.M. Tellichenko. Moscow University Press, Moscow (in Russian). pp. 66–79.

Singh, R.N. (1961). *The Role of Blue-green Algae in Nitrogen Economy of Indian Agriculture.* ICAR, New Delhi.

Srinivasan, S., and Ponnaya, J.H.S. (1978). Blue-green algae as a biofertiliser—Tamil Nadu experience. FAI Seminar, New Delhi.

Stewart, W.D.P. (1970). Algal fixation of atmospheric nitrogen. *Plant and Soil,* **32,** 555–588.

Stewart, W.D.P. (1971). Physiological studies on nitrogen fixing blue-green algae, *Plant and Soil.,* sp. vol. **377,** 391.

Stewart, W.D.P. (1974). Blue green algae. In *Biology of Nitrogen Fixation.* Ed. A Quispel. North Holland Publishing Co., Amsterdam. pp. 202–287.

Subramanyam, R., Relwani, L.L., and Manna, G.B. (1964). Observations on the role of blue-green algae on rice yield compared with that of conventional fertilisers. *Curr. Sci.,* **33,** 485–486.

Talpasayi, E.R.S. (1967). Localization of ascorbic acid in heterocysts of blue-green algae. *Curr. Sci.,* **36,** 190–191.

Thomas, J., and David, K.A.V. (1972). Site of nitrogenase activity in the blue-green algae *Anabaena* sp. L. 31. *Nature,* London. **238,** 219–221.

Venkataraman, G.S. (1972). *Algal Biofertilisers and Rice Cultivation,* Today and Tomorrow's Printers and Publishers, New Delhi.

Venkataraman, G.S., and Kaushik, B.D. (1980). Save on N fertilisers by the use of algae in rice fields. *Indian Farming,* October, 27–30.

Venkataraman, G.S., and Neelakantan, S. (1967). Effect of the cellular constituents of the nitrogen fixing blue-green algae, *Cylindrospermum muscicola* on the root growth of rice seedlings. *J. Gen. Appl. Microbiol.,* **13,** 53–61.

Watanabe, A. (1967). The blue-green algae as the nitrogen fixers. *Proc. IX Int. Cong. Microbiol.,* USSR Academy of Sciences, Moscow. pp. 77–85.

Watanabe, A., Shirota, M., Endo, H., and Yamamoto, Y. (1969). An observation of the practical applications of nitrogen fixing blue-green algae for rice cultivation, *Proc. Global Impacts of Applied Microbiology,* Bombay. Eds. Y.M. Freitas and F. Fernandes. pp. 53–64.

6

Azolla

Azolla is a floating freshwater fern and is ubiquitous in distribution. There are six species of *Azolla* — *A. caroliniana, A. nilotica, A. filiculoides, A. mexicana, A. microphylla,* and *A. pinnata.* The common species of the fern occurring in India is *A. pinnata.* It grows in ditches and stagnant water along with other water weeds such as *Lemna* and *Spirodela.* Under ideal conditions, *Azolla* multiplies vegetatively and growth is prolific. Sexual reproduction has been reported but is not the usual mode of multiplication. The fern usually forms a green mat over water which often becomes reddish due to the accumulation of anthocyanin pigments.

The plant has a floating branched stem, deeply bilobed leaves, and true roots which penetrate the body of water. The leaves are arranged alternately on the stem. Each leaf has a dorsal and a ventral lobe. The dorsal fleshy lobe is exposed to air and contains chlorophyll. It has an algal symbiont (*Anabaena azollae*) within a central cavity. The ventral lobe is thin, is partly submerged in water, and lacks chlorophyll. The alga fixes atmospheric nitrogen and is present at all stages of growth and development of the fern. There are multicellular epidermal hairs lining the cavities which house the algal symbiont and these hairs may be involved in the transport of nutrients between the two symbionts (Peters, 1977).

The importance of *Azolla* as an organic input in rice cultivation was first demonstrated in North Vietnam in 1957. Subsequently, its potentiality has been recognized in the United States, Indonesia, Japan, the Philippines, and China (Talley *et al.,* 1977).

Survival of *Azolla*

Survival of *Azolla* after a drought period is associated with the production of sexual organs since plants die due to desiccation. The plant produces macrosporocarps (male) as well as microsporocarps (female). *Azolla* plants have a main rhizome bearing alternate secondary and tertiary branches. Sporocarps are initiated at the place of attachment of branches and replace the lower lobe of the first leaf of a branch. The dorsal lobe covers the sporocarp. The sporocarps occur in pairs, both male and female or male plus female side by side. Macrospocarps are small, oval-shaped, with pointed ends measuring 0.75–1.0 mm in length and 0.5 mm in breadth. They are yellowish-green especially at the tip, which becomes brown and hard due to lignification and tannin deposits. It is through the macrocarp tip that vegetative cells of *Anabaena* get into the plant and establish symbiosis. A mature microsporocarp is actually larger than a macrosporocarp, is globular, and measures about 2 mm in length and 1.5 mm in breadth. As many as 120 or more microsporangia may develop inside a single microsporocarp. Within each microsporangium 32–64 microspores develop. On the other hand, a mature macrocarp contains a single functional macrospore.

The micro- and macrosporocarps which are seasonally produced decay and sink to the bottom of a pond or any body of water in which *Azolla* grows. The decay and rupture of these sporocarps results in a meshed consortium described as macrosporangium complex. A mature microspore does not get freed from this macrosporangium complex and therefore development of macro and microgametophytes takes place in close proximity, which makes matters easy for fertilization. The macrosporophyte (female) develops an archegonium (female apparatus) in which the egg cell (macrospore) is situated. The microsporophyte formed from a microspore also remains entangled with its appendages and develops an antherdium (the male apparatus). Fertilization of the egg cell with a spermatozoid (antherozoid) from the antherdium results in the formation of a zygote or embryo.

The development of the embryo takes place in the macrosporic complex and only when the seedling emerges with its cotyledons can the unaided eye recognize the juvenile *Azolla* seedling with its rhizoidal development. The bilobed leaf formation takes place and the mature plant develops in about 21 days. The life cycle of *Azolla* is shown in Figs. 13 and 14.

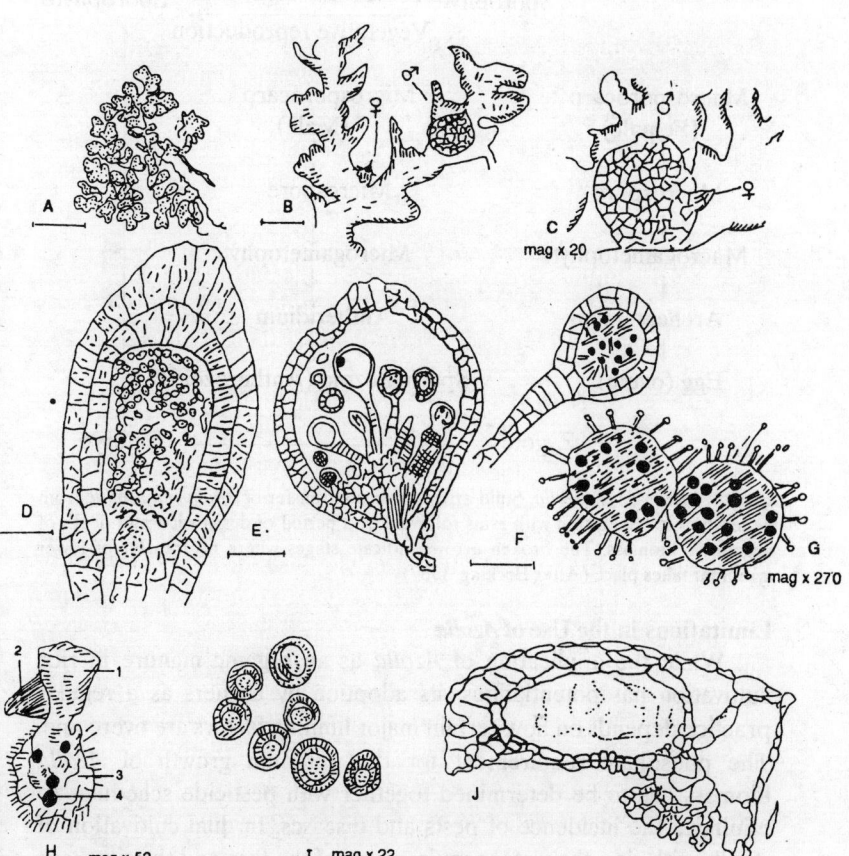

Fig. 13. A—*Azolla pinnata* showing the main rhizome, alternate branching, and the leaves, bar = 0.5 cm. B—Macrosporocarp (female) and microsporocarp (male) of *A. filiculoides* on two different branches, bar = 1 mm. C—A pair of sporocarps, macro and micro, in the axil of the lower lobe of *A. filiculoides* × 20. D—Young developing macrosporocarp where the *Anabaena* filaments fill the cavity with a basal developing megaspore; bar = 40 μ. E—Longitudinal section through a young microsporocarp of *A. filiculoides* showing number of stalked microsporangia on a basal placenta; bar = 160 μ. F—A microsporangium with microspores amidst developing massulae. G—Free massulae of *A. filiculoides* with anchor-like projections called 'glochidia' which help in the attachment to macrospore, facilitating fertilization. The microspores are embedded in the massulae; × 270, H—An *Azolla* seedling (1) emerging from a fertilized megaspore (2) of the megasporic complex which includes adhering massulae (3) with microspores (4) × 52. I—Very young seedlings of *Azolla* freely floating on water; × 22. J—A section through an older dorsal leaf lobe of *Azolla* showing *Anabaena azollae* filaments in the leaf cavity. (After Becking, 1987)

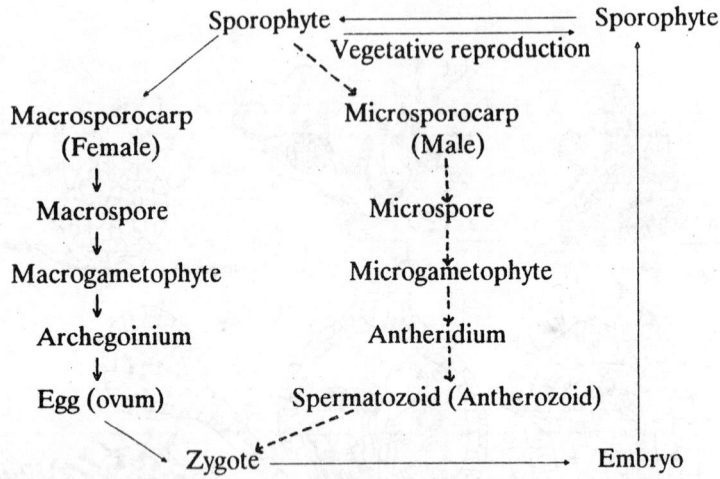

Fig. 14: Life cycle of *Azolla*. Solid arrows indicate transfer of *Anabaena azollae* from generation to generation with rains followed by a period of desiccation and death of vegetative biomass. The broken arrows indicate stages where no transfer of lower symbiont takes place (After Becking, 1987)

Limitations in the Use of *Azolla*

While the application of *Azolla* as an organic manure in rice cultivation has potentialities, its adoption by farmers as a regular practice depends on how certain major limiting factors are overcome. The phosphate requirement for the optimum growth of *Azolla* biomass has to be determined together with pesticide schedules to minimize the incidence of pests and diseases. In dual cultivation of *Azolla* with rice, the water requirements of the fern and the rice have to be borne in mind in situations where water is scarce. If incorporation of *Azolla* is advocated in a given situation, maintenance of separate ponds to raise the *Azolla* biomass is necessary. This obviously requires land which otherwise could be used for crop cultivation. The requirement of biomass to the tune of 10 t/ha of fresh weight with the attendant problem of autolysis and the labour-intensive nature of the entire operation renders the practice suitable only for developing nations where labour is relatively cheap. Multiplication of *Azolla* depends upon vegetative propagation and spore production by sexual reproduction is more an exception than a rule. Research in understanding factors promoting spore production may perhaps make the practice a lot easier by use of a small mass of spores to develop a nursery of *Azolla* instead of resorting to use of large quantities of fresh biomass. Transportation adds to the expense of the operation in situations where nurseries of *Azolla* are located away from cultivators' fields.

Use of *Azolla* in China

According to an FAO report (1977) the optimum temperature for growth of *Azolla* in China is 20°–28°C with a maximum limit of 35°C. The optimum pH is between 6 and 7. In China, many small nurseries are prepared and *Azolla* is initially grown on them for 4 weeks. The nurseries are covered with plastic sheetings when temperature is low. The fields are prepared for rice cultivation and flooded with water followed by seeding with *Azolla* at the rate of 7.5 t/ha. After 5–10 days, the water in the field is drained off and the *Azolla* mat (now approximately 22.5 t/ha) is ploughed into soil by a tractor. This procedure may be repeated by flooding the field with water followed by draining water and ploughing in *Azolla* plants into soil.

Azolla can also be grown simultaneously with rice seedlings after transplantation. In such cases, the practice is to bury the fern into soil by hand and the procedure is repeated as often as required to prevent choking of rice plants due to mat formation of *Azolla* resulting in O_2 starvation of rice roots.

In China, the nitrogen requirement of rice is met by *Azolla* to the extent of 50 per cent although phosphorus is applied at 150–225 kg/ha as superphosphate (24–36 kg $P_2 O_5$ or 11–16 kg P/ha).

Use of *Azolla* in India

Work done at the Central Rice Research Institute, Cuttack (Singh, 1977a, 1977b, 1977c; Pande, 1979), has revealed the following: (1) Standing water 5–10 cm deep and the application of superphosphate at 4–8 kg/ha are essential for rapid growth of *Azolla*. (2) *Azolla* nurseries in small plots (50–100 sq. m) are preferable to large plots to avoid wind erosion. Concrete tanks are also suitable for this purpose. (3) *Azolla* inoculum at 0.1 to 0.4 kg/sq. m is most desirable for the rapid multiplication of the fern in nurseries for production of 8–10 t/ha green matter in 20 days. (4) A pH of 8.0 is ideal and acidic soils (below pH 4.6) are not suitable unless lime is used to correct pH. (5) Water temperature in the range of 14°–30°C is ideal. (6) Use of carbofuran at 1–2 kg/ha prevents the rapid spread of insect parasites and the consequent destruction of *Azolla* nurseries. (7) Harvested *Azolla* accumulated as heaps decomposes rapidly in 7–10 days. (8) The composition of *Azolla* is approximately 94 per cent water, 1 per cent of P, K, Ca, Mn, and Fe and 5 per cent N. (9) It is necessary to plan a series of *Azolla* nurseries several weeks ahead of rice plantings (Plate 4).

Two methods of *Azolla* application have been recommended in India — as a green manure by incorporating in fields prior to rice planting and by dual cropping with rice when the fern grows side by side with the main crop for some time. In the first method, *Azolla* is grown on the flooded field for 2–3 weeks, the water drained, and the green manure incorporated in soil by ploughing followed by rice planting within a week's time. In the dual culture, 0.1 to 0.5 kg/sq. m (fresh weight) is inoculated a week after planting rice seedlings. Sooner or later, an *Azolla* mat is formed. At this stage, water is drained and *Azolla* incorporated in soil. Several high-yielding rice varieties have been used (IR 8, Vani, Supriya, Ratna, Jaya, Kalinga 2, Pusa 2–21, CR 1005, CR 191–5, CR 188–10, SG 1) to test the effect of *Azolla* inoculation on grain yield (Singh, 1977a, 1977b, 1977c; Pande, 1979; Lumpkin and Plucknett, 1982).

In these experiments, it has been shown that incorporation of 10 t fresh *Azolla*/ha is as efficient as basal application of 25–30 kg N/ha. By increasing *Azolla* from 5 to 20 t/ha, a linear response on grain yield could be obtained. The practice of incorporation of *Azolla* in soil appears to be more beneficial than dual culture. In farmers' fields, it has been shown that the use of 20 kg N/ha as ammonium sulphate with *Azolla* is equivalent to the use of 40 kg N/ha as ammonium sulphate. These results point out the feasibility of using *Azolla* in combination with fertilizer nitrogen to step up rice yields (Tables 30 and 31).

Studies in the United States of America

In the rice-growing regions of California, two species of *Azolla* — *A. filiculoides* and *A. mexicana* — can be grown. During the fallow season of November to April the frost-tolerant *A. filiculoides* can be grown for incorporation, whereas in summer, both species can be grown as companion crops with rice.

It has been observed that *A. filiculoides* completely covers the water surface in 15 days and by 35 days a biomass of 1700 kg dry wt/ha containing 52 kg N/ha could be developed. *Azolla* is readily decomposed to ammonia which is available for the rice plants. It has also

Table 30: Average yield of rice (kg/ha) in India with the application of *Azolla* as an organic nitrogeneous fertilizer

Soil type: Centre: Variety: Basal dose of NPK:	Alluvial Tiabar Manoharsali 0–40–40	Laterite Kharagpur Rama 0–30–30	Laterite Bhubaneswar Rama 0–10–50	CRRI Supriya 0–30–30
Control	2800	2479	2937	2747
5 tons of fresh *Azolla* (inc. before planting)	2900	3390	3479	3092
10 tons of fresh *Azolla* (inc. before planting)	3480	3754	4000	3295
1 ton of fresh *Azolla* after planting (inc. after 20 days) + P_2O_5 at 10 kg/ha	3000	3052	3600	3081
5 tons of *Azolla* + 30 kg N/ha	3360	3562	3762	3421
10 tons of *Azolla* + 30 kg N/ha	3360	4144	4041	3427
30 kg N/ha	2880	3735	3375	3031
60 kg N/ha	3120	4185	4200	3247
CD at 5% level	242	147	358	361

Source: Pande, 1979.

been observed that nitrogen contents of rice receiving *A. filiculoides* and *A. mexicana* are 10 and 35 kg/ha respectively higher than controls. An application of 30 kg P/ha in the form of triple superphosphate one day after inoculation or 15 kg P/ha as split treatment after inoculation is necessary to successfully grow *Azolla* with rice. The release of nitrogen to rice plants takes place after death and decomposition of *Azolla* cover. The results obtained in California on the efficacy of *Azolla* on the yield of rice are shown in Fig. 15. (Talley *et al.*, 1977; Talley and Rains, 1980).

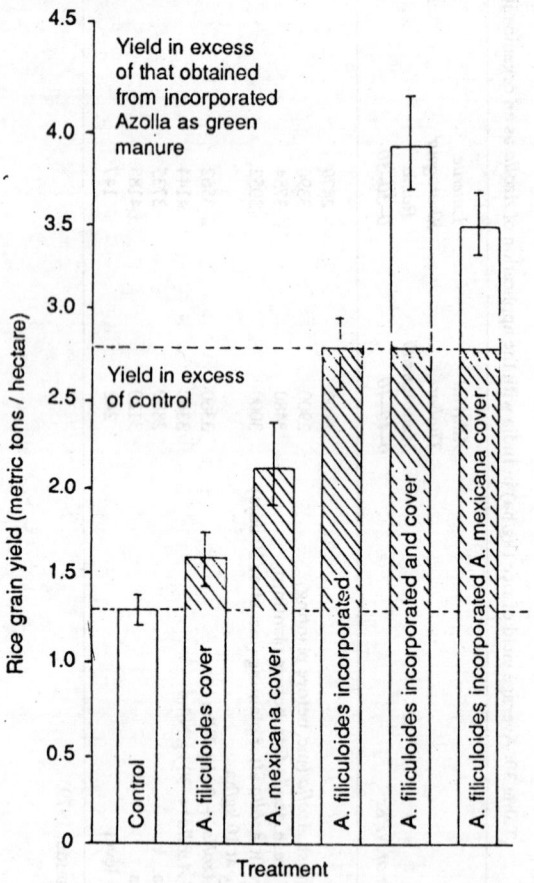

Fig. 15. Effect of *Azolla* on the yield of rice in California

Table 31: Effect of *Azolla* on grain yield of rice under farmer's field conditions in India

Location	Grain yield (kg/ha)		
	40 kg N/ha	*20 kg N/ha (Azolla) +20 kg N (ammonium sulphate)*	*40 kg N/ha (ammonium sulphate)*
Keshpur	4091	4435	4132
Kanderpur	3678	4153	4644
Athanga	3420	3859	3580
Nakhara	2814	3217	3543
Ananthpur	2524	3067	2063
Jagannathpur	4948	4923	5923
Mean	3578	3942	3980

Source: Pande, 1979.

In Other Countries

Azolla pinnata was grown in 400,000 ha in Vietnam providing nitrogen equivalent to 5 t/ha of rice (Tran and Dao, 1973). It is now a common practice to grow *Azolla* with rice in Thailand (Moore, 1969), Indonesia (Saubert, 1949), China (Lin, 1976), and the Philippines (Watanabe *et al.*, 1977).

REFERENCES

FAO (1977). *China: Recycling of Organic Wastes in Agriculture.* Food and Agricultural Organization of the UN, Rome.

Lin, Pin-tung (1976). Progress in the trial of an alternative to chemical fertilizer and its extension work. *Sino-Amer. Tech. Coop. Assn.,* **21(4)**, 1–3.

Moore, A.W. (1969). *Azolla*: Biology and Agronomic significance, *Bot. Rev.* **35**, 17–34.

Pande, H.K. (1979). Organic resource management *Azolla*: Their potential role in developing Indian agriculture. Paper presented at the FAI seminar, Fertilizer Association of India, New Delhi.

Peters, G.A. (1977). The *Azolla-Anabaena azoliae* symbiosis. In *Genetic Engineering for Nitrogen Fixation.* Ed. A. Hollaender. Plenum Press, New York. pp. 231–258.

Saubert, G.G.P. (1949). Provisional communication on the fixation of elementary nitrogen by a floating fern. *Ann. Roy. Gar. Buitenzorg.* **51**, 177–197.

Singh, P.K. (1977a). Azolla plants as fertilizer and feed, *Indian Farming,* **27**, 19–21.

Singh, P.K. (1977b). Multiplication and utilization of fern *Azolla* containing nitrogen-fixing algal symbiont as a green manure in rice cultivation. *Il Riso,* **26(2)**, 125–136.

Singh, P.K. (1977c). Effects of *Azolla* on the yield of paddy with and without application of N-fertilizer. *Curr. Sci.,* **46**, 642–644.

Talley, S.N., and Rains, D.W. (1980). *Azolla* as a nitrogen source for temperate rice. In *Nitrogen Fixation,* Vol. II. Eds. W.E. Newton and W.H. Orme-Johnson. University Park Press, Baltimore. pp. 311–320.

Talley, S.N., Talley, B.J., and Rains, D.W. (1977). Nitrogen fixation by *Azolla* in rice fields. In *Genetic Engineering for Nitrogen Fixation.* Ed. A Hollaender. Plenum Press, New York. pp. 259–281.

Tran Quang and Dao The Tuan (1973). *Azolla*: A green manure. *Agric. Prob.,* Vol. 4, Vietnamese Studies, **38**, 119–127.

Watanabe, I., Espinas, C.R., Berja, N.S., and Alimagno, B.V. (1977). Utilization of the *Azolla-Anabaena* complex as a nitrogen fertilizer for rice. IRRI Research Paper Series No. 11.

Lumpkin, T.A., and Plucknett, D.L. (1982). *Azolla as a Green Manure,* Westview Tropical Agricultural Series, Westview Press, Boulder, Co.

7

Green Manure

Rice (*Oryza sativa*) is the mainstay of the diet of one half of the world population. There are about 143 million ha of rice cultivation in the world of which 75 per cent are in lowlands which remain flooded during most part of the year. The flooded rice soils provide a congenial microhabitat for a variety of nitrogen-fixing microorganisms to thrive with the result that without the addition of any chemical fertilizer, rice can be grown year after year with minimum but constant yields. Nevertheless, the fertilizer-responsive new dwarf rice varieties have contributed to bumper yields due to the application of high amounts of chemical nitrogenous fertilizers. However, all the applied chemical fertilizer nitrogen is not fully utilized in lowland rice soils. The present evidences point to the fact that ammonia volatilization, nitrification and denitrification processes, and leaching of nitrogen in sandy porous soil could be of some relevance in minimizing the utilization of added chemical nitrogen. It is estimated that flooded rice crops use only 20–40 per cent of added nitrogen. This calls for intensive research on better fertilizer use efficiency by innovative technologies coupled with integrated nutrient management practices involving judicious combination of organic and inorganic sources of plant nutrients (De Datta and Patrick, 1986).

Source of Natural Nitrogen in Rice Soils

Lowland rice soils have all sorts of nitrogen-fixing micro-organisms, both heterotrophic and autotrophic. The photosynthetic autotrophs, notably the blue-green algae, are an important source of biologically fixed nitrogen and this aspect has been covered in an

earlier chapter. The *Azolla anabaena* symbiosis which affords potentialities as an organic manure for rice has also been dealt with in an
earlier chapter. Together, the nitrogen-fixing microorganisms and
associations can contribute up to 40 kg N/ha under ideal agroclimatic
conditions to the wetland rice ecosystem and this fact has been clearly
established. There is yet another source of biologically fixed nitrogen
under lowland rice ecosystem which comes under the general
category of 'legume green manure', and the potentialities of this
biofertilizer input in rice cultivation is discussed here.

Legume Green Manures

As the name denotes legume green manure comes from freshly
collected green materials of selected herbs, shrubs, and trees which
are rich in nitrogen and easily decomposable. The fresh green matter
can be collected from species of plants grown specially for this
purpose or from naturally growing shrubs and trees whose leaves are
collected, transported, and incorporated to rice fields prior to transplantation of seedlings.

Allen and Allen (1981) listed nine genera of legumes which have
been used as green manure crops in wetland rice cultivation: *Aeschynomene*, *Astragalus*, *Crotalaria*, *Indigofera*, *Lathyrus*, *Pongamia*,
Tephrosia, *Trifolium*, and *Sesbania*. They also listed the names of 39
genera whose species are being used as general green manures in
plantation crops: *Arachis*, *Atylosia*, *Cajanus*, *Calpogonium*, *Canavalia*,
Cassia, *Cochlianthus*, *Cullen*, *Derris*, *Dipogon*, *Dolichos*, *Dunbaria*,
Erythrina, *Flemingia*, *Gliricidia*, *Kummerowia*, *Lablab*, *Lespedeza*,
Leucaena, *Lupinus*, *Mastersia*, *Melilotus*, *Mimosa*, *Mucuna*, *Ormocar-
pum*, *Pachyrhizus*, *Parkia*, *Phaseolus*, *Pisum*, *Psophocarpus*, *Ptero-
loma*, *Peueraria*, *Shuteria*, *Stylosanthes*, *Tetragonolobus*, *Trigonella*,
Uraria, *Vicia*, and *Vigna*. The potentialities of these legumes in rice
cultivation have however not been assessed. Vachhani and Murty
(1964) evaluated about 50 green manure species in India for their
nitrogen accumulation. Similarly, Meelu and Morris (1986) have
reviewed the green manuring research in the Philippines. In China,
green manuring has been practised for over 2300 years.

Stem Nodulating Green Manure Species

There are three genera of legumes which are known to bear
nodules on stems. They are *Aeschynomene*, *Sesbania*, and *Neptunia*,
of which the former two are being used as green manures. In the

genus *Aeschynomene,* which has 150–250 species ranging from herbs to small and medium-sized trees, about half the species are semi-aquatic. Among these, several workers have reported the stem nodulating habit in *A. indica, A. aspera, A. elephroxylon, A. villosa, A. evenia, A. paniculata, A. afaspera,* and other species in India, Mali, Ghana, Venezuela, Brazil, United States, Japan, Zimbabwe, Jawa, South Africa, Zambia, South America, Puerto Rico, Argentina, and Trinidad. In India, *A. indica* and *A. aspera* have received major attention (Arora, 1954; Subba Rao *et al.,* 1980; Subba Rao and Yatazawa, 1984).

The genus *Sesbania* has about 170 species which are annual to perennial herbs and slender fast-growing trees widespread in the warmer latitudes of both the hemispheres. *Sesbania rostrata* is an annual plant which thrives well in flooded soils of the Sahel region of West Africa and has nitrogen-fixing stem as well as root nodules. Because of this property, *S. rostrata* has attracted the attention of rice agronomists all over the world (Dreyfus and Dommergues, 1981a; Dreyfus *et al.,* 1985). The nitrogen fixation potential of *S. rostrata* is higher than that of soybean and the nitrogen contribution has been estimated at 200 kg N_2/ha in 50 days (Rinaudo *et al.,* 1983). However, the basic question whether *S. rostrata* by virtue of its stem nodulating habit is a superior green manure crop over other species of *Sesbania* which do not bear stem nodules is yet to be answered by extensive field trials. The results of a field trial carried out at the Agricultural University of Coimbatore, India, is given in Table 32.

The species of *Rhizobium* inducing stem as well as root nodulation in *S. rostrata* has been designated as *Azorhizobium caulinodans.* It is capable of fixing high levels of nitrogen (1500 nM C_2H_2/mg protein/hour) in pure culture in the presence of an unusually high level of oxygen. Stem nodulation is profuse up to 50 g/plant and acetylene reduction activity corresponds to 550–600 μM C_2H_2 reduced per hour. One interesting feature is that nodulation is insensitive to the presence of combined nitrogen in soil (Dreyfus and Dommergues, 1981b; Rinaudo *et al.,* 1982).

Whether the occurrence of nodules on stem of *S. rostrata* offers special advantage over root-nodulated species such as *S. sesban* was investigated by ^{15}N direct isotope dilution method and the difference method (Ndoye and Dreyfus, 1988). It was calculated that 93–109 kg N_2/ha and 7–18 kg N_2/ha would be fixed in 60 days by *S. rostrata* and

S. sesban, respectively, indicating the high nitrogen-fixing potential of the stem nodulating legume.

Table 32: Comparison of effects of *Azolla* and *Sesbania* on grain yield of rice (var. IR 50)

Treatments	Grain yield (kg/ha)	Straw yield (kg/ha)
Control	1480	3905
A. microphylla	2315	4885
A. filiculoides	2030	4555
S. rostrata	2350	6550
S. aculeata	2155	5695
S. speciosa	1945	6285
60 kg N/ha	2975	5610
60 kg N/ha + A. microphylla	3045	6255
60 kg N/ha + A. filiculoides	4105	6945
60 kg N/ha + S. rostrata	3930	4175
60 kg N/ha + S. aculeata	4370	5285
60 kg N/ha + S. speciosa	4310	6710
CD at 5% level	521.52	1369.68

Source: Prof. S. Kannaiyan, personal communication.

Benefits by Increased Rice Yield Due to N Value of Added Green Manure

The nitrogen content of a green manure species may serve as a guide to denote its potential as a green manure crop. Several workers have reported the nitrogen contents of green manure crops (Bhardwaj *et al.,* 1981; Ghose *et al.,* 1956; Watanabe, 1984). They vary but in terms of kg/ha they are as follows: *Astragalus sinicus, 108–123; Canavalia ensiformis, 98; Cassia mimosoides, 97; Crotalaria anagyroides, 98; C. juncea, 105–129; Dolichos biflorus, 89; Sesbania aculeata, 96–122; S. sesban, 100–202;* and *S. rostrata, 267.* One way of evaluating the benefits is to compare the increase in yield of rice by green manuring with the yield obtained by the use of chemical nitrogen fertilizer. From several published reports, the mean benefits could be generalized as equivalent to that derived by 30–80 kg N/ha. With *S. rostrata,* yield increase by application of a 52-day-old crop of the green manure to soil before rice seedling transplantation was of the order of 3.7 t/ha, whereas with 60 kg N/ha of chemical fertilizer, the increase was only 1.7 t/ha (Rinaudo *et al.,* 1981).

Benefits Other Than Increased Yield of Rice

The nitrogen content of rice grain and organic matter content of soil have been found to increase by green manuring (Tiwari *et al.,* 1980; Sanyasi Raju, 1952). Other soil properties which are improved by green manuring are the availability of zinc and the hydraulic conductivity, water holding capacity, and aggregate stability of the soil (Biswas *et al.,* 1970). Similarly, the loss of nitrogen by denitrification, volatilization, or leaching during the fallow period of rice cultivation is also prevented (Lowendorf, 1982).

The Use of *Astragalus*, *Sesbania* and *Aeschynomene* as Green Manure in China

Astragalus sinicas originated in China and its cultivation is known for over 1000 years. Fresh biomass of the plant may reach anywhere from 22.5 to 75 t/ha. This green manure crop is suitable for the temperate season's rice because of its tolerance for low temperature and its short (25–35 days) growth period. It has high nitrogen-fixing capacity (up to 270 kg N/ha) with low lignin and C/N content and is therefore most suitable for decomposition. One kg N containing fresh biomass of *Astragalus* is believed to increase rice yield by 12–16 kg with residual increases in soil organic matter status. The seeds of *Astragalus* are usually broadcast between two rows of rice during heading of the late rice crop so as to extend the growth period of *Astragalus*. The rice plant canopy helps in providing shade for the germination and survival of *Astragalus* seedlings. To improve germination, water is drained from the standing rice crop and when the green manure stands reach the flowering stage, the biomass is incorporated into the soil before beginning a new crop of rice (Liu Chung Chu, 1987).

Sesbania cannabina is the widely distributed summer green manure followed by *S. aculeata, S. aegyptica, S. paludosa, S. grandiflora, S. speciosa,* and *S. sesban*. Apart from improving soil organic matter, incorporation of 7.5–15 t/ha of *Sesbania* green matter increased rice grain yield from 10 to 46 per cent over controls. *Sesbania* seed is broadcast into rice fields even before the rice harvest and the green manure crop grows under the rice canopy. Alternatively, *Sesbania* seedlings may be planted after the harvest of rice when the field is drained and prepared for the next rice crop. A third method is to intercrop *Sesbania* with rice either by direct seeding of *Sesbania* seeds or by transplanting seedlings.

Aeschynomene indica is being recently used as green manure whose biomass often reaches 15,000 kg/ha after one month's growth. Direct seeding or intercropping is practised (Liu Chung Chu, 1987).

Green Manuring in India

The art of green manuring has been known for a long time to Indian farmers, especially in the southern parts of India. The following leguminous crops have been often used in rice cultivation (the vernacular name is indicated in parenthesis): *Crotalaria juncea* (sannhemp); *Sesbania aculeata bispinosa* (Dhaincha); *Phaseolus trilobus* (pillipesara); *Vigna mungo* (mung); *V. unguiculata* (cowpea); *Cyamopsis tetragonoloba* (gaur); *Melilotus alba* (sengi); *Lathyrus sativus* (khesari), and *Trifolium alexandrinum* (berseem). In southern India, leaves of the following tree species and herbs are often used as leaf green manure: *Thespesia populena, Cassia auriculata, Pongamia glabra, Melia azadirachta, Calatropis gigantea, Jatropha gossipifolia, J. glandulifera, Gliricidia maculata, Tephrosia purpurea, T. candida, Cassia tora,* and *Ipomea carnea* (Abdul Samad and Sahadevan, 1952; Sanyasi Raju, 1952).

The technique of green manuring used in Chingleput and North Arcot districts of Tamil Nadu in South India consists of sowing rice seed by drill under semi-dry conditions after the onset of the southwest monsoon. The green leaf manure is brought from outside weeks before sowing or at the sowing time and ploughed in when the northeast monsoon arrives. At this time, the low-lying tanks get filled with rain water and this water serves to irrigate the rice fields. Alternatively, sowing of a green manure crop and rice is advocated followed by trampling of the green manure crop when the rice crop is 2 months old. With this practice, using sannhemp, 42 per cent increase in the yield of rice was obtained in field experiments (Subramaniam and Dorai Raj, 1952).

The preferred green manure species in northern India is *S. aculeata,* which is sown after wheat in April. The biomass turned into soil in standing water after about 8 weeks of growth followed by transplantation of rice seedlings.

It has been observed that green manuring with sannhemp, dhaincha, pillipesara, and cowpea not only increased the yield of rice from 180 to 207 per cent over no manure treatments, but also improved per cent nitrogen of soil from 0.08 to anywhere between 0.12 and 0.14 (Sanyasi Raju, 1952). In an alkali soil, field experiments with dhaincha have clearly shown that with no additions of fertilizer nitrogen, incorporation of 65-day-old green manure increased yields of rice from 2.64 t/ha to 5.64 t/ha (Dargan *et al.,* 1975). The Indian experience with dhaincha has been that rice plantings can be done immediately after incorporating the green manure in soil (Bhardwaj, 1982).

Limitations in the Use of Green Manure

The practice of green manuring is labour intensive and the effect is not as dramatic as that of chemical fertilizers. It is not always possible to set apart land for 6–8 weeks exclusively for growing green manure species at all locations. Limitations of labour, water, and green manure seed add to the constraints for adopting the practice of green manuring on a large scale. Research on green manure species is sporadic and lacks imaginative planning. The case for revival of green manuring is due to the identification of root as well as stem nodulating species of legumes as exemplified by the use of *S. rostrata* and *Aeschynomene* spp. (Plate 5). There is therefore great scope to intensify location-specific research efforts to improve the technology of green manruing in rice cultivation in the light of scarcity and high cost of chemical fertilizers.

REFERENCES

Abdul Samad, A., and Sahadevan, P.C. (1952). Manuring for rice in Malabar. *Madras Agric. J.* **39,** 160–172.

Allen, O.N., and Allen, E.K. (1981). *The Leguminosea. A Source Book of Characteristics, Uses and Nodulation.* The University of Wisconsin Press, Madison, Wise.

Arora, N. (1954). Morphological development of the root and stem nodules of *Aeschynomene indica* L. *Phytomorphology,* **4,** 211–216.

Bhardwaj, K.K.R. (1982). Effect of the age and decomposition period of dhaincha on the yield of rice. *Indian J. Agron.,* **27,** 284–285.

Bhardwaj, S.P., Prasad, S.N., and Singh, G. (1981). Economizing N by green manure in rice wheat rotation. *Ind. J. Agric. Sci.,* **51,** 86–90.

Biswas, T.D., Roy, M.R., and Sahu, B.N. (1970). Effect of different sources of organic manures on the physical properties of the soil growing rice. *J. Ind. Soc. Soil Sci.,* **18,** 233–242.

Dargan, K.S., Chillar, R.K., and Bhardwaj, K.K.R. (1975). In alkali soils green manuring for more paddy. *Indian Farming,* **25(3),** 13–15.

deBruijn, F.J., Pawlowski, K, Ratet, P., Hilgert, U., Wong, C.H., Schneider, M., Meyer, Z.H., and Schell, J. (1988). Molecular genetics of nitrogen fixation by *Azorhizobium caulinodans* ORS 571, a diazotrophic stem nodulating symbiont of *Sesbania rostrata.* In *Nitrogen Fixation: One Hundred Years After.* Gustav Fischer, Stuttgart. pp. 351–355.

De Datta, S.K., and Patrick Jr., W.H. (1986). *Nitrogen Economy of Flooded Rice Soils,* Martinus Nijhoff Publishers, Boston.

Dreyfus, B.L., and Dommergues, Y.R. (1981a). Stem nodules on the tropical legume *Sesbania rostrata*. In *Current Perspectives in Nitrogen Fixation.* Ed. A.H. Gibson. Aust. Acad. Sci., *Canberra.* p. 615.

Dreyfus, B.L., and Dommergues, Y.R. (1981b). Nitrogen fixing nodules induced by *Rhizobium* on the stem of the tropical legume *Sesbania rostrata. FEMS Microbiol. Lett.,* **10,** 313–317.

Dreyfus, B., Rinaudo, G., and Dommergues, Y.R. (1985). Observations on the use of *Sesbania rostrata* as green manure in paddy fields. *Mircen J.,* **1,** 111–121.

Ghose, R.L.M., Ghatge, M.B., and Subramanyan, V. (1956). *Rice in India.* ICAR, New Delhi.

Liu Chung-Chu (1987). Integrated green manure use in rice fields in South China. In *The Role of Green Manure Crops in Rice Farming Systems.* Proc. Symp. Int. Rice Research Institute, Manila, Philippines.

Lowendorf, H.S. (1982). Biological nitrogen fixation in flooded rice fields. *Cornell Int. Agric. Mimeogr.,* 96.

Meelu, O.P., and Morris, R.A. (1986). Green manuring research in the Philippines — A review. *Philipp. J. Crop. Sci.,* **11,** 53–59.

Ndoye, I., and Dreyfus, B. 1988. N2 fixation by *Sesbania rostrata* and *Sesbania sesban* estimated using ^{15}N and total N difference methods. *Soil Biol. Biochem.,* **20,** 209–213.

Rinaudo, G., Dreyfus, B., and Dommergues, Y.R. (1981). *Sesbania rostrata* green manure on the nitrogen content of rice crop and soil. *Soil Biol. Biochem.,* **15,** 111–113.

Rinaudo, G., Dreyfus, B., and Dommergues, Y.R. (1982). Influence of *Sesbania rostrata* green manure on the nitrogen content of the rice crop and soil. *Soil Biol. Biochem.,* **15,** 111–113.

Sanyasi Raju, N. (1952). Role of organic manures and inorganic fertilizers in soil fertility. *Madras Agric. J.,* **39,** 130–147.

Subba Rao, N.S., and Yatazawa, M. (1984). Stem nodules. In *Current Developments in Biological Nitrogen Fixation.* Ed. N.S. Subba Rao. Oxford and IBH Publishing Co. Pvt. Ltd., New Delhi. pp. 101–110.

Subba Rao, N.S., Tilak, K.V.B.R., and Singh, C.S. (1980). Root nodulation studies of *Aeschynomene aspera. Plant and Soil,* **56,** 491–494.

Subramaniam, M.K.V., and Dorairaj, K. (1952). Green manuring for semi-dry paddy. *Madras Agric. J.,* **39,** 157–159.

Tiwari, K.N., Pathak, A.N., and Hari Ram (1980). Green manuring in combination with fertilizer nitrogen on rice under double cropping system in an alluvial. *Soil J. Ind. Soc. Sci.,* **28,** 162–169.

Vachhani, M.V., and Murty, K.S. (1964). *Green Manuring for Rice. Bull. No. 4,* Central Rice Research Institute, Cuttack, India.

Watanabe, I. (1984). Use of green manure in North East Asia. In *Organic Matter and Rice.* The International Rice Research Institute, Los Banos, Philippines. pp. 229–234.

8

Phosphate-solubilizing Microorganisms

Next only to nitrogen, phosphorus is a vital nutrient for plants and microorganisms. The inorganic forms of the element in soil are compounds of calcium, iron, aluminium, and fluorine. The organic forms are compounds of phytins, phospholipids, and nucleic acids which come mainly by way of decaying vegetation. Therefore, soils containing high organic matter are also rich in organic forms of phosphorus.

Superphosphate (single or triple) is one of the common forms of phosphatic fertilizer. The triple superphosphate contains two-and-a-half times the P_2O_5 content of single superphosphate. Rock phosphate is one of the basic raw materials for phosphatic fertilizer production and 100 million tons of rock phosphate deposists are available in India, although hardly one sixth of them are sufficiently enriched with P_2O_5 to be of any use for conversion into superphosphate. Furthermore, direct application of rock phosphate is limited to acidic soils. These considerations together with the cost involved in transportation and pulverization of the rock phosphate for agricultural use pose problems for rapid agronomic utilization of the raw material directly on the farm.

Solubilization of Phosphates by Microorganisms·

Several soil bacteria, particularly those belonging to the genera *Pseudomonas* and *Bacillus,* and fungi belonging to the genera *Penicillium* and *Aspergillus* possess the ability to bring insoluble phosphates in soil into soluble forms (Table 33) by secreting organic acids such as

Table 33: Microorganisms and sources of phosphate which are involved in phosphate solubilization

Microorganisms	Phosphate sources
Bacteria	**Mineral**
Bacillus sp., *B. pulvifaciens*, *B. megaterium*,	Tricalcium phosphate
B. circulans, *B. subtilis*, *B. mycoides*,	Calcium phosphate
B. mesentericus, *B. fluorescence*,	Iron phosphate
B. circulans	hydroxyapatite
Pseudomonas sp., *P. putida*, *P. liquifaciens*,	Fluorapatite
P. calcis, *P. rathonia*	Rock phosphate
Escherichia freundii, *E. intermedia*	
Xanthomonas spp.	**Organic**
Flavobacterium spp.	
Brevibacterium spp.	Calcium phosphate
Serratia spp.	Calcium glycero-phosphate
Alcaligenes spp.	Phytin
Achromobacter spp.	Lecithin
Aerobacter aerogenes	Hexose monophosphatic ester
Erwinia spp.	Phenyl phosphate
Nitrosomonas spp.	
Thiobacillus thiooxidans	Other organic phosphates
Fungi	
Aspergillus sp., *A. niger*, *A. flavus*,	
A. fumigatus, *A. terreus*, *A. awamori*	
Penicillium sp., *P. lilacinum*, *P. digitatum*	
Fusarium sp., *F. oxysporum*	
Curvularia lunata	
Humicola sp.	
Sclerotium rolfsii	
Phythium sp.	
Acrothecium sp.	
Phoma sp.	
Mortierella sp.	
Paecilomyces sp.	
Cladosporium sp.	
Rhizoctonia sp.	
Cunninghamella sp.	
Rhodotorula sp.	
Candida sp.	
Schwanniomyces occidentalis	
Oideodendron sp.	
Pseudogymnoascus sp.	
Actinomycetes	
Streptomyces sp.	

Source: Several published reports.

formic, acetic, propionic, lactic, glycolic, fumaric, and succinic acids (Plate 6). These acids lower the pH and bring about the dissolution of bound forms of phosphate (Table 34). Some of the hydroxy acids may chelate with calcium and iron resulting in effective solubilization and utilization of phosphates (Garretsen, 1948; Sen and Paul, 1957; Sperber, 1957; Katznelson and Bose, 1959; Louw and Webley, 1959; Subba Rao and Bajpai, 1965; Chhonkar and Subba Rao, 1967; Sethi and Subba Rao, 1968; Gaur and Ostwal, 1972; Ostwal and Bhide, 1972).

Table 34: Solubilization of $Ca_3(PO_4)_2$ by fungi associated with legume root nodules

Fungus	P_2O_5, mg in 50 ml medium (av. of 3 replicates)	P_2O_5 mg over control	% solubilized	pH of filtrate
Control (uninoculated)	2.76	—	—	6.7
Penicillium lilacinum (1)	8.66	+5.90	25.96[*]	6.0
P. lilacinum (2)	11.63	+8.87	39.02[*]	4.7
Aspergillus sp.	6.80	+4.04	17.77[*]	5.5
A. flavus	6.75	+3.99	17.55[*]	6.8
A. niger (1)	8.43	+5.67	24.94[*]	1.8
A. niger (2)	7.28	+4.52	19.88[*]	2.9
A. terreus	4.83	+2.07	9.10[**]	8.6
A. nidulans (1)	1.42	−1.34	0.0	7.6
A. nidulans (2)	2.91	+0.15	0.60	8.7
A. nidulans (3)	1.61	−1.15	0.0	8.4
Curvularia lunata	1.61	−1.15	0.0	8.0
Alternaria tenuis	2.07	−0.69	0.0	8.3
Fusarium sp.	1.61	−1.15	0.0	8.0
Rhizoctonia solani	1.05	−1.77	0.0	8.1
Trichoderma viride	2.07	−0.69	0.0	7.4

Source: Chhonkar and Subba Rao, 1967.
[*]Significantly different at 0.01 level.
[**]Significantly different at 0.05 level.

Isolation of Phosphate-solubilizing Microorganisms

A known quantity of soil or rhizosphere sample (1 g) is suspended in a known volume of sterile water and serial dilutions of the suspension made in sterile water blanks. Appropriate dilutions are plated on phosphate-containing solid media (see Appendix) for obtaining microorganisms capable of dissolving phosphates. The plates are incubated for 4–5 days. Transparent zones of clearing around microbial colonies indicate the extent of phosphate solubilization (Sundara Rao and Sinha, 1963). Such cultures are isolated and identified and the extent of solubilization determined quantitatively.

Quantitative Measurement of Phosphate Solubilization in Culture Medium

Selected cultures are grown in 50–100 ml aliquots of Pikovskyaya's liquid medium (see Appendix) for 6–17 days at 28°C (± 2). In the case of fungi, the culture is filtered using Whatman No. 42 filter paper. Due to pigments, the filtrate may often be coloured, in which case 1–2 g of activated charcoal is added and shaken until the filtrate becomes colourless. Bacterial cultures are filtered through Whatman No. 1 paper to remove insoluble phosphate and centrifuged at 10,000 rpm for 10–15 minutes. Filtration and centrifugation may be repeated until a clear solution is obtained which is finally made up to a known volume (50–100 ml).

To a 10 ml aliquot of the neat filtrate. 2.5 ml of Barton's reagent (see Appendix for details) is added and the volume made up to 50 ml. After 10 minutes, the resultant colour is read in a colorimeter using 430 μ wavelength.

A standard curve is prepared by dissolving 0.2195 g KH_2PO_4 in water and the solution made up to 1 litre (1 ml = 59 ppm phosphorus). Further dilution of 10 ml into 250 ml is made so as to give 1 ml = 2 ppm P. Aliquots of 2, 3, 4, 5, 6, 8, 10, 15, and 20 ml of the 2 ppm stock solution are taken in 50 ml volumetric flasks, 2.5 ml of Barton's reagent added, and the volume made up to 50 ml with water. After 10 minutes, using a filter the colour developed is read in a colorimeter. A standard graph is then prepared from which P values for experimental samples are calculated (Koening and Johnson, 1942).

Agronomic Aspects

Selected bacteria capable of high phosphate solubilization (e.g., *Pseudomonas* sp., *B. megaterium* var. *phosphaticum*) are grown in Pikovskaya's broth for 7–18 days at 28°C (± 2°C) and mixed in suitable sterilized carrier (such as peat soil, lignite powder). The mixture is cured for a week at 28°C (± 2°C) in large trays covered with loosely fitting empty trays. The inoculant is then packed at the rate of 300 g per plastic packet and stored at 15°–20°C until use. Normally, the inoculant is used as early as possible (within a month) to inoculate seeds in the same way as *Rhizobium* inoculants are used for seed inoculation. Much more research work needs to be done on the survival of phosphate-solubilizing microorganisms in carrier-based inoculants on the lines of *Rhizobium* inoculants. A carrier based preparation under the name 'Microphos' has been developed recently at the microbiology Division, Indian Agricultural Research Institute, New Delhi by Dr. A.C. Gaur.

Table 35: Phosphobacterin inoculation experiments in India

Location	Crop	No. of field trials	% increase over control	No. of expts. showing significant increases
Delhi	Berseem	6	10–20	4
Alluvial soil	Maize	1	20–30	1
Karnal	Wheat	3	16–37	1
Alluvial impregnated	Maize	2	14.0	1
with salt	Paddy	3	—	Nil
Pusa (Bihar)	Gram	1	—	Nil
Calcareous soil	Urid	3	16–19	1
	Wheat	1	—	Nil
	Maize	1	—	Nil
	Paddy	1	—	Nil
Wellington	Potato	1	—	Nil
Acid soil	Wheat	1	—	Nil
Nagpur	Arhar	1	—	Nil
Black cotton soil				
Indore	Paddy	2	19–31	1
Black cotton soil				
Simla	Wheat	1	—	Nil
Acid soil				
Rajendranagar	Paddy	5	12–14	1
(Hyderabad)	Paddy	1	—	Nil
Bapatla, Ranchi	Soybean	1	—	Nil
Acid soil (limed)	Groundnut	2	—	Nil
	Total	37		10

Source: Sundara Rao, 1968.

In Russia a commercial biofertilizer under the name 'phospho-bacterin' was first prepared by incorporating *B. megaterium* var. *phosphaticum* and widely used in Russia and other East European countries with yield increases of 5–10 per cent over corresponding controls. Several field trials have also been conducted by the Indian Agricultural Research Institute using phosphobacterin on wheat, berseem, maize, arhar, and rice. The results (Table 35) show that in different agroclimatic conditions 10 out of 37 field experiments showed significant increase in yield over uninoculated controls. Further work at the field level is needed to evaluate the role of phosphate-dissolving microorganisms in phosphate uptake and yield of crop plants.

Recently, emphasis has been placed on the possibility of greater utilization of indigenously available rock phosphate resources by the action of phosphate-solubilizing microorganisms. In this connection, field experiments have been carried out in India using culture suspensions of *B. polymyxa, B. circulans, P. striata,* and *Aspergillus awamori* with and without superphosphate or rock phosphate on the yield of wheat and rice (Gaur *et al.,* 1980). The results demonstrated that significant increase in grain yield was possible when wheat was inoculated with *P. striata* in the presence of rock phosphate at 100 kg P_2O_5/ha. Similarly, grain yield significantly increased when rice (paddy) was inoculated with *B. polymyxa* in the presence of rock phosphate.

Table 36: Some results of work in India on the influence of inoculation with phosphate-solubilizing bacteria on the yield of crops

Microorganisms	Details of study	Reference
Bacillus polymyxa B. pulvifaciens	*B. polymyxa* in the presence of rock phosphate significantly increased grain and straw yield and P uptake of wheat whereas *B. pulvifaciens* did not.	Gaur and Ostwal, 1972
Pseudomonas striata	With superphosphate and rock phosphate significantly increased yield of wheat.	Gaur et al., 1980
B. polymyxa	With rock phosphate significantly increased the yields of rice.	Gaur et al., 1980
P. striata	With rock phosphate and superphosphate significantly increased potato yield.	Gaur and Negi, personal communication

In another experiment, using *P. striata* as the test organism, field trials were conducted to test inoculation effects on the yield of potato (Gaur and Negi, personal communication). The seed tubers were inoculated with a peat-based culture and experiments done with and without rock phosphate, superphosphate, or combinations of both. Even simple inoculation of tubers increased yield significantly, which was further improved in the presence of superphosphate at 50 kg P_2O_5/ha. These results have been summarized in Table 36. *Pseudomonas* spp. have been recognized as potent plant growth promoting rhizobacteria (PGPR) which are deleterious to seed borne rhizosphere inhabiting pathogens and hence contributed to increased yield of potato in Netherlands (see Chapter 13). Therefore, the beneficial effects of *Pseudomonas* inoculation have also to be examined in the light of such observations.

REFERENCES

Chhonkar, P.K., and Subba Rao, N.S. (1967). Phosphate solubilization by fungi associated with legume root nodules. *Can. J. Microbiol.*, **13**, 749–753.

Garretsen, F.C. (1948). The influence of microorganisms on the phosphorus uptake by the plant. *Plant and Soil*, **1**, 51–81.

Gaur, A.C., and Ostwal, K.P. (1972). Influence of phosphate dissolving bacilli on yield and phosphate uptake of wheat crop. *Indian J. Exp. Biol.*, **10**, 393.

Gaur, A.C., Ostwal, K.P., and Mathur, R.S. (1980). Save superphosphate by using phosphobacteria. *Kheti*, **32**, 23–25.

Katznelson, H., and Bose, B. (1959). Metabolic activity and phosphate dissolving ability of bacterial isolates from wheat root, rhizosphere and non-rhizosphere soil. *Can. J. Microbiol.*, **5**, 79–85.

Koening, H.A., and Johnson, C.R. (1942). Method for estimating phosphorus. *Indust. Eng. Chem.* (Anal Ed.), **14**, 155.

Louw, H.A., and Webley, D.M. (1959). A study of soil bacteria dissolving certain mineral phosphate fertilizers and related compounds. *J. Appl. Bact.*, **22**, 227–233.

Ostwal, K.P., and Bhide, V.P. (1972). Solubilization of tricalcium phosphate by soil *Pseudomonas*. *Indian J. Exp. Biol.*, **10**, 153.

Sen, A., and Paul, N.B. (1957). Solubilization of phosphates by some common soil bacteria. *Curr. Sci.*, **26**, 222.

Sethi, R.P., and Subba Rao, N.S. (1968). Solubilization of tricalcium phosphate and calcium phytate by soil fungi. *J. Gen. Appl. Microbiol.*, **14**, 329–331.

Sperber, J.I. (1957). Solution of mineral phosphates by soil bacteria, *Nature*, Lond., **180**, 994–995.

Subba Rao, N.S., and Bajpai, P.D. (1965). Fungi on the surface of legume root nodules and phosphate solubilization. *Experientia*, **21**, 386–387.

Sundara Rao, W.V.B. (1968). Phosphorus solubilization by microorganisms. *Proc. All India Symp. on Agricultural Microbiology*, Univ. Agric. Sci., Bangalore, pp. 21–29.

Sundara Rao, W.V.B., and Sinha, M.K. (1963). Phosphate dissolving organisms in the soil and rhizosphere. *Ind. J. Agric. Sci.*, **33**, 272–278.

9

Mycorrhizal Fungi

'Mycorrhiza' (meaning fungus root) is the term commonly used to denote the symbiotic association between plant roots and fungal mycelia (Plate 7). There are two primary types of mycorrhizal fungal associations with plant roots — the ectotrophic or ectomycorrhiza and the endotrophic or endomycorrhiza. Mycorrhizal plants increase the surface area of the root system for better absorption of nutrients from soil especially when the soils are deficient in phosphorus. The ectomycorrhizal associations exist primarily in the families Pinaceae, Fagaceae, Betulaceae, and Saliceae and the few genera of other families such as *Eucalyptus, Casuarina, Tilia,* and *Arbutus.* Several members of the Ceasalpiniaceae and Dipterocarpaceae also carry ectomycorrhiza. The fungal partner of the symbiosis in ectomycorrhiza belongs to Basidiomycetes and Ascomycetes although few members of Endogonaceae also infect roots (Trappe, 1962; Harley, 1969; Hacskaylo, 1971; Marks and Kozlowski, 1973; Mikola, 1981). In ectomycorrhizae (Fig. 16) the fungus completely encloses each feeder rootlet in a sheath or mantle of fungal hyphae and hyphal branches penetrate the space between the cells of the root cortex (intercellular). Endomycorrhizae, however, are prevalent in representative species of most families of angiosperms, in conifers except pinaceae, and in certain pteridophytes and bryophytes. Some orchids of the genera *Neottia, Limodorum, Epipogon, Vanilla,* etc. are dependent on endomycorrhizal fungi for growth which get into the plant system when seed germinates. The orchid fungi may be from Basidimycetes (e.g., *Fomes, Corticium*) or from Fungi imperfectii (e.g., *Rhizoctonia*). Mycorrhizal orchids depend on the fungus for nutritional requirements in juvenile stage of growth. In endomycorrhizae of orchids, the fungal hyphae enter the cells of the root (intracellular) and are often distintegrated and thus contribute to the nutritional

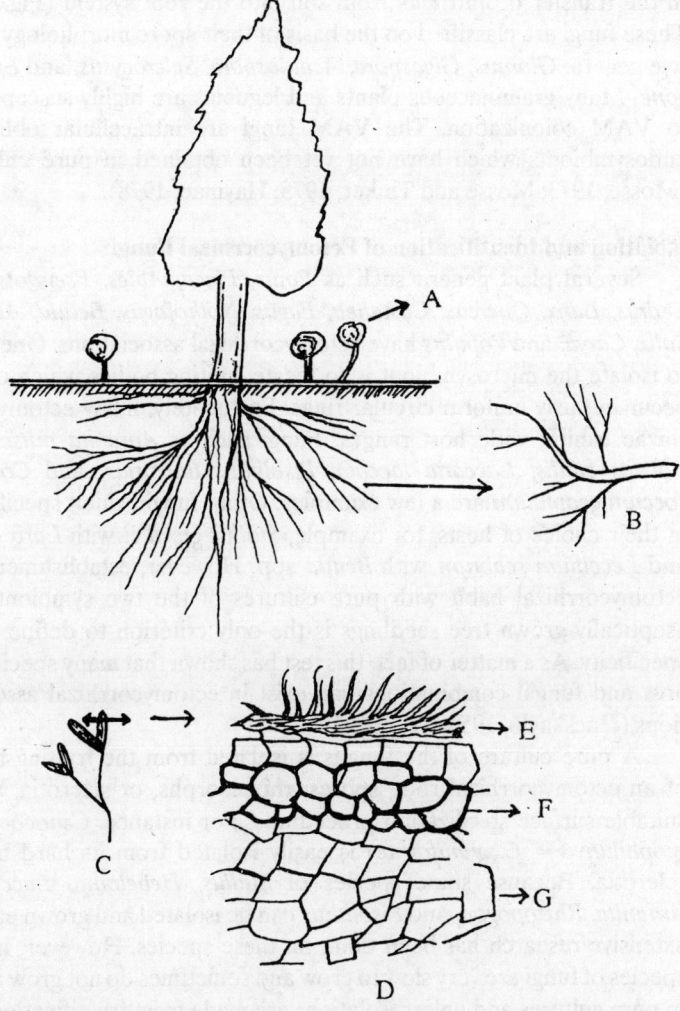

Fig. 16. Diagrammatic representation of a typical ectomycorrhizal association with a forest tree (e.g., pine). A—Fruiting bodies of an ectomycorrhizal fungus on the soil surface whose mycelia surround the roots; B—A portion of the finer root system with dichotomously branching feeder roots; C—Feeder roots having a fungal mantle outside; D—Transverse section of a feeder root showing the fungal mantle E and the intercellular 'Harting net' F followed by uninfected cortical cells of the root G. Diagram not to scale.

requirements of the host. Yet another class of endomycorrhizae are known as vesicular-arbuscular mycorrhiza (VAM), which possess special structures known as vesicles and arbuscules, the latter helping in the transfer of nutrients from soil into the root system (Fig. 17). These fungi are classified on the basis of their spore morphology into five genera: *Glomus, Gigaspora, Acaulospora, Sclerocystis,* and *Endogone.* Many graminaceous plants and legumes are highly susceptible to VAM colonization. The VAM fungi are intracellular obligate endosymbionts which have not yet been obtained in pure culture (Mosse, 1973; Mosse and Tinker, 1975; Hayman, 1978).

Isolation and Identification of Ectomycorrhizal Fungi

Several plant genera such as *Pinus, Picea, Abies, Pseudotsuga, Cedrus, Larix, Quercus, Castanea, Fagus, Nothofagus, Betula, Alnus, Salix, Carya,* and *Populus* have ectomycorrhizal associations. One way to isolate the microsymbiont is to locate fruiting bodies which often occur in fairly uniform circular rings. Fortunately, many ectomycorrhizae exhibit wide host ranges. Fungi such as *Amanita muscaria, Boletus edulis, Laccaria laccata, Pisolithus tinctorius,* and *Coenococcum geophilum* are a few examples. Other fungi exhibit specificity in their choice of hosts, for example, *Suillus grevillei* with *Larix* spp. and *Leccinum scabrum* with *Betula* spp. However, establishment of ectomycorrhizal habit with pure cultures of the two symbionts in aseptically grown tree seedlings is the only criterion to define host specificity. As a matter of fact, this test has shown that many species of host and fungal combinations can exist in ectomycorrhizal associations (Hacskaylo, 1953; Trappe, 1969).

A pure culture of the fungus is isolated from the fruiting body of an ectomycorrhizal root, spores, rhizomorphs, or sclerotia, after suitable surface sterilization procedures. For instance, *Cenococcum geophilum* (= *C. graniforme*) is easily isolated from its hard black sclerotia. Because some species of *Suillus, Hebeloma, Laccaria, Amanita, Rhizopogon,* and *Pisolithus* can be isolated and grown easily, extensive research has been done on these species. However, many species of fungi are very slow to grow and sometimes do not grow at all in pure cultures and unless isolations are made from fructifications, it becomes difficult to identify the species (Mikola, 1981).

Physiology and Function of Ectomycorrhizal Fungi

Ectomycorrhizal fungi do not generally secrete cellulolytic or lignolytic enzymes and they depend on the carbon skeletons supplied

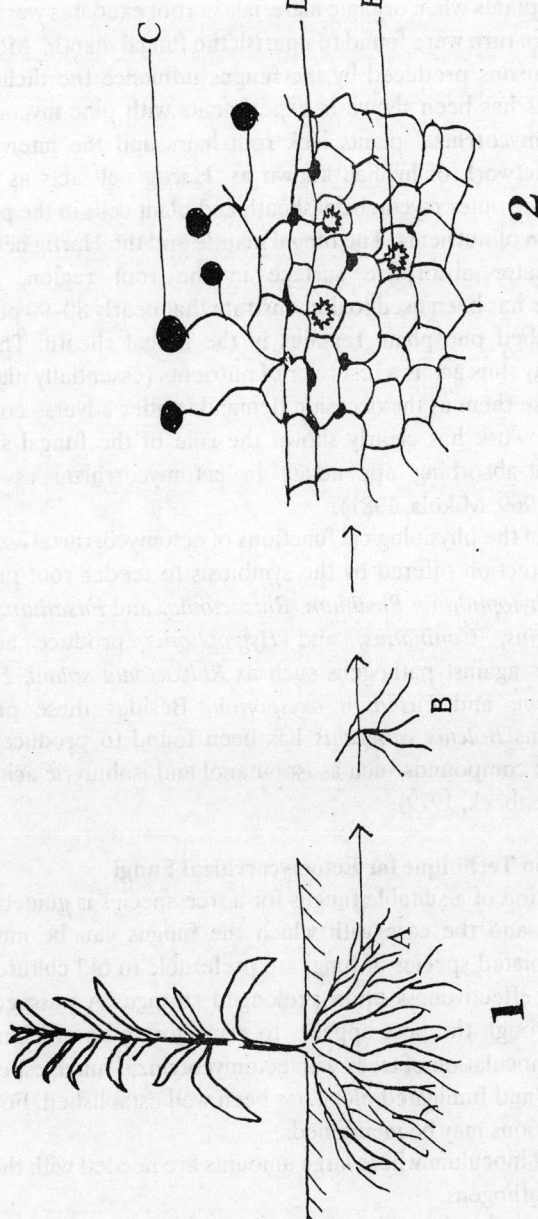

Fig. 17. VA mycorrhizal association with a graminaceous plant (e.g., pearl millet) is shown in (1). A portion of the root system (A) is enlarged (B). Its transverse section (2) reveals external mycelium of the fungus having spores (C) in the soil. Inside the root cortex are shown intracellular vesicles (D) and arbuscules (E). Diagram not to scale.

by the host plant. This has been shown in experiments by feeding $^{14}CO_2$ to plants when organic materials in root exudates were labelled and they in turn were found to nourish the fungal mantle. Metabolites such as auxins produced by the fungus influence the dichotomy of rootlets as has been shown in experiments with pine mycorrhiza. In general, mycorrhizal plants lack root hairs and the internal inter-cellular network of hyphae known as 'Hartig net' acts as a liaison between the outer mycorrhizal sheath and plant cells in the process of absorption of nutrients. The fungal mantle and the Hartig net serve to offer greater absorptive surface in the root region. Labelled phosphate has been used to demonstrate that nearly 80–90 per cent of the absorbed phosphate remains in the fungal sheath. The fungal sheath may thus act as a reservior of nutrients (essentially phosphate) and release them as the occasion demands under adverse conditions. Extensive work has clearly shown the role of the fungal sheath as a nutrient-absorbing appendage in ectomycorrhizal associations (Harley, 1969; Mikola, 1981).

One of the physiological functions of ectomycorrhizal association is the protection offered by the symbiosis to feeder root pathogens such as *Phytophthora, Phythium, Rhizoctonia,* and *Fusarium.* Species of *Lactarius, Cortinarius,* and *Hygrophorus* produce antifungal substances against pathogens such as *Rhizoctonia solani, Phythium debaryanum,* and *Fusarium oxysporum.* Besides these protective mechanisms *Boletus variegatus* has been found to produce volatile fungistatic compounds such as isobutanol and isobutyric acid (Marx, 1972; Schonbeck, 1979).

Inoculation Technique for Ectomycorrhizal Fungi

Selection of a suitable fungus for a tree species is guided by host specificity and the ease with which the fungus can be multiplied. Freshly isolated species of fungi are preferable to old cultures which lose their effectiveness upon prolonged storage. A passage of the fungus through the host appears to reinvigorate its efficiency. The need for inoculation of trees with ectomycorrhizal fungi, especially in new areas and fumigated plots, has been well established. Four types of inoculations may be mentioned:

1) Soil inoculum where large amounts are needed with the risk of carrying pathogens.

2) Mycorrhizal seedlings from nursery interplanted in seed beds.

3) Spores and sporocarps of fungi serving as inocula which are labour intensive and dependent on natural occurrence of fruiting bodies.

4) Pure cultures as inoculum, which is ideal but is time consuming and probably expensive.

All these inoculation methods are practised. With *Pisolithus tinctorius,* natural collection of spores with abundant fruiting bodies known as 'puff balls' and subsequent inoculation of $5.5 \times 10^8 - 1.3 \times 10^{10}$ spores/sq. m of soil surface in nurseries of the southern United States, especially after mixing with wood pulp suspended in water (hydromulch), has been quite effective (Marx, 1981). Successful ectomycorrhizal establishment of *Pinus radiata* in Australia was achieved with basidiospores of *Rhizopogon luteolus* coated to seeds before sowing. Even freeze-dried spores produced mycorrhizal association (Theodorou, 1967, 1971; Theodorou and Bowen, 1970, 1973). Pulverized sporocarps of *R. luteolus* have been used with success to inoculate *P. radiata* nurseries in South Africa (Donald, 1975).

Inoculation studies with pure cultures of *Pisolithus tinctorius* have been done extensively in the United States Forest Service Institute for Mycorrhizal Research and Development, Athens, Georgia (Marx, 1981). *Pisolithus tinctorius* can be readily isolated from sporocarps and quickly grown in culture. The entire feeder root system of seedlings inoculated with the pure culture of the fungus gets colonized. Other added advantages of this fungus are that it readily forms ectomycorrhizae with nearly 48 species of trees, can withstand environmental stresses, and is distributed worldwide. The fungus is grown for 3–4 months in 2 jars containing sterilized peat moss-vermiculite substrate moistened with modified Melin-Norkrans nutrient solution (Marx, 1969).

At the end of the growth period, the left-over nutrient in the inoculum is washed away in running tap water and the suspension of fungal mat is spread in soil at the rate of about 1 litre/sq. m and incorporated 8 to 10 cm into the soil before the seed is sown. The inoculum from jars can be dried to 12 per cent moisture in a forced air oven and the dried inoculum is superior to wet inoculum. The inoculum can be stored at 5°–25°C for 7–9 weeks and at 30°C for 7 weeks. The inoculum is known to survive in soil for 30 days even in the absence of the host. A peat moss-vermiculite mixture in containers can serve as an inoculum substrate as well as potting mixture for seedlings. Such 'containerized seedlings' inoculated with *P. tinctorius* have proved successful in *Pinus, Pseudotsuga, Tsuga,* and *Quercus.* Similarly, such containerized seedlings inoculated with *Laccaria laccata, Cenococcum geophilum,* and *Hebeloma crustruliforme* have successfully established ectomycorrhizae on species of *Pinus, Tsuga, Picea, Larix,* and *Pseudotsuga* (Molina and Trappe, 1982).

Occurrence and Distribution of VAM

The VA type of endomycorrhiza is prevalent in most angiosperms, gymnosperms, pteridophytes, and bryophytes but absent in Pinaceae, Betulaceae, Ericales and Orchidaceae. Some species like *Eucalyptus, Leucaena,* and *Casuarina* have both VAM and ectomycorrhizae. Dense VAM infections are common in most species of leguminosea and graminae. Most of the economically important crops such as sorghum, barley, upland rice, cassava, onions, cowpea, strawberries, apple, rubber, coffee, tea, papaya, and oil palm are infected by VAM fungi. Except under waterlogged conditions, VAM fungi are virtually worldwide in temperate, tropical, and arctic regions. They flourish in rainforests, open woodlands, scrub, savanna, grasslands, heaths, sand dunes, and semideserts. There are fossil records which bear resemblance to VAM fungal spores. Highly fertile soils generally show less VAM fungal populations and pesticide treatment tends to decrease their numbers (Hayman, 1982).

Ecology of VAM Fungi in Soil

Even though any VAM fungus can infect any host plant species, there can be soils or plant species more suitable for a given species of VAM fungus, depending on soil pH, fertility status of soil, and pesticide applications. Therefore, the 'specificity' between the two symbionts is non-existent, although the competitive ability of a given VAM fungal inoculum to out perform native strains may influence the establishment of a suitable VAM fungus in the root. The per cent infection in a given root need not necessarily be the index of its effectiveness on the host (growth response). It is not clear whether the quantum of mycelial growth outside the root is more important than the number of vesicles or arbuscules. As a matter of fact, facile techniques are unavailable to quantify the extent of fungal mycelial ramifications in the rhizosphere.

Physiology of VAM Fungus Host Interaction

Apart from the well-known effect of VAM fungal associations on phosphate uptake (Gray and Gerdemann, 1969) reports show that Zn uptake is enhanced in peaches (Gilmore, 1971; La Rue *et al.*, 1975) and maize, wheat, and potatoes (Swaminathan and Verma, 1979). Similarly, the uptake of sulphur is enhanced by VAM fungal infection in red clover and maize (Gray and Gerdemann, 1973). Cytokinins and chlorophyll contents of plants have been found to increase by VAM fungal association (Allen *et al.*, 1980).

There are indications to show that VAM fungal associations with plant roots can help plants to overcome water stress by stomatal regulation in citrus (Levy and Krikun, 1980).

It is generally believed that the VAM fungus depends upon the supply of carbohydrates from the host as shown by $^{14}CO_2$ experiments (Ho and Trappe, 1973). However, under poor light and temperature conditions, the fungus may tilt the balance from symbiosis to slight parasitism (Hayman, 1974). More details on this subject can be had from the book on VA Mycorrhiza edited by Powell and Bagyaraj (1984).

Isolation and Identification of VAM Fungal Spores

Since VAM fungi are obligate endosymbionts and have not been cultured the only means of identifying them is to collect resting spores from soil and determine the morphological characteristics. By staining roots following appropriate methods, the morphology of vesicles and arbuscules can be understood, which also serves as a diagnostic characteristic to define species. The soil near the root system is collected and an aqueous suspension passed through different sieves to collect spores of different sizes (Gerdemann and Nicolson, 1963). Vesicles are normally oval, occasionally round, and sometimes irregularly lobed. They serve as storage organs. Arbuscules are like haustoria of parasitic fungi and are believed to transfer nutrients, especially phosphate. Cushion-like structures known as 'appresoria' are formed at points of entry of the fungal mycelium into the root hair and they serve to connect the external hyphae in soil with internal hyphae in the root. The external hyphae bear large resting spores in soil (Fig. 17). The external hyphae are sometimes so voluminous that they contribute to soil aggregation properties.

Classification of VAM Fungi

VAM fungi are classified in the family Endogonaceae, order Mucorales, and class Zygomycetes of the Phycomycete group. There has been confusion about the taxonomy of VAM fungi and at present the scheme of Gerdemann and Trappe (1974) is followed, which is based on the size, shape, and colour of spores, presence or absence of stalk for attachment of spores, wall thickness, types of layers of the spore wall, cytoplasmic structure of the spore contents, the method of spore germination, and the presence or absence of spores and sporocarps as diagnostic characteristics for speciation. For example, 50 μ diameter spore is classified as *Glomus microcarpus* whereas 100 to 200 μ spore may belong to *Glomus mosseae, Gigaspora cladospora,* and *Glomus caledonius.* Spores measuring 200 to 400 μ or even 1 mm are considered *Gigaspora margarita* and *Gigaspora* spp. Spores of *Glomus* spp. have single stalk, whereas those of *Gigaspora* have bulbous stalk and *Acaulospora* spores are sessile. The colour of spores is yellow, red, grey, amber, or shades of these colours. The spore wall may be simple to reticulate.

Inoculum Production of VAM Fungi

After the wet-sieving procedure, individual types of living spores (10–20) can be identified and collected in bulk in a watch glass for initially infecting seedlings grown in sterilized soil in funnels. These spores are easily seen and handled under a binocular stereo microscope using a capillary tubing. The spores may be surface-sterilized by being immersed in 2 per cent (wt/vol.) chloramine T and 200 ppm streptomycin for 15 minutes followed by successive washings in sterile water (Hayman, 1982). When the required species multiply on the roots, the authenticity of the species must be checked microscopically. Once this is assured, the entire root system is finely chopped with adhering soil and used as the inoculum for scaling up inoculum production on living roots of test hosts grown in pots containing sterilized soil. As a matter of fact, different species of VAM fungi are maintained in this way, care being taken to check purity of species periodically. Onions, sorghum, and other grasses are suitable hosts to multiply VAM fungal inocula and the plants are grown in 1:1 sand-soil mixture to obtain good root growth. The pots are kept in the greenhouse adequately separated so that there is no contamination between the species during watering. Such root-based VAM fungal cultures are now being commonly used as inoculum in the form of seed pellets or granules, or as such in plastic bags (Fig. 18).

The quality and quantity of VAM fungal inocula produced by the pot culture method are subject to variation by external contamination and the inocula are not always free of other microorganisms vitiating experimental results. To overcome these defects, VAM fungi have been grown in root-organ cultures (Mosse and Hepper, 1975;

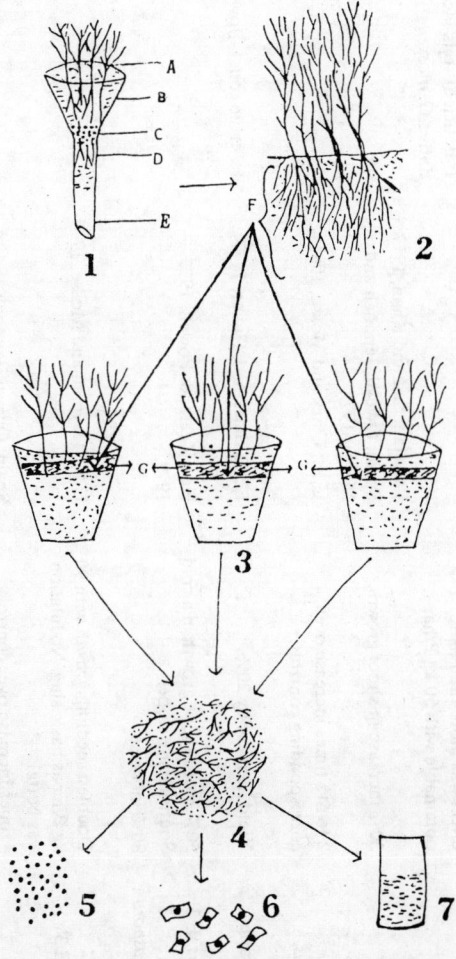

Fig. 18. Root-based inoculum production method for VAM fungi — A funnel-plant system (1) supports the growth of test seedlings (A) on a sand + soil mixture (B) containing 20–30 spores of a selected VAM fungus (C) held by a piece of glass wool (D) in the bottom of a large funnel (E). After a few weeks of growth the plants are removed from the funnel (2) and the root system checked microscopically for fungal colonization. Later, the root system together with adhering soil is macerated to form the starter inoculum, which is placed at 5 per cent level, one inch below the soil (G) in big pots (3) supporting the growth of test plants. After 3–4 months the root system with soil is macerated to constitute the bulk inoculum (4). This bulk inoculum may be dispensed for field application in the form of granular preparation (5) or pelleted with seed and an inert material (6) or packaged in polythene pouches as semi-wet inoculum

Table 37: Results of field experiments on the effect of VAM fungal inocula on yield of various plants

Plant inoculated	Inoculant	Results obtained	Country and reference	Remarks
Maize, wheat	Glomus mosseae	Doubled shoot dry weight and effect was more than that obtainable with 50 kg P/ha.	Pakistan: Khan, 1972, 1975	Experiment done on P-deficient soils lacking native G. mosseae
Barley	G. mosseae	"	Pakistan: Saif and Khan, 1977	"
Barley	G. mosseae	30% increase in shoot growth.	Spain: Owusu Bennoah and Mosse, 1979	
Barley	G. mosseae, G. fasciculatus, G. caledonius	2 to 6½ times increase over corresponding controls.	U.K.: Clark and Mosse, 1981	
Potatoes	VAM from barley fields	Yield increase by 20%.	U.K.: Black and Tinker, 1977	Infertile soil, fallow for 2 years
White clover	G. fasciculatus 'E 3'	50% more shoot growth in a cold South-facing slope.	New Zealand: Powell, 1977, 1979	
White clover	G. tenuis, Gigaspora margarita	80% increase.		
White clover	G. mosseac, G. fasciculatus 'E 3'	Doubled seedling growth with 90 kg P/ha as basic slag. Nodulation was better.	U.K.: Hayman and Mosse, 1979	
Lucerne	G. caledonius	4 times increase over controls.	Spain: Owusu Bennoah and Mosse, 1979	
Cowpea	G. fasciculatus	More growth in the presence of rock phosphate.	Nigeria: Islam et al., 1980	Transplanted seedlings

Table 38: Results of field experiments carried out by US workers on the effect of VAM fungal inocula on the yield of citrus, peach, and soybean in fumigated soils

Plant inoculated	Inoculant	Results obtained	Location and reference
Citrus	Glomus mosseae	Increased growth up to 150% depending on citrus varieties.	California: Hattingh and Gerdemann, 1975
Citrus	G. fasciculatus	Increased growth by 70 to 300%, depending on citrus species.	California: Kleinschmidt and Gerdemann, 1972
Peach	VAM fungi	Nursery seedlings had more Zn in their tissues upon inoculation	California: La Rue et al, 1975
Soybean	Endogone	Nodulating isoline of soybean increased by 53%, whereas no such increases secured in non-nodulating isoline.	Florida: Schenck and Hinson, 1973

Miller-Wideman and Watrude, 1984) and in solution cultures (Crush and Hay, 1981; Ḩowler *et al.*, 1982; Elmes and Mosse, 1984; Mosse and Thompson, 1984). Aeroponic and membrane system cultures of a plant and a selected VAM fungus have been grown to produce better spore counts on roots (Sylvia and Hubbell, 1986).

Field Experiments with VAM Fungi

Field experiments carried out in various parts of the world have shown beneficial effects of VAM inoculation on cereals, potato, clovers, lucerne, and cowpea (Table 37). Plant protectants, especially fungicides, are known to effect fungal growth in soils. Therefore, beneficial responses to fresh VAM applications in fumigated soils have been demonstrated in citrus, peach, and soybean (Table 38).

Interaction of Nodulated Legumes with VAM Fungi

When a species of *Rhizobium* and a VAM fungus are co-inoculated, the growth of the legume is enhanced in many legumes such as clovers, groundnut, soybean, pigeon pea, and chick-pea. This additive effect is demonstrated to a greater degree in phosphate deficient soil as shown in field experiments with cowpea (Islam *et al.*, 1980).

Future Directions

The impediments in the speedy application of mycorrhiza to improve plant growth are the relatively slow growth of ectomycorrhizal fungi and the very obligate nature of VAM fungi which limit large-scale production of inocula. If spores of VAM fungi can be made to grow and produce large mycelia in nutrient media, it is likely that dual inoculation of N_2-fixing bacteria and VAM fungi either by seed pelleting or furrow application with seeds can be practised on a wider scale.

By genetic engineering, if nitrogen fixation genes (nif genes) can be transferred to VAM fungi, the opportunity for biological nitrogen fixation and phosphate mobilization can be combined in one microorganism. This biotechnological possibility is still in the realm of speculation and perhaps may become a reality in the not too distant future.

REFERENCES

Allen, M.F., Moore, T.S., and Christensen, M. (1980). Phytohormone changes in *Bouteloua gracilis* infected by vesicular-arbuscular mycorrhizae. I. Cytokinin increases in the host plant. *Can. J. Bot.,* **58,** 371–374.

Black, R.L.B., and Tinker, P.B. (1977). Interaction between effects of vesicular-arbuscular mycorrhiza and fertilizer phosphorous on yields of potatoes in the field. *Nature,* **267,** 510–511.

Clark, C., and Mosse, B. (1981). Plant growth responses of barley at two soil p levels. *New Phytol.,* **87,** 695–703.

Crush, J.R., and Hay, M.J.M. (1981). A technique for growing mycorrhizal clover in solution culture. *N.Z.J. Agric. Res.,* **24,** 371–372.

Donald, D.G.M. (1975). Mycorrhizal inoculation of pines. *S. African Forestry J.,* **92,** 27–29.

Elmes, R.P., and Mosse, B. (1984). Vesicular-arbuscular endomycorrhizal inoculum production. II. Experiments with maize (*Zea mays*) and other hosts in nutrient flow culture. *Can. J. Bot.* **62,** 1531–1536.

Gerdemann, J.W., and Nicolson, T.H. (1963). Spores of mycorrhizal *Endogone* species extracted from soil by wet sieving and decanting. *Trans. Brit. Mycol. Soc.,* **46,** 235–244.

Gerdemann, J.W., and Trappe, J.M. (1974). *The Endogonaceae in the Pacific North West.* Mycologia Memoir No. 5.

Gilmore, A.E. (1971). The influence of endotrophic mycorrhizae on the growth of peach seedlings. *J. Amer. Soc. Hort. Sci.,* **96,** 35–38.

Gray, L.E., and Gerdemann, J.W. (1969). Uptake of phosphorus-32 by vesicular arbuscular mycorrhizae. *Plant and Soil,* **30,** 415–422.

Gray, L.E., and Gerdemann, J.W. (1973). Uptake of Sulphur-35 by vesicular-arbuscular mycorrhizae. *Plant and Soil,* **39,** 687–689.

Hacskaylo, E. (1953). Pure culture synthesis of pine mycorrhizae in terralite. *Mycologia,* **45,** 971–975.

Hacskaylo, E. (1971). *Mycorrhizae.* USDA Forest Service Misc. Pub. No. 1189.

Harley, J.L. (1969). *The Biology of Mycorrhiza.* 2nd Ed. Leonard Hill, London.

Hattingh M.J., and Gerdemann, J.W. (1975). Inoculation of Brazilian sour orange seed with an endomycorrhizal fungus. *Phytopathology,* **65,** 1013–1016.

Hayman, D.S. (1974). Plant growth responses to vesicular arbuscular mycorrhiza. VI. Effect of light and temperature, *New Phytol.,* **73,** 71–80.

Hayman, D.S. (1978). Endomycorrhizae, In *Interactions between Non-pathogenic Soil Microorganisms and Plants.* Eds. Y.R. Dommergues and S.V. Krupa. Elsevier, Amsterdam. pp. 401–442.

Hayman, D.S. (1982). Practical aspects of vesicular-arbuscular mycorrhiza. In *Advances in Agricultural Microbiology.* Ed. N.S. Subba Rao. Oxford and IBH Publishing Co. Pvt. Ltd., New Delhi. pp. 325–373.

Hayman, D.S., and Mosse, B. (1979). Improved growth of white clover in hill grasslands by mycorrhizal inoculation. *Ann. Appl. Biol.,* **93,** 141–148.

Ho, I., and Trappe, J.M. (1973). Translocation of ^{14}C from *Festuca* plants to their endomycorrhizal fungi. *Nature, New Biol.,* **244,** 30–31.

Howler, R.H., Asher, C.J., and Edwards, D.C. (1982). Establishment of an effective endomycorrhizal association on cassava in flowing solution culture and its effects on phosphorus nutrition. *New Phytol.,* **90,** 229–238.

Islam, R., Ayanaba, A., and Sanders, F.E. (1980). Response of cowpea (*Vigna unguiculata*) to inoculation with VA mycorrhizal fungi and to rock phosphate fertilization in some unsterilized Nigerian soils. *Plant and Soil.,* **54,** 107–117.

Khan, A.G. (1972). Occurrence of Endogone spores in West Pakistan soils. *Trans. Brit. Mycol. Soc.,* **56,** 217–224.

Khan, A.G. (1975). The effect of vesicular arbuscular mycorrhizal associations on growth of cereals. II. Effects on wheat growth. *Ann. Appl. Biol.,* **80,** 27–36.

Kleinschmidt, G.D., and Gerdemann, J.W. (1972). Stunting of citrus seedlings in fumigated nursery soils related to the absence of endomycorrhizae. *Phytopathology,* **62,** 1447–1453.

La Rue, J.H., McClellan, W.D., and Peacock, W.L. (1975). Mycorrhizal fungi and peach nursery nutrition. *Calif. Agric.,* **29,** 6–7.

Levy, Y., and Krikun, J. (1980). Effect of vesicular arbuscular mycorrhiza on *Citrus jambhiri* water relations. *New Phytol.,* **85,** 25–31.

Marks, C.G., and Kozlowski, T.T. (Eds). (1973). *Ectomycorrhizae—Their Ecology and Physiology,* Academic Press, New York.

Marx, D.H. (1969). The influence of ectotrophic mycorrhizal fungi on the resistance of pine roots to pathogenic infections. I Antagonism of mycorrhizal fungi to root pathogenic fungi and soil bacteria *Phytopathology,* **59,** 153–163.

Marx, D.H. (1972). Ectomycorrhizae as biological deterrents to pathogenic root infections. *Annv. Rev. Phytopath.,* **10,** 429–454.

Marx, D.H. (1981). Ectomycorrhizal fungus inoculations: A tool for improving forestation practices, In *Tropical Mycorrhiza Research.* Ed. P. Mikola. Oxford Univ. Press, Oxford. pp. 13–71.

Mikola, P. (Ed.) (1981). *Tropical Mycorrhiza Research.* Oxford University Press, Oxford.

Miller-Wideman, M..A., and Watrude, L.S. (1984). Sporulation of *Glomus mosseae* in root cultures of tomato. *Can. J. Microbiol.,* **30,** 642–646.

Molina, R., and Trappe, J.M. (1982). Applied aspects of ectomycorrhizae, In *Advances in Agricultural Microbiology.* Ed. N.S. Subba Rao. Oxford and IBH Publishing Co. Pvt. Ltd., New Delhi. pp. 305–324.

Mosse, B. (1973). Advances in the study of vesicular arbuscular mycorrhiza, *Ann. Rev. Phytopathol.,* **11,** 171–196.

Mosse, B., and Hepper, C. (1975). Vesicular arbuscular mycorrhizal infections in root organ culture. *Physiol. Plant Pathol.,* **5,** 215–223.

Mosse, B., and Thompson, J.P. (1984). Vesicular arbuscular endomycorrhizal inoculum production. I. Exploratory experiments with beans (*Phaseolus vulgaris*) in nutrient flow culture. *Can. J. Bot.,* **62,** 1523–1530.

Mosse, B., and Tinker, P.B. Ed. (1975). *Endomycorrhizas,* Academic Press, London.

Owusu Bennoah, E., and Mosse, B. (1979). Plant growth responses to vesicular arbuscular mycorrhiza. XI. Field inoculation responses in barley lucerne and onion. *New Phytol.,* **83,** 671–679.

Powell, C. Li. (1977). Mycorrhizas in hill country soils. III. Effect of inoculation on clover growth in unsterile soils, *N.Z.J. Agric. Res.,* **20,** 343–348.

Powell, C. Li. (1979). Inoculation of white clover and rye grass seed with mycorrhizal fungi., *New Phytol.,* **83,** 81–85.

Powell, C. Li., and Bagyaraj, D.J. Eds. (1984). VA Mycorrhiza CRC Press, Florida, USA.

Saif, S.R., and Khan, A.G. (1977). The effect of vesicular arbuscular mycorrhizal associations on growth of cereals. III. Effects of barley growth. *Plant and Soil,* **47,** 17–26.

Schenck, N.C., and Hinson, K. (1973). Response of nodulating and non-nodulating soybeans to a species of *Endogone mycorrhiza. Agron. J.,* **65,** 849–850.

Schonbeck, F. (1979). Endomycorrhiza in relation to plant diseases, In *Soil-borne Plant Pathogens.* Eds. B. Schippers and W. Grams. Academic Press, New York. pp. 271–280.

Swaminathan, K., and Verma, B.C. (1979). Responses of three crop species to vesicular arbuscular mycorrhizal infection on zinc deficient Indian soils. *New Phytol.,* **82,** 481–487.

Sylvia, D.M., and Hubbell, D.H. (1986). Growth and sporulation of vesicular arbuscular mycorrhizal fungi in aeroponic and membrane systems. *Symbiosis,* **1,** 259–267.

Theodorou, C. (1967). Inoculation with pure cultures of mycorrhizal fungi of radiata pine growing in partially sterilized soil. *Austral. Forestry,* **31,** 303–309.

Theodorou, C. (1971). Introduction of mycorrhizal fungi into soil by spore inoculation of seed. *Austral. Forestry,* **35,** 17–22.

Theodorou, C., and Bowen, G.D. (1970). Mycorrhizal responses to radiata pine in experiments with different fungi. *Austral. Forestry,* **34,** 183–191.

Theodorou, C., and Bowen, G.D. (1973). Inoculation of seeds and soil with basidiospores of mycorrhizal fungi. *Soil Biol. Biochem.,* **5,** 765–771.

Trappe, J.M. (1962). Fungus associates of ectotrophic mycorrhizae, *Bot. Rev.,* **28,** 538–606.

Trapper, J.M. (1969). Studies on *Cenococcum graniforme.* I. An efficient method for isolation from Sclerotia. *Can. J. Bot.,* **47,** 1389–1390.

10

Organic Matter and Composting

Dead and decaying parts of plants and animals contribute to the primary sources of organic matter in soil. In order of abundance, the insoluble chemical constituents of organic matter are celluloses and lignin while the soluble constituents are composed of sugars, amino acids, and organic acids. Other constituents are fats, oils, waxes, resins, pigments, proteins, and minerals.

Soil microorganisms thrive on the above-mentioned ingredients of organic matter in soil by feeding readily on soluble resources and rather slowly on insoluble forms. Essentially, the carbon content of the protoplasm of microorganisms is derived from organic substrates by a process known as 'assimilation'. Not all the carbon in the organic matter is assimilated into the microbial protoplasm but depending on the nature of the microflora and the oxygen status of soil, the element is also released as carbon dioxide. For instance, fungi release less CO_2 and incorporate more carbon in their tissues, whereas in certain aerobic bacteria, the reverse is true. Under anaerobic conditions, due to incomplete degradation of organic matter, methane (CH_4) and hydrogen (H_2) are evolved. In waterlogged situations, in addition to several intermediate organic acids, CH_4, H_2, and CO_2 are generated due to microbial activity. The dominant organic acids generated are acetic, formic, and butyric acids but lactic and succinic acids are also known to appear in lesser quantities. The magnitude of CO_2 formation is often taken as an index of organic matter decomposition. Because of the biochemical diversity of organic matter, other parameters are also used to measure organic matter decomposition — O_2 uptake, loss of weight, and quantitative measurement of the disappearance of an added known substrate. In the process of carbon assimilation, other nutrients such as N, P, K, and S are also taken up by the microbial cell and the entire process is often termed 'immobilization', which results in the reduction of readily available nutrients in soil for absorption by plants.

In the literature on organic matter, the term 'mineralization' is often used to denote the conversion of organic complexes of an element to its inorganic state. The process is opposite in magnitude to immobilization and results in the accumulation of ammonium and nitrates. When fresh plant residues reach soil immobilization is not fast but mineralization gradually increases depending upon temperature, oxygen supply, water content, hydrogen ion concentration, inorganic nutrients, C/N ratio of the organic matter, and the nature of microflora, among which the nitrogen content of residues or the initial C/N ratio of the organic matter is an important factor. Leguminous plant residues which have high nitrogen encourage the growth of microorganisms by supplying readily available nitrogen and hence accelerate decomposition. Similarly, addition of ammonium or nitrate to nitrogen-deficient cereal straw residues serves a similar purpose to accelerate microbial activity and hence accelerate substrate decomposition.

Residues of younger plants with more soluble nutrient materials are more easily metabolized than branches of older trees with relatively higher woody tissues containing lignin. On the contrary, cellulose being easily susceptible to microbial attack, most of its constituents are easily metabolized by microorganisms. Filamentous fungi degrade cellulose in acidic soils while in neutral and alkaline pH levels, a variety of microorganisms act on cellulose. Examples of celluloytic microorganisms are *Chaetomium* and *Trichoderma* (fungi), *Cellulomonas* and *Clostridium* (bacteria), and *Nocardia* and *Streptomyces* (actinomycetes). Cellulose has a number of glucose molecules in a linear chain held together by B-linkages at carbon atoms 1 and 4 of the glucose units. The first step is the enzymatic hydrolysis of the cellulose polymer by cellulase complex which converts the polymer into the glucose monomer. The cellulase complex consists of three types of enzymes — C_1, C_x, and B-glucosidase. The second step involves metabolization of simple sugars to CO_2 (aerobic) or organic acids and alcohols followed by CH_4 and CO_2 (anaerobic) with a simultaneous incorporation of carbon into the microbial protoplasm (Allison, 1973; Alexander, 1977).

Humus, an organic fraction of soil, is a product of microbial activity in soil through successive immobilization and mineralization processes. In this way, the original plant residues repeatedly undergo changes and constitute the organic fractions of soil. Humus is in a dynamic state and contains amino acids, purines, pyrimidines, aromatic substances, uronic acids, amino sugars, pentoses, hexoses, sugar alcohols, methyl sugar, and aliphatic acids. Barring amino acids and aliphatic acids, which are soluble, the remaining nutrients of the humus are in a bound form and can be brought into solution by alkali. The age of humus can vary from 1000 to 2860 years, based on radiocarbon dating techniques. The three major fractions of humus are fulvic acid, humin, and humic acid, of which humic acids are regarded as the oldest and most persistent. Some fungi such as *Penicillium* and *Aspergillus* and also a few actinomycetes produce dark humus-like substances (amino acids, peptides, and polyphenols) which serve as structural bases for humic substance formation (Flaig, 1966; Hughes and Rose, 1971; Gray and Williams, 1971).

Isolation of Microorganisms

The different groups of microorganisms such as fungi, bacteria, and actinomycetes which possess the ability to degrade cellulose can be isolated by an enrichment technique using appropriate media (see Appendix). Aliquots of 100 ml media for each group of microorganisms are distributed in several 250 ml conical flasks plugged with cotton and autoclaved at 121°C for 20 minutes. They are inoculated with dilutions of soil or other appropriate samples such as excreta of animals, paper mill effluents, or compost materials. Sterile filter paper strips are hung from cotton plugs in such a way that a portion of the filter paper is immersed in the liquid medium (broth) in the flask. At the end of 1 week incubation (28°C ± 2°C), the filter paper and 10 ml broth are transferred into freshly prepared and autoclaved broth. After repeated (about five) transfers, the medium will be sufficiently enriched for plating on standard media (see Appendix) using appropriate dilutions.

Individual colonies of fungi, bacteria, and actinomycetes are picked up and transferred to test tubes. They are further purified by streaking on respective media and identified.

Screening Isolates for Cellulase Production

Three types of media—Czapek, asparagine, and Mandel and Reese media (see Appendix)—with cellulose as the sole source of carbon can be used for determining the extent of cellulase production by fungi. For bacteria and actinomycetes other media listed in the Appendix may be used with cellulose as the sole source of carbon.

Aliquots of 100 ml of each medium are distributed in 250 ml flasks, autoclaved at 121°C for 20 minutes, and inoculated with selected microorganisms. The flasks are transferred to rotary shakers (180 rpm) and incubated at 30° ± 1°C.

After incubation for known periods, samples of 20 ml are removed aseptically. The unused cellulase and mycelium are separated by centrifuging the sample at 10,000 rpm for 20 minutes at room temperature. To the clear light yellow supernatant, 1 per cent methiolate (1 ml per 100 ml of extract) is added and this could be stored in a refrigerator without appreciable loss of enzyme activity. This extracellular supernatant fluid is used as a crude enzyme extract for determining cellulase activity.

The procedure for determining cellulase activity (Reese and Mandel, 1963) consists of estimating the reducing sugars formed by the action of cellulases on carboxy methyl cellulose. The assay mixture consists of 2.0 ml of the enzyme solution in 18 ml of 1 per cent carboxy methyl cellulose in McIlvaine's citrate phosphate buffer (pH 6.0). After the reaction mixture is incubated at 40°C for 60 minutes, the reducing sugars (as glucose) are determined using the method outlined by Nelson (1944). The following reagents and standard solution of glucose are prepared:

1. Copper reagent A

Na_2CO_3 (anhydrous)	25 g
Na-K-tartarate	25 g
$NaHCO_3$	20 g
Na_2SO_4 (anhydrous)	200 g
Distilled water (final volume)	1000 ml

2. Copper reagent B

Fifteen grams of copper sulphate ($CuSO_4 \cdot 5H_2O$) is dissolved in 100 ml distilled water and acidified with one or two drops of concentrated sulphuric acid.

3. Arsenomolybdate

Twenty-five grams of ammonium molybdate [$(NH_4)_2 MoO_4 4H_2O$] is dissolved in 450 ml of distilled water and 21 ml of concentrated sulphuric acid is added. Three grams of sodium arsenate ($Na_2 HASO_4 \cdot 7H_2O$) is dissolved in 25 ml of distilled water. The solutions are mixed and placed in an incubator at 37°C for 48 hours.

4. Standard solution of glucose

One gram of Analar anhydrous glucose is dissolved in 100 ml of 0.2 per cent benzoic acid in a volumetric flask. This stock solution gives 10 mg glucose per ml. Aliquots of 0.25, 0.50, 0.75, 1.00, 1.25, and 1.50 ml of the above stock solution are transferred into 100 ml volumetric flasks separately and the volume made up to 100 ml with 0.2 per cent benzoic acid. They give corresponding value of 25, 50, 75, 100, 125, and 150 μg of glucose per ml respectively.

To 1.0 ml aliquots of each concentration of glucose, 2 ml alkaline copper reagent mixture (25 ml of copper reagent A + 1 ml of copper reagent B mixed just before use) is added. The solutions are mixed and boiled for 20 minutes on a water bath. The tubes are cooled and 2 ml of the arsenomolybdate reagent is added to each tube. Upon shaking, the mixture gives blue colour with effervescence. The mixture is then diluted to 25 ml with distilled water and the resulting blue colour is read at 540 mμ in a colorimeter. A standard curve is prepared by plotting optical density on the X-axis and the concentration of glucose on the Y-axis. By extrapolation, the reducing sugar content of experimental samples could be calculated with the aid of the standard curve which is an indication of cellulase activity.

Measurement of Carbon Dioxide Evolution in Soil

The amount of CO_2 evolved by a given sample of soil gives an approximate indication of microbial activities (Gaur et al., 1971). Conical flasks of 1000 ml capacity are filled with 100 g soil and adjusted to 33 per cent of their water-holding capacity. A test tube containing 10 ml of N/10 NaOH solution is hung in each flask with the help of a thread as shown in (Fig. 19). The flasks are closed with rubber stoppers and sealed with molten wax and incubated at 30°C ($\pm$ 1°C). The CO_2 evolved is absorbed by the alkali in the test tube and measured titrimetrically at desired intervals. In the initial stages diurnal measurements of CO_2 evolution are taken, followed by estimation at weekly intervals. After each estimation, the alkali in the test tube is replaced with a fresh aliquot, the rubber stopper replaced and sealed with molten wax.

During each estimation, the contents of the test tube are quantitatively transferred to a flask followed by the addition of 5 ml of saturated solution of $BaCl_2$ to precipitate as $BaCO_3$. The residual amount of NaOH in the flask is measured by titrating against N/10

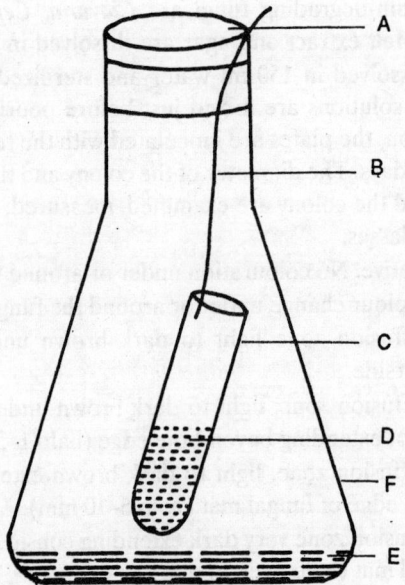

Fig. 19. A method for measuring CO_2 evolution by soil samples — A. rubber stopper; B. thread; C. test tube; D. N/10 NaOH; E. soil; F. flask.

HCl using 2–3 drops of phenolphthalein as the indicator. The reactions involved are as follows:

$$2NaOH + CO_2 \rightarrow Na_2CO_3 + H_2O$$
$$Na_2CO_3 + BaCl_2 \rightarrow BaCO_3 + 2NaCl$$

The calculations are done as follows: 1 ml of N/10 HCl = 1 ml of N/10 NaOH + 2.2 mg of CO_2. If the original volume in the flask is 10 ml and the unutilized NaOH is 5 ml, the utilized NaOH would be 5 ml; the amount of CO_2 evolved is $5 \times 2.2 = 11$ mg CO_2. The carbon mineralized is 3 mg.

Measurement of Lignin Degradation

According to Bavendamm (1927), lignin and tannic acid are closely related substances and therefore the evidence for tannic acid degradation could be taken for lignin degradation. Tannic acid degradation is shown by the formation of a brown zone around the fungal colony due to the decomposition products of tannic acid.

A medium containing 1.5 per cent malt extract, 0.5 per cent tannic acid, and 2 per cent agar is used for primary screening of fungi.

Examples of lignin-degrading fungi are *Clavaria, Cephalosporium,* and *Humicola.* Malt extract and agar are dissolved in 850 ml water; tannic acid is dissolved in 150 ml water and sterilized at 121°C for 15 minutes. The solutions are mixed just before pouring the plates. After solidification, the plates are inoculated with the test fungus and incubated for six days. The diameter of the colony and the brown zone developed around the colony are examined, measured, and classified under different classes:

Class 0. Negative. No colouration under or around the inoculum.

Class I. No colour change under or around the fungal mat.

Class II. Diffusion zone light to dark brown under inoculum visible from underside.

Class III. Diffusion zone, light to dark brown under most of the fungal mat, but not extending beyond the edge (halo 1–5 mm).

Class IV. Diffusion zone, light to dark brown extending a short distance from the edge of fungal mat (halo 6–10 mm).

Class V. Diffusion zone very dark extending considerably beyond the edge of fungal mat (halo over 10 mm).

The ability of an organism to utilize lignin as a source of carbon can be tested by growing the organism on a solid medium containing lignin as a sole source of carbon (Day *et al.,* 1949). The composition of the lignin medium is outlined in the Appendix. The diameter of the colony in millimetres after 6 days on solid medium and dry weight of mycelium in milligrams in liquid medium after every week are taken as parameters. The residual lignin is quantitatively measured colorimetrically using tyrosine reagent (Berk and Schroeder, 1942).

The following reagents and standard solution are prepared:

1) Tyrosine reagent (Lignin reagent)

Sodium tungstate ($Na_2WO_42H_2O$)	100 g
Phosphomolybdic acid	20 g
Orthophosphoric acid (H_3PO_4), 85%	50 ml

The solution is refluxed for 2 hours, cooled, and diluted to 1000 ml with distilled water.

2) Saturated sodium carbonate solution.

Two hundred grams of Na_2CO_3 are dissolved in 500 ml of warm distilled water and made up to one litre. One gram of lignin is dissolved in 1000 ml of distilled water to give a standard solution of 1000 μg of lignin per ml. Aliquots of 10, 20, 30, 40, 50, 60, 70, 80, and 90 ml are pipetted into 100 ml volumetric flasks and the volume is made up to 100 ml to give 100, 200, 300, 400, 500, 600, 700, 800, and 900 μg of lignin per ml, respectively.

One ml of a standard solution is taken in a test tube. To this 2 ml of lignin reagent is added and mixed well. After 5 minutes, 10 ml of concentrated sodium carbonate is added, mixed well, and allowed to develop the colour. When blue colour develops the optical density is measured at 700 mμ in a colorimeter and a standard curve is prepared by plotting optical density on the X-axis and the concentration of lignin on the Y-axis. By extrapolation, the lignin content of experimental samples could be calculated with the aid of the standard curve.

Organic Matter and Biological Nitrogen Fixation

It has been shown that the application of specific calcium and sodium humate increases the number of nodules, nodule weight, and yield of pea (*Pisum sativum*), berseem (*Trifolium alexandrinum*), and dhaincha (*Sesbania aculeata*) (Bhardwaj and Gaur, 1968; Gaur *et al.*, 1968; Gaur and Bhardwaj, 1971). It has also been demonstrated that when soybean seeds are pelleted with calcium humate and grown in a saline and alkaline soil the number of nodules and dry weight yield increase (Iswaran and Chhonkar, 1971). In general, addition of farmyard manure improves the root nodulation status of leguminous plants and the number of *Azotobacter* cells in soil (Reports of ICAR coordinated research project on organic matter decomposition).

Composting in India

Quite a good deal of work on practical composting has been done by many earlier workers in India who describe the advantages or disadvantages of the different composting processes practised in rural India (Fowler, 1930; Howard, 1935; Acharya, 1939, 1949). The native method of preparing farmyard manure by composting on the farm is often crude and unscientific. The two recommended methods are the 'Indore method' (aerobic) and the 'Bangalore method' (initially aerobic but later anaerobic).

In the Indore method, a pit (3 feet deep and 6–8 feet wide) is dug near a cattle shed on a site free from waterlogging. Plant residues are cut into shreds and used as beds for cattle in sheds. After use, the wet beds along with excreta are removed and heaped in a layer (3–5 m) in the pit. Over this layer, sufficient quantity of cattle dung is spread. Water is sprinkled to maintain optimum moisture and the process of layering and spreading cowdung is repeated so that layers are formed one above the other till the residues reach one foot above the ground level. To avoid rains soaking the pit, a protective shed may be erected over the pit. The residues are turned every fortnight, and a good quality compost is ready in 16 weeks.

In the Bangalore method, greater conservation of nutrients is attempted by an anaerobic process. The heaps are prepared as outlined in the Indore process, except that each heap in a pit is sealed with plaster of mud, which increases the temperature inside the plastered pit due to anaerobic fermentation. By this process, a nitrogen-rich compost is formed in 32 weeks (ICAR, 1964).

Composting in China

In field sites, aquatic weeds or green manure crops (0.75 t), rice straw (0.15 t), animal dung or pig excreta (1.0 t), and silt (7.50 t) are used in composting in circular or rectangular pits dug in a corner of a field. The pits are filled in layers with chopped or shredded crop residues, each layer being 15 cm thick. The upper layer is plastered with mud and covered with a water column 3–4 cm deep (FAO, 1977), creating anaerobic conditions and thus reducing nitrogen losses. In a month's time the material is turned over and superphosphate (0.020 t) is added. This is followed by two subsequent turnings and the manure (8 t) is ready in 12 weeks with a C/N ratio of 15 to 20 and organic matter content of 7.8–10.3 per cent.

In certain locations, mechanically ground mud mixed with pig excreta (1:1) or ash mixed with 40 per cent night soil or pig excreta is stored in a shed until use.

In other locations, liquid manure containing pig droppings and washings from the sty are kept in a cement pit to which weeds and aquatic plants are also added. Alternatively, night soil and urine are kept in closed tanks and allowed to ferment for 2–3 weeks. The resulting liquid manures are used as top dressing.

In a process called 'high temperature compost' crop wastes (4 parts) and a mixture of human as well as animal excreta (1 part) are alternately piled up in a heap. Keeping the moisture level at an optimum level, a number of hollow bamboo poles are driven into the heap and the heap sealed with mud. The bamboo poles are immediately removed. After about 2 days, when the temperature reaches 60°–70°C, the holes are sealed with mud. At the end of 2 weeks, the mud plaster is broken and the heap is turned by adding fresh liquid excreta followed by resealing with mud plaster. At the end of 8 weeks, a high quality compost is produced.

In some places, dry soil is spread periodically on the floor of stables to absorb liquid excreta. After several months, a type of compost called 'earth compost' is formed which can be used for crop cultivation.

In other places, city garbage (70–80 per cent) and night soil (20–30 per cent) are mixed in heaps and bamboo poles are placed horizontally at regular intervals which are also connected to a vertically placed bamboo pole in the centre which ensures all-round aeration. The heap is sealed and bamboo poles are taken out leaving holes for aeration. Within 2 days, the temperature of the heap attains 50°–55°C which destroys the pathogens during subsequent days. This type of compost is ready in 3–4 months.

Acceleration of Composting by Adding Microorganisms

Composting involves microbiological processes which go on naturally with the help of native cellulolytic microorganisms in compost pits. A question has often been asked whether addition of laboratory-grown cultures of cellulolytic microorganisms enhances the rate of microbiological processes in composting. The results of a study undertaken at IARI (Yadav, 1977) using efficient cellulolytic microorganisms such as *Trichoderma viride*, *Chaetomium abuanse*, *Myrothecium roridum*, *Aspergillus niger*, *A. terreus*, *Cellulomonas* sp., and *Cytophaga* sp. are shown in Table 39. The initial C/N ratio of the material mixture of wheat straw and jamun (*Eugenia jambolina*) leaves was 75. After 4 months of incubation the C/N ratio in the control series (without inoculum) was lowered to 47 while the C/N ratio of *Cellulomonas* treatments were 16 to 18 depending on the isolates. When *T. viride* was used, the resulting C/N ratio of the compost was 17 and 18. The loss of weight (Plate 6) and humic acid content was also highest with *Cellulomonas* and *T. viride*. A pot culture experiment with wheat and mung crops using the compost prepared with isolates of *Cellulomonas* and *T. viride* proved to be of good quality. These results and other experiments in compost pits (Table 40) show that addition of selected cellulose decomposers accelerate the microbiological activities in composting resulting in the alteration in C/N ratio, weight, and humic acid contents to the beneficial side.

Table 39: Evaluation of efficient cellulolytic isolates in composting (mean of three replications)

Treatment	Strain number	Organic carbon %	Total nitrogen %	C/N ratio	Moisture %	Humic acid %	Loss of weight %
Analyses in the beginning		53.08	0.700	75.83	45.00		
Analyses after 4 months:							
Control (uninoculated)	CONT	49.11	1.050	46.83	55.00	4.00	35.71
Cellulomonas	CAB 3	37.82	2.400	15.76	60.00	9.50	69.57
Cellulomonas	GB 3	40.97	2.317	17.69	58.80	8.60	63.29
Cellulomonas	BHB 1	40.54	2.325	17.44	59.20	8.40	65.00
Cytophaga	BHB 2	48.25	1.485	32.47	58.93	6.60	50.00
Trichoderma viride	BF 8	38.21	2.217	17.69	58.60	8.30	62.86
T. viride	BHF 5	38.82	2.250	17.03	57.00	7.90	66.71
Chaetomium	BHF 3	48.84	1.433	34.09	57.00	8.10	51.14
C. abianse	COF 4	47.62	1.250	38.09	56.00	7.50	47.71
Myrothecium roridum	BHF 4	47.17	1.130	41.74	55.07	6.30	41.43
Aspergillus niger	GF 5	48.83	1.255	38.51	57.20	7.30	45.71
A. terreus	BF 2	48.04	1.257	45.47	56.40	6.40	42.86
Mixture of bacteria	MB	40.31	1.933	20.86	56.60	7.30	57.71
Mixture of fungi	MF	39.52	1.742	22.63	56.20	7.60	56.29
Mixture of bacteria + fungi	MBF	41.78	1.642	25.10	55.80	6.90	53.43

Source: Yadav, 1977.

Table 40: Effect of inoculation by cellulolytic fungi on composting in pits

Treatment	Sampling intervals in months								
	1			2			3		
	C%	N%	C/N	C%	N%	C/N	C%	N%	C/N
Control	35.9	1.14	31.4	30.9	1.33	22.4	28.2	1.41	20.0
Aspergillus sp. (IF$_1$)	29.8	1.26	23.6	27.6	1.09	25.3	27.6	1.63	16.8
Aspergillus sp. (IF$_1$)	32.4	1.40	23.1	28.7	1.47	19.5	25.2	1.33	18.9
Aspergillus sp. (RF$_2$)	33.7	1.68	20.6	25.2	1.49	16.9	23.6	1.65	14.3
Penicillium sp. (RF$_2$)	25.9	1.33	19.6	24.8	1.47	16.8	23.9	1.61	14.8

Source: Dr. A.C. Gaur, personal communication.

Initial C/N ratio 45.7.

Weight of raw materials = 32 kg/pit.

Anaerobic Fermentation of Human, Animal, and Agricultural Wastes

In rural areas, crop residues and animal wastes can be collected and used for the generation of methane as fuel. This practice has recently been promoted vigorously in India, China, Taiwan, Korea, Uganda, and Bangladesh. It has the twin advantages of minimizing pollution and using the residual slurry as fertilizer. Experiments in designing a simple cowdung gas plant were initiated at the Indian Agricultural Research Institute in 1939 and since then research on all aspects of biogas technology has been continuously carried out. Similar work has been started by the Khadi and Village Industries Commission of India. Cattle dung is a good medium for anaerobic fermentation in specially designed and inexpensively fabricated gobar gas plants. On a small farm, individual small plants can provide enough gas for cooking and leave residues as fertilizer for crops. The composition of the gas is approximately 55–60 per cent CH_4, 5–10 per cent H_2, and 30–35 per cent CO_2 (Acharya, 1961; Idnani and Varadarajan, 1974).

Other organic matter with potential for methane production are crop wastes (sugarcane residues and crop stubbles), animal wastes (dung, urine, poultry droppings, goat droppings, slaughterhouse wastes, fish wastes, tannery wastes, and wool industry residues), human refuse, agro-industry by-products (oil cakes, bagasse, rice bran, wastes from tobacco and vegetables, pressmud from sugar factories, tea and cotton wastes), and wastes of forest and marine origin. The starter microorganisms for anaerobic organic matter fermentation are provided by adding cowdung slurry to the bulk of chopped or shredded residues.

Under anaerobic conditions, organic matter is decomposed by primary as well as secondary microorganisms. The primary colonizers initially convert the complex carbohydrates and proteins into simple carbon sources. The genus *Clostridium* predominant in anaerobic surroundings degrades cellulose to organic acids (acetic, formic, lactic, succinic, and butyric acids) and alcohols. Methane bacteria such as *Methanococcus, Methanosarcina, Methanobacillus,* and *Methanobacterium* which are secondary colonizers break down organic acids into CH_4 and CO_2. Experiments have been carried out to trace the pathway of methane production by using single as well as mixed cultures of methane bacteria which have served to depict the following typical reactions: (1) $CO_2 + 4H_2 \rightarrow CH_4 + 2H_2O$;

(2) $4HCOOH \rightarrow CH_4 + 3CO_2 + 2H_2O$; (3) $CH_3COOH \rightarrow CH_4 + CO_2$; and (4) $2CH_2CH_2OH \rightarrow 3CH_4 + CO_2$ (Barker, 1956; Wolfe, 1971; Alexander, 1977).

REFERENCES

Acharya, C.N. (1939). Comparison of different methods of composting waste materials. *Ind. J. Agric. Sci.,* 9, 817–833.

Acharya, C.N. (1949). Preparation of compost manure from town wastes. Misc. Bull. Imp. Coun. Agric. Res., 60, 3rd Edition.

Acharya, C.N. (1961). Preparation of fuel gas and manure by anaerobic fermentation of organic material, ICAR Tech. Bull. Series No. 15. Krishi Bhavan, New Delhi.

Alexander, M. (1977). *Introduction to Soil Microbiology,* 2nd Ed. John Wiley and Sons, New York.

Alison, F.E. (1973). *Soil Organic Matter and Its Role in Crop Production.* Elsevier, Amsterdam, London and New York.

Barker, H.A. (1956). *Bacterial Fermentations.* John Wiley and Sons, New York.

Bavendamm, M. (1927). Neve Untersuchungen Uber die Lebensbedingingungen Holzzerstorender pilze Ein Beitrag zur Immunitalsfrage. *Ber. Deut. Bot. Ges.,* 45, 357–367.

Berk, A.A., and Schroeder, W.C. (1942). Determination of tannin substances in boilers water. *Ind. Eng. Chem.,* 14, 456–459.

Bhardwaj, K.K.R., and Gaur, A.C. (1968). Humic acid in relation to bacterial inoculation of crops. *Agrochimica,* 12, 100.

Day, W.C., Pelczar, H.J. Jr., and Gottlieb, S. (1949). The biological degradation of lignin, I. *Arch. Biochem.,* 23, 360–369.

FAO (1977). China: Recycling of Organic Wastes in Agriculture. *Soils Bull.* 40. FAO, Rome.

Flaig, W. (1966). *The Use of Isotopes in Soil Organic Matter Studies.* Pergamon Press, New York.

Fowler, G.J. (1930). Recent experiments on the preparation of organic manure: A review. *Agric. Livestock Indian,* 7, 711–717.

Gaur, A.C., and Bhardwaj, K.K.R. (1971). Influence of sodium humate on the crop plants inoculated with bacteria of agricultural importance. *Plant and Soil,* 35, 613–621.

Gaur, A.C., Mathur, R.S., and Bhardwaj, K.K.R. (1968). Some aspects of influence of humic substances on soil microflora. *Proc. Natl. Acad. Sci. India,* 38(a), 25.

Gaur, A.C., Sadasivam, K.V., Vimal, O.P., and Mathur, R.S. (1971). A study of decomposition of organic matter in an alluvial soil: CO_2 evolution, microbiological and chemical transformations. *Plant and Soil,* 34, 17–28.

Gray, T.R.G., and Williams, S.T. (1971). Microbial productivity in soil. In *Microbes and Biological Productivity.* Eds. D.E. Hughes and A.H. Rose. Cambridge University Press, London. pp. 255–286.

Howard, A. (1935). The waste products in agriculture. *J. R. Soc. Arts,* 84, 120.

Hughes, D.E., and Rose, A.H. (Eds.) (1971). *Microbes and Biological Productivity.* Cambridge University Press, London.

ICAR (1964). *Handbook of Manures and Fertilizers.* ICAR, New Delhi.

Idnani, M.A., and Varadarajan, S. (1974). Preparation of Fuel Gas and Manure by Anaerobic Fermentation of Organic Material, ICAR Tech. Bull. (Agric.) No. 46, Krishi Bhavan, New Delhi..

Iswaran, V., and Chhonkar, P.K. (1971). Action of sodium humate on nodulation and dry matter accumulation by soybean in saline and alkaline soils. *Trans. Intl. Symp. Humus et Planta V*, pp. 613–615.

Nelson, N. (1944). A photometric adaptation of the Somogyi method for determination of glucose. *J. Biol. Chem.*, 153, 375–380.

Reese, E.T., and Mandel, (1963). Enzymatic hydrolysis of cellulose and its derivatives. *Meth. Carbon Chem.*, 4, 139–142.

Wolfe, R.S. (1971). Microbial fermentation of methane. *Adv. Microb. Physiol.*, 6, 107–146.

Yadav, K.S. (1977). Studies on cellulolytic and lignolytic microorganisms. Ph.D. thesis, IARI, New Delhi.

11

Inoculants for Nodulated Leguminous Trees

The family Leguminosae is ubiquitous in distribution with an estimated 18,000–19,000 species in about 750 genera from the three subfamilies Mimosoideae, Caesalpinioideae, and Papilionoideae. Of these species only about 16 per cent have been examined for nodulation and of those which were examined nearly 95 per cent of Mimosoideae, 28 per cent of Caesalpinioideae and 90 per cent of Papilionoideae possess root nodules (Allen and Allen, 1981). Even though woody and tree species are represented in all the three subfamilies, the bulk of the tree species come from Caesalpinioideae and Mimosoideae barring about 1000 tree species which come from Papilionoideae. Sprent and associates in Scotland and Brazil have been carrying out extensive studies on nodulation of woody species (Faria *et al.*, 1984, 1985, 1986, 1987a, 1987b; Sprent, 1985; Sprent and Raven, 1985; Sprent *et al.*, 1987). They have updated our knowledge on nodulation in legumes (Table 41). According of Faria *et al.*, (1989), 57 per cent of the legume genera, comprising 3395 species (20 per cent of Leguminosae), have been examined for nodulation. Of the examined species, only 23 per cent have been found to possess nodules in Caesalpinioideae. In these studies, some earlier findings have been confirmed, others disputed, and many additions made. From these studies on root nodulation of woody leguminous species from South-east Brazil, Sprent and associates have added 56 new nodulated species to Papilionoideae, 40 to Mimosoideae, and 12 to Caesalpinioideae. These authors emphasize that the parameters intended for studies on annual legumes do not necessarily hold good for woody species. First, there is the problem of recognition of nodules in woody species which are often black, irregular in shape, and sometimes resembling calluses or tumours. Second, nodules of tree legumes have a great variety of structure and shape arising out of determinate or indeterminate type of growth and these character-istics are of taxonomic importance. The general mode of infection of roots appears to be through root epidermis or wherever there is a potential for the emergence of lateral roots. Nodules may therefore be formed even on older roots. Persistent infection threads were observed in several species of trees of the subfamily Caesalpinioideae and some species of Papilionoideae, but none from Mimosoideae. In these cases, infection spreads in the developing nodule by movement of rhizobia intercellularly rather than by infection threads. Faria *et al.* (1986) believe that infection threads may have evolved in infected cells 'in primitive tree species and later extended to early stages of the infaction process including entry into root hairs'.

Table 41: Summary of nodulation status in Leguminosae as revised by Sprent and associates in Edinburgh

Subfamily	Known no. of species	No. of species examined for nodulation	No. of species found to be nodulated
Papilionoideae	13,000	2730 (21)	2648 (97)
Mimosoideae	2713	454 (17)	408 (90)
Caesalpinioideae	1900	323 (17)	74 (23)

The figures in parentheses represent percentage of species –

The deep root system coupled with extensive lateral root formations enables tree species such as *Acacia* and *Prosopis* to tap nutrients. For instance, even though they are non-nodulating *A. albida* or *Cercidium* grow excellently in dry areas of Africa (Wickens, 1967; Sprent, 1985, 1986, 1987). Trees such as *Tamarindus indica* and *Ceratonia siliqua* grow and survive for over 100 years in spite of the fact that they remain non-nodulated. Apparently, nodulating habit is not critical for survival even in environments containing extremely low levels of nitrogen. Even in sparsely nodulating trees, it is extremely difficult to pinpoint the total biomass of nodules in a given tree species and estimate the amount of nitrogen fixed by the active nodule mass. Many studies have been done on acetylene reduction measurements of tree species to quantify the amount of nitrogen fixed by expressing the data in terms of μmol/hour/g fresh or dry weight of nodules or per plant. The results showed low values for fixation (Nakos, 1977; Monk et al., 1981; Hingston et al., 1982; Roskoski and Van Kessel, 1985). The exception was Leucaena leucocephala, which showed a fixation of 110 kg N/ha in a low rainfall area in Tanzania (Hoberg and Kvarnstrom, 1982).

Only two reports are available on the estimation of nitrogen fixed by woody species by measurements of natural abundance of ^{15}N. Prosopis sp. was found to fix 25–30 kg N/ha/yr in a ground cover in Tanzania where the root system penetrated to a depth of 4–5 m and produced nodules only near the water table (Rundel et al., 1982; Hoberg, 1986). The amount of nitrogen fixed by this species has been assessed in field plots by the ^{15}N and difference methods (Sanginga et al., 1988a, 1988b, 1988c). In six months, Rhizobium inoculation with strain IRc 1050 showed a nitrogen fixation level of 98 kg/ha, whereas with strain IRc 1045 the enhanced fixation was of the order of 134 kg/ha, which represented 34–39 per cent of plant nitrogen. Rhizobium inoculation increased nodule mass, shoot dry matter, and nitrogen content in plots receiving no fertilizers. Application of ammonium sulphate appears to depress nitrogen fixation. One of the important conclusions drawn from this experiment was that inoculation with specific and effective rhizobia increased the early growth of plants through biological nitrogen fixation.

The effects of Leucaena growth on the subsequent maize crop was investigated by Sanginga et al., (1988b) in field experiments in Nigeria. Leucaena residues served as nitrogen source and yielded about 3.5 t/ha maize when the average yield of about 40 t/ha can be obtained by the application of 100 kg N/ha of nitrogenous fertilizer in Nigeria and other African countries. Maize contained significantly more nitrogen in plots fertilized by Rhizobium-inoculated Leucaena residues than in plots receiving residues from uninoculated plants. About 300 kg N/ha could be recovered from Leucaena prunings but the utilization of residues was poor because of their low C/N ratio (hence poor mineralization) when compared to 80 kg N/ha in the form of ammonium sulphate. In plots where the prunings were removed, the leaf litter, decaying roots, and nodules contributed nitrogen equivalent of 32 kg/ha.

Indirect Measurements to Assess Nitrogen Input by Nodulated Leguminous Tree Species

Among the nodulated tree species which have so far been investigated, black locust (Robinia pseudoacacia) merits consideration. In

the United States, catalpa (*Catalpa* spp.) growing with black locust
had larger diameter and height than pure stands of catalpa grown on
the same area (Ferguson, 1922; Cope, 1929; McIntyre and Jeffries,
1932). The level of soil nitrogen appears to be improved by black
locust stands (Mattoon, 1930; Ike and Stone, 1958). In conifer stands,
mixed planting with black locust is recommended only when conifers
grow for 5–8 years so that the tree legume does not overgrow the non-
legume (Kellogg, 1936). Superior growth of *Quercus rubra, Liquidambar styraciflua, Liriodendron tulipifera* (Yellow poplar), and *Juglans
regia* (black walnut) was observed in areas previously planted with
black locust for 23 years (Carmean *et al.*, 1976). Severely eroded soils
have been relcaimed by plantings of black locust (Seidel and
Brinkman, 1962; Ashby and Baker, 1968; Brown, 1973). The merits of
black locust lie in the fact that the litter decompose rapidly and hence
improve soil structure. Vegetative propagation from root suckers
helps the plant to establish rapidly and for the same reason, it
becomes difficult to eradicate plantings once they are established.
Robinia stands have been reported to accumulate in soil as much as 44
kg/ha/yr (Ike and Stone, 1958).

In the third world countries where fertilizers are unavailable for
forest management, various nitrogen-fixing trees are being planted for
fuel, furniture, or paper pulp, or just to reclaim denuded land. There
are governmental as well as private non-profit-making cooperative
agencies devoted to this task. The following species have been commonly used for planting depending upon the situation: *Prosopis* spp.
*Acacia nilotica, Dalbergia sisso, Pongamia glabra, Pterocarpus indicus,
Leucaena leucocephala* (fixing about 500 kg N/ha/yr), *A. auriculiformis, A. mangium, Calliandra calothyrsus, Sesbania bispinosa,
Albizia* spp., and others. In mixed cropping system or as ground
cover, legumes such as *Stylasanthes, Calopogonium, Centrosema,* and
Pueraria have been used in tree plantations.

Indirect Measurements to Assess Nitrogen Input by Leguminous Herbs and Shrubs in Forest Management

Several herbaceous and shrubby legumes have been used in
temperate regions as cover crops or green manure in plantations of
tree species such as sycamore (*Platanus occidentalis*), pine (*Pinus*
spp.), Douglas fir (*Pseudotsuga meziesii*), yellow poplar (*Liriodendron
tulipifera*), hairy vetch (*Vicia villosa*), alfalfa (*Medicago sativa*), ladino
clover (*Trifolium repens* var. *latum*), arrowleaf clover (*T. vesiculosum*), red clover (*T. pratense*), crimson clover (*T. incarnatum*), white

dutch clover (*T. repens*), sub-clover (*T. subterraneum*), lespedeza (*L. cuneata* and *L. striata*), birdsfoot trefoil (*Lotus corniculatus*), lupines (*Lupinus* spp.), hairy indigo (*Indigofera pseudotinctoria*), partridge pea (*Cassia fasciculata, C. nictitans*), and others. (Stone, 1955; Pechmann and Wutz, 1960; Bengtson and Mays, 1978; Gordon *et al.*, 1979; Gordon and Wheeler, 1983).

These legumes are grown for two to three years and then ploughed back into the soil before tree planting. Interplanting as understorey and planting into an established forest plantation, known as underplanting, is also in vogue, in which case the benefit of the legume would last until canopy shading prevents sunlight from reaching the herbaceous plants. The results of some case studies may throw further light on the possible benefits of these practices.

In northern Alabama, USA, Haines *et al.*, (1978) and White (1978) did studies in which *Trifolium subterraneum, T. vesiculosum, T. incarnatum, Vicia villosa,* and *Vicia* spp. were established for six years as interplants with sycamore (*Platanus occidentalis*). Sycamore plantation without interplantings of legumes served as control. The results on the total height (m) and diameters (cm) revealed that the volume index of sycamore significantly increased from 208 to 520 in legume intercropping as against 106 in controls. Apparently the biologically fixed nitrogen and consequent improvement in the soil structure may have favoured the girth and height improvement in sycamore. The highest figure was obtained with *T. vesiculosum*. The whole leaf nitrogen concentration was 1.37 per cent in controls, whereas it reached 1.78 per cent in sycamore grown in association with *V. villosa*.

Monterey pine (*Pinus radiata*) is the main forest species of New Zealand, covering 4000 ha of new plantings and 500,000 ha of existing forest plantings. Lupins (*Lupinus* spp.) contribute over 400 kg N/ha/yr to the pine plantations (Silvester *et al.*, 1979) by way of improved soil nutritional status, which was reflected in the foliage nitrogen concentration and growth rate of the pine. In terms of basal area (sq. m/ha), the growth rate of pine was 9.71 in the absence of lupin, which was increased by lupin growth alone, by fertilizer application of 112 kg N/ha/yr as urea, and by N fertilizer plus lupin growth to the extent of 11.34, 11.92, and 13.07, respectively. The results suggest that lupin growth alone contributed to a fertilizer nitrogen equivalent of 112 kg N/ha/yr and the green manuring effect was accentuated by fertilizer application (Jackson, 1976).

Table 42: Caesalpinioid tree species known to have ectomycorrhizae and the general nodulation/rhizobial status of the genera to which the species belong, as cited by Allen and Allen (1981) and Harley and Smith (1983)

Genera (No. of species)	Habit	Habitat	No. of species examined and reported to possess nodules	No. of species examined and reported to have no nodules	Nature of Rhizobium	Species reported to possess ectomycorrhizae
Afzelia Sm, syn. Pahudia (30)	Trees	Tropical Asia, Africa	No report	2	No report	A. africana, A. quanzensis, A. bella
Aldina Endl. (12)	Trees	Venezuela, Guiana, Northern Amazon	No report	No report	No report	No mention of species
Anthonotha Beauv., syn. Macrolobium (15)	Trees	Sierra Leone, Congo basin	No report	No report	No report	A. macrophylla
Bauhinia L. (550–575)	Trees	India, Sri Lanka,	1	26	No report	No mention of species
Brachystegia Benth (70)	Trees	Africa	No report	8	No report	B. laurentii
Cassia L. (600)	Trees, shrubs, herbs	Tropical	44	55	Slow-growing cowpea Soybean lupin type	No mention of species
Eperua Aubl (14)	Trees	Tropical South America	1	3	No report	No mention of species

Gilbertiodendron J. Leonard (26)	Trees	Africa	1	No report	No report	No report	*G. dewevrei* symbiose with 5 species of ectomycorrhizae
Julbernardia Pellegr. (9–11)	Trees	Tropical West Africa	No report	No report	1	No report	*J. serretii*
Monopetalanthus Harms (8–10)	Trees	Tropical West Africa	No report	No report	No report	No report	No mention of species
Mora Schomb, ex Benth, syn. *Dimorphanda* (10)	Trees	West Indies, Tropical, Central and South America	1	No report	2	No report	*M. excelsa,* *M. gonggrijpii*
Paramacrobium J. Leonard. syn. *Macrolobium* (1)	Trees	Tropical Africa	No report	No report	No report	No report	*P. coeruleum,* *P. fragrans* syn. *M. coeruleum*
Swartzia Schreb. (130)	Trees	Tropical Mexico, West Indies, Central and South America	7	Cowpea miscellany	No report		No mention of species

Mycorrhizal Associations with Nodulated Woody Legumes

Not many nodulated or non-nodulated tree species have been observed for the occurrence of mycorrhiza. Even in those species which have been examined for mycorrhizal habit, the investigations have been rather superficial. Allen and Allen (1981) and Harley and Smith (1983) list the following tree species from Caesalpinioideae as possessing ectomycorrhizal associations: *Afgelia africana, A. quanzensis,* and *A. bella; Anthonotha macrophylla; Brachystegia laurentii; Eperua bijuga* and *E. grandiflora; Gilbertiodendron dewervei; Julbernardia serretii; Monopetalanthus* sp.; *Mora excelsa* and *M. gouggrijpii;* and *Paramaclobium coeruleum.* A brief outline of symbiotic features of even the few caesalpinioid tree species so far examined (Table 42) as mentioned by Allen and Allen (1981) reflects that our knowledge of these symbioses is scarce and worthy of the attention of future research workers. The information cited by Allen and Allen (1981) and Harley and Smith (1983) come from three Italian reports made by Fassi and Fontana (Cited by Harley and Smith, 1983). The genera *Acacia* (Mimosoideae) and *Robinia* (Papilionoideae) are two instances of trees whose species have been mentioned by Harley and Smith (1983) as ectomycorrhizal but they also cite other papilionoid shrubs (*Burtonia, Brachysema, Chlorizema, Daviesia, Dillurynia, Eutaxia, Gompholobium, Jacksonia, Mirbelia, Oxylobium, Platylobium, Pultenaea, Viminaria*) and herbs (*Hardenbergia, Kennedya, Vicia*) as examples of other legumes having ectomycorrhizae.

The results of a survey carried out recently from a semiarid region in Bangalore (Table 43) demonstrate the widespread occurrence of VAM fungi in roots of natural stands of leguminous as well as non-leguminous trees.

Rhizobia Associated with Tree Legumes

Rhizobium isolates from tree species are generally slow growing and have been assigned to the genus *Bradyrhizobium* (Barnet *et al.,* 1985). Wide variations in rhizobial specificity have been observed in isolates from tree legumes when examined by conventional cross-inoculation grouping (Basak and Goyal, 1975; Dobereiner, 1984) or by numerical taxonomy (Lieberman *et al.,* 1985). For instance, rhizobia from *Entada polyphylla, Acacia molissima,* and *Albizia lebbek* cross-inoculated with three to six other species while rhizobia from *Leucaena leucocephala, Mimosa laticifera,* and *Pithecolobium* sp. cross-inoculated with one other species. On the contrary, rhizobia from *Mimosa scabrella*, *Adenanthera perigrina*, and *Prosopis juliflora*, which are important woody species, exhibited no cross-inoculation features (Dobereiner, 1984). Even though these studies are by no means exhaustive or conclusive, the message is clear that there is an urgent need to have a culture collection of rhizobia from tree species and to conduct careful studies under pot-culture conditions.

Table 43: A profile of the colonization of VAM fungi in roots of some tree species of collected from a semiarid region near Bangalore

Tree species	Total root pieces examined	Infection (%)	Vesicles (%)	Arbuscules (%)
Azadirachta indica	23	47.0	0.0	0.0
Dalbergia sisso	20	50.0	5.0	0.0
Wrightia tinctoria	22	0.0	0.0	0.0
Ficus religiosa	22	45.0	0.0	0.0
F. bengalensis	22	0.0	0.0	0.0
F. glomerata	20	0.0	0.0	0.0
F. mysorensis	22	0.0	0.0	0.0
Santalum album	21	95.0	28.5	38.1
Prosopis juliflora	19	47.0	0.0	0.0
Acacia ampliceps	21	23.8	0.0	0.0
A. holeserecea	21	66.6	0.0	0.0
A. auriculiformis	21	57.0	4.8	0.0
A. stenophylla	20	95.0	25.0	25.0
A. nilotica	21	95.0	53.0	4.8
Eucalyptus hybrid	22	81.8	13.6	9.0

Nodulation in *Parasponia* species belonging to the family Ulmaceae is one standing example of a non-leguminous plant known to nodulate with *Rhizobium* or *Bradyrhizobium* (see Trinick and Hadobas, 1989). Mention may also be made with caution of root nodulation of five species of the genera *Tribulus* and *Zygophyllum* by *Rhizobium* in the family Zygophyllaceae. Even though the isolates from *Tribulus* nodulated *Vigna* spp., no test has been done to verify nodulation of *Tribulus* and hence this instance of nodulation remains equivocal (athar and Mamood, 1981). Since *Parasponia* is a pioneer plant capable of quick growth and high nitrogen fixation, exploitation of this nitrogen-fixing tree in agroforestry has been recommended (Trinick and Hadobas, 1989).

Inoculation with *Rhizobium* and VAM Fungi

In pot trials, the interaction of three effective strains of *Rhizobium* (Lcn-1, Lc-3, and Tal-582) with three species of VAM fungi

(*Acaulospora* sp., *Gigaspora margarita,* and *Glomus fasciculatum*) on symbiotic parameters of *L. leucocephala* was investigated at three levels of phosphorus (0, 50, and 100 kg P_2O_5/ha). The interaction effects were measured on nodulation, dry weight of shoot, and uptake of nitrogen and phosphorus at 50 days and 100 days of plant growth in unsterilized soil. The per cent of VAM colonization was measured at appropriate intervals. In general, *Rhizobium* and mycorrhizal inoculation enhanced growth and nutrient uptake over control even though the effects of phosphorus were not consistent. However, applications of phosphorus with *Rhizobium* and VAM fungi significantly increased nodulation, dry weight of shoot, and nitrogen and phosphorus uptake. The colonization of VAM fungi in roots was also enhanced by *Rhizobium* as well as VAM inoculation (Nalini and Subba Rao, unpublished). Similar results on the beneficial effect of *G. fasciculatum* inoculation on *L. leucocephala* nodulation have also been reported by Manjunath *et al.,* (1984).

Inoculation with VAM fungi is known to benefit tree species. For example, *Acacia holosericea* was benefitted under semiarid conditions when inoculated with VAM fungi (Cornet *et al.,* 1982). This effect may be due to better nutrient uptake or drought resistance since it has been reported that mycorrhizal inoculation improves plant growth more under dry conditions than under wet conditions (Nelsen and Safir, 1982; Fitter, 1985). However, experiments on tropical trees with regard to protection offered by VAM on drought resistance are scarce. VAM inoculation of *L. leucocephala* has been shown to improve growth in exotic plantations and agroforestry systems of subhumid tropics (Huang *et al.,* 1985). Several *Acacia* spp. are very dependent on VAM fungi for their phosphorus nutrition (Jasper *et al.,* 1989). In a recent study, experiments were carried out to compare the drought resistance of VAM in VAM fungi-inoculated *L. leucocephala* and *A. nilotica* plants under controlled conditions (Michelsen and Rosendahl, 1990). The VAM inoculum used was a mixture of *Glomus etunicatum, G. mossae,* and *G. occultum.* VAM inoculation as well as phosphorus application increased the total biomass by 82 per cent in *L. leucocephala* and 66 per cent in *A. nilotica.* While this increment was significant in high water regime for both the tree species, it was significant for *L. leucocephala* under drought strees (115 per cent improvement) but not for *A. nilotica* (66 per cent improvement). Drought treatment suppressed nodulation in *A. nilotica* but did not do so in *L. leucocephala.* The authors concluded that as far as *Leucaena* was concerned VAM inoculation under drought conditions was beneficial in both normal and phosphorus-amended conditions.

Stylosanthes and *Leucaena* are known to respond favourably to VAM inoculation when soil phosphorus is low (Mosse, 1981; Habte and Manjunath, 1987). In a recent study in potted *L. leucocephala* plants, the response of the plant to VAM inoculation and rock phosphate application was investigated (Manjunath *et al.*, 1989). VAM colonization increased as the rock phosphate level was enhanced in soil. Inoculation with *G. aggregatum* significantly increased the uptake of Cu, P, and Zn as well as dry matter yields at all the levels of rock phosphate. In developing countries such as India, indigenous rock phosphates are available for tree cultivation but the study shows that large quantities are needed to attain growth similar to that obtainable with soluble phosphate source (KH_2PO_4).

Suggested Methods for Inoculating Leguminous Tree Seedlings in Nurseries

To date, legume (*Rhizobium*) inoculants for leguminous plants are in the form of agar-based cultures, peat-based moist powder, lignite-based moist powder, and free-flowing granular inoculants. Any one of these forms of culture can be used to inoculate seedlings grown in polythene pouches in nurseries. However, it should be remembered that free-flowing granular inoculants prepared in 2 per cent perlite (a form of exploded sand) mixed with 2 per cent sodium alginate and 0.1 M $CaCl_2$ has shelf life of one year or more at room temperature (S.V. Hegde, personal communication). Such a culture ought to be of great value for inoculating nursery stands at distant places. Peat- or lignite-based inoculant have short shelf life extending to five months. If such cultures are used, it is necessary to use the material for inoculation at an early date, to avoid the loss of viable rhizobia.

The soil medium in each polybag used for planting tree seedlings has to be mixed at the rate of 5–10 per cent with the inoculant, and the seed or transplanted seedlings placed in the polybags.

Dual Inoculation

VAM cultures are available as soil-cum-root bit mixtures in selected agricultural universities and research institutions in India. Soilrite (trade name) is an inert material supplied by Karnataka Explosives (18, Crescent Road, Bangalor-560001) for growing seedlings. It has been found by many workers that Soilrite is suitable for growing test plants to prepare mass cultures of root- and soil-based

VAM cultures. To prepare VAM inoculum with a known species of VAM fungus (e.g., *G. fasciculatum*), it is necessary to grow a suitable host plant (e.g., pearl millet, *Pennisetum americanum,* or any other suitable grass) in Soilrite substratum for 2–3 months in pots which has been mixed with the selected VAM fungus. At the end of the growth period, the tops of the plants are removed and the remaining soil in pots and roots are pulverized and partly dried. Since Soilrite substratum is a sterile, inert material, the chances of contamination with other microorganisms are minimized. The final powdered material enriched with the selected VAM fungus can be stored in polythene bags for use in nurseries. The material contains spores and propagules of fungal mycelia vegetating on root pieces. Since VAM fungi are obligate symbionts capable of growing only on host plant roots, the current method of choice to prepare VAM inoculum is to grow the fungi on live plant roots.

If VAM culture is co-inoculated with appropriate *Rhizobium* culture for a given leguminous tree species, it is necessary to obtain a culture of VAM fungus culture found to be dominant on roots of the particular tree legume. The Soilrite-based VAM fungal inoculum recommended for the selected tree species can be used by mixing 5 per cent of the inoculum into polythene pouches already inoculated with the specific *Rhizobium*. Such inoculation is known as dual inoculation. Experiments have clearly established that in *L. leucocephala,* a fast-growing leguminous tree species recommended for wasteland reclamation, dual inoculation with VAM and *Rhizobium* is superior to inoculation with *Rhizobium* alone. This being the case, the technology has to be propagated at the nursery level by dual inoculation of seedlings so that the juvenile plants are better equipped to manage themselves for both nitrogen and phosphorus, which are essential for tree growth.

Haustorial Links

Sandalwood (*Santalum album*), which grows extensively in forests of the Indian peninsula, is a root parasite (Barber, 1903). Sandal roots establish haustorial connections with the neighbouring plant species, obtain nourishment, and grow to maturity yielding the commercially valuable sandalwood and oil. There are several leguminous as well as non-leguminous hosts of the sandal tree (Table 44). Many are nodulating legumes and *Casuarina,* an actinorhizal plant, is also a host (Narasimhan, 1918). Till now haustorial establishment on roots was known and described. However, in a recent study (Subba Rao *et al.*, 1990), direct establishment of haustorial connections between roots of sandal and nodules of pigeon pea (*Cajnus cajan*) and *Pongamia glabra* have been observed and the consequent effect on symbiotic parameters measured in pot trials. In pigeon pea more than 75 per cent of nodules had haustorial connections. Many were single but some were multiple connections between roots and nodules. In *Pongamia*, haustorial connections in young nodules could be visually distinguished, whereas in older multilobed nodules, the flask-shaped haustorial connection was evident only on sectioning. The dry weight of parasitized nodulated plants was reduced with a consequent increase in the biomass and nitrogen content of sandal. Similar haustorial links between roots of sandalwood plant and *Casuarina equisetifolia* have also been noticed (Subba Rao and Yadav, unpublished).

Table 44: Leguminous plants and trees which are known to serve as hosts for the sandal tree (*Santalum album* Linn)

Acacia caesia Wall	*Castanospermum australe* A cunn.
A. catechu Willd	*Clitoria ternatea* Linn.
A. concinna DC.	*Dalbergia latifolia* Roxb.
A. ferruginea DC	*D. paniculata* Roxb.
A. intesia Willd.	*D. scandense* Roxb.
A. leucophloea Willd	*D. sisso* Roxb.
A. pinnata Willd.	*Dolichos lablab* Linn.
A. suma kurz.	*Erythrina stricta* Roxb.
A. sundra DC	*Leucaena glauca* Benth
Adenanthera pavonia Linn.	*Parkia biglandulosa* wight and Arn.
Albizzia amara Biov.	*Parkinsonia aculeata* Linn.
A. lebbek Benth.	*Peltophorum ferrugineum* Benth
A. odoratissima Benth.	*P. indicum*
Bauhinia racemosa Lam.	*Pithecolobium dulce* Benth
Butea frondosa Roxb.	*P. saman* Benth
Caesalpinia bonducella Fleming	*Pongamia glabra* Vent.
Canavalia ensiformis DC	*Prosopis spicigera* Linn.
Cassia auriculata Linn.	*Pterocarpus marsupium* Roxb.
C. fistula Linn.	*Pterolobium indicum* A. Rich.
C. siamea Lam.	*Tamarindus indica* Linn.

REFERENCES

Allen, E.N., and Allen, O.N. (1981). *The Leguminosea: A Source Book of Characteristics, Uses and Nodulation.* The University of Wisconsin Press, Madison, Wisc.

Ashby, W.C., and Baker, M.B., Jr. (1968). Soil nutrients and tree growth under black locust and shortleaf pine overstories in strip mine plantings. *J. Forestry,* **66**, 67–71.

Athar, M., and Mamood, A. (1981). Extension of *Rhizobium* host range to zygophyllaceae. In *Current Perspective in Nitrogen Fixation.* Eds. A.H. Gibson and W.E. Newton. Australian Academy of Science, Canberra. p. 481.

Barber, C.A. (1903). Report on spike disease in sandal wood trees Coorg. *Indian Forester,* **29**(1), 21–31.

Basak, M.K., and Goyal, S.K. (1975). Studies on tree legumes. I. Nodulation pattern and characterization of the symbiont. *Ann. Arid Zone,* **14**, 367–370.

Barnet, Y.M., Catt, P.E., and Hearne, D.H. (1985). Biological nitrogen fixation and root nodule bacteria (*Rhizobium* sp. and *Bradyrhizobium* sp.) in two rehabilitating sand dune areas planted with *Acacia* spp. *Austral. J. Bot.,* **33**, 595–599.

Bengtson, G.W., and Mays, D.A. (1978). Growth and nutrition of loblolly pine on coal mine spoil as affected by nitrogen and phosphorus fertilizer and cover crops. *Forest Sci.,* **24**(3), 389–409.

Brown, J.H. (1973). Height growth prediction for black locust on surface-mined areas in West Virginia. Bull. No. 617, West Virginia University Agricultural Experimental Station. pp. 11.

Carmean, W.H., Clark, F.B., Williams, R.D., and Hannah, P.R. (1976). Hardwoods planted in old-fields favoured by prior tree cover. USDA Forest Service Research Paper NC-134, pp. 16.

Cope, J.A. (1929). Concerning black locust in New York. *J. Forestry,* **27**, 828.

Cornet, F., Diem, H.G., and Dommergues, Y.R. (1982). Effect de l' inoculation avec *Glomus mossae* sur la croissance d'*Acacia holosericea* en pepiniere et apres transplantation sur la terrain. In *Les Mycorrhizes: Biologie et Utilisation.* Eds. S. Gianinazzi, V. Gianinazzi-Pearson and S. Trouvelot. INRA Press, Paris, pp. 287–293.

Dobereiner, J. (1984). Nodulacao e fixacao de nitrogenic em leguminosas florestais *Pesq. agropec. bras* 19 s/n, 83 pages.

Faria, S.M. de, Franco, A.A., Jesus, R.M. de, Menandro, M.S., Baitello, E.S.F., Mucci, J., Dobereiner, J., and Sprent, J.I. (1984). New nodulating legume trees from South-east Brazil. *New Phytol.,* **98**, 317–327.

Faria, S.M. de, Lewis, G.P., Sprent, J.I., and Sutherland, J.M. (1989). Occurrence of nodulation in the Leguminosae. *New Phytol.,* **111**, 607–619.

Faria, S.M. de, Lima, H.C. de, and Campelo, E.F.C. (1985). A morfologia dos nodulos radiculares na taxonomia da tribo Dalbergieae. *Proc. xxxvi Cong. Nacional de Botanica,* 20–26 January 1985, Parana, Ed. J. Dobereiner, Braz. Acad. Sci., Brazil.

Faria, S.M. de, Sutherland, J.M., and Sprent, J.I. (1986). A new type of infected cell in root nodules of *Andira* spp. (Leguminosae). *Plant Sci.,* **45**, 143–137.

Faria, S.M. de, Lima, H.C. de, Franco, A.A., Mucci. E.S.F., and Sprent, J.I. (1987a). Nodulation of legume trees from SE Brazil. *Plant and Soil,* **99**, 347–356.

Faria, S.M. de, McInroy, S.G., and Sprent, J.I. (1987b). The occurrence of infected cells, with persistent infection threads in legume root nodules. *Can. J. Bot.,* **65**, 553–558.

Ferguson, J.A. (1922). Influence of locust on the growth of catalpa. *J. Forestry,* **20,** 318–319.

Fitter, A.H. (1985). Functioning of vesicular-arbuscular mycorrhizas under field conditions. *New Phytol.,* **99,** 257–265.

Gordon, J.C., and Wheeler, C.T. (Eds.) (1983). *Biological Nitrogen Fixation in Forest Ecosystems: Foundations and Applications..* Martinus Nijhoff/Dr. W. Junk Publishers, The Hague.

Gordon, J.C., Wheeler, C.T., and Perry, D.A. (Eds.) (1979). *Symbiotic Nitrogen Fixation in the Management of Temperate Forests.* Forest Research Laboratory, Oregon State University, Corvallis, Ore.

Habte, M., and Manjunath, A. (1987). Soil solution phosphorus status and mycorrhizal dependency in *Leucaena leucocephala. Appl. Environ. Microbiol.,* **53,** 797–801.

Haines, S.G., Haines, L.W., and White, G. (1978). Leguminous plants increase sycamore growth in northern Alabama. *Soil Sci. Soc. Amer. J.,* **42,** 130–132.

Harley, J.L., and Smith, S.E. (1983). *Mycorrhizal Symbiosis.* Academic Press, New York.

Hingston, F.J., Malajczuk, N.A., and Grove, T.S. (1982). Acetylene reduction (N_2 fixation) by Jarrah forest legumes following fire and phosphate application. *J. Appl. Ecol.,* **19,** 631–641.

Hoberg, P. (1986). Nitrogen fixation and nutrient relations in savanna woodland trees (Tanzania). *J. Appl. Ecol.,* **23,** 675–685.

Hoberg, P., and Kvarnstrom, M. (1982). Nitrogen fixation by the woody legume *Leucaena leucocephala* in Tanzania. *Plant and Soil,* **66,** 21–27.

Huang, R.S., Smith, W.K., and Yost, R.S. (1985). Influence of vesicular-arbuscular mycorrhiza on the growth, water relations and leaf orientation in *Leucaena leucocephala* (Lam) de Wit. *New Phytol.,* **99,** 229–243.

Ike, A.F., and Stone, E.L. (1958). Soil accumulation under black locust. *Soil Sci. Soc. Amer. Proc.,* **22,** 346–349.

Jackson, D.S. (1976). Nitrogen and soil moisture in coastal sand forest. In *Forest Research Annual Report 1975,* Publication of New Zealand Forest Service Wellington. pp. 39–41.

Jasper, D.A., Abbot, L.K., and Robson, A.D. (1989). Acacias respond to addition of phosphorus and inoculation with VA mycorrhizal fungi in soil stockpiled during mineral sand mining. *Plant and Soil,* **115,** 99–108.

Kellogg, L.F. (1936). Failure of black locust-coniferous mixtures in the central states. USDA Forest Service Central States Forest Experimental Station Note No. 15. pp. 4.

Lieberman, M.T., Mallony, L..M., Simkins, S., and Alexander, M. (1985). Numerical taxonomic analysis of cross-inoculation patterns of legumes and Rhizobium. *Plant and Soil,* **84,** 225–244.

Manjunath, A., Bagyaraj, J., and Gopala, G.H.S. (1984). Dual inoculation with VA mycorrhiza and *Rhizobium* is beneficial to *Leucaena. Plant and Soil,* **78,** 445–448.

Manjunath, A., Hue, N.V., and Habte, M. (1989). Response of *Leucaena leucocephala* to vesicular-arbuscular mycorrhizal colonization and rock phosphate fertilization in an oxisol. *Plant and Soil,* **114,** 127–133.

Mattoon, W.R. (1930). Black locust. *J. Forestry,* **28,** 763–769.

McIntyre, A.C., and Jeffries, C.D. (1932). The effect of black locust on soil nitrogen and growth of catalpa. *J. Forestry,* **30,** 22–28.

Michelsen, A., and Rosendahl, S. (1990). Propagule density of VA mycorrhizal fungi in semi-arid bushland in Somalia. In *Proc. IInd Eur. Symp. Mycorrhizae*, Prague. Elsevier, Dusseldort.

Monk, D., Pate, J.S., and Loneragen, W.A. (1981). Biology of *Acacia pulchella* R. Br. with special reference to symbiotic nitrogen fixation. *Austral. J. Bot.*, **29**, 592–599.

Mosse, B. (1981). *Vesicular-arbuscular Research for Tropical Agriculture*. Research Bulletin 194. College of Tropical Agriculture and Human Resources, University of Hawaii, Honolulu. pp. 82.

Nakos, G. (1977). Acetylene reduction (N_2-fixation) by nodules of *Acacia cynophylla*. *Soil Biol. Biochem.*, **9**, 131–137.

National Academy of Sciences (1977). *Leucaena: Promising Forage and Tree Crop for the Tropics*. National Academy of Sciences, Washington, DC. pp. 115.

Narasimhan, M.J. (1918). A preliminary study of root nodules of *Casuarina*. *Indian Forester*, **44**, 265–268.

Nelsen, C.E., and Safir, G.R. (1982). Increased drought tolerance of mycorrhizal onion plants caused by improved phosphorus nutrition. *Planta*, **154**, 407–413.

Pechmann, H. von, and Wutz, A. (1960). Do mineral fertilizers and planting of lupins have any effect on the properties of wood of spruce and pine. *Forstwissenschaftliches Centralblatt.*, March/April, 91–105.

Roskoski, J.P., and Van Kessel, S. (1985). Annual seasonal and diurnal variation in nitrogen fixation activity by *Inga jinicuil* Schl., a tropical leguminous tree. *Oikos*, **44**, 306–310.

Rundel, P.W., Nilsen, E.T., Sharifi, M.R., Virginia, R.A., Jarrell, W.M., Kohl, D.H., and Shearer, G.B. (1982). Seasonal dynamics of nitrogen cycling for a *Prosopis* woodland in the Sonaran desert. *Plant and Soil*, **67**, 343–349.

Sanginga, N., Mulongoy, and Ayanaba, A. (1988a). Nodulation and growth of *Leucaena leucocephala* (Lam.) de Wit as affected by N fertilizer. *Plant and Soil*, **112**, 129–135.

Sanginga, N., Mulongoy, and Ayanaba, A. (1988b). Nitrogen contribution of *Leucaena/Rhizobium* symbiosis to soil and a subsequent maize crop. *Plant and Soil*, **112**, 137–141.

Sanginga, N., Mulongoy, and Ayanaba, A. (1988c). Nitrogen fixation of field-inoculated *Leucaena leucocephala* (Lam.) de Wit estimated by ^{15}N and the difference methods. *Plant and Soil*, **117**, 269–274.

Seidel, K.W., and Brinkman, K.A. (1962). Mixed or pure walnut plantings on strip mined land in Kansas? USDA Forest Service Central States Forest Experimental Station Technical Paper 187. pp. 10.

Silvester, W.B., Carter, D.A., and Sprent, J.I. (1979). Nitrogen input by *Lupinus* and *Coriaria* in *Pinus radiata* forest in New Zealand. In *Symbiotic Nitrogen Fixation in the Management of Temperate Forests*. Eds. J.C. Gordon, C.T. Wheeler and D.A. Perry. Forest Research Laboratory, Oregon State University, Corvallis, Ore. pp. 253–265.

Sprent, J.I. (1985). Nitrogen fixation in arid environments. In *Plant for Arid Lands*. Eds. G.E. Wickens, J.R. Goodin and D.V. Field. George Allen and Unwin, London. pp. 215–229.

Sprent, J.I. (1986). Potentials for nitrogen fixing legume trees in the tropics. *Intl. Tree Crops J.*, **4**, 47–51.

Sprent, J.I. (1987). Opportunities for the exploitation of nitrogen fixation in *Report of the EEC Workshop*, Dublin, March 4–6.

Sprent, J.I., and Raven, J.A. (1985). Evolution of nitrogen fixing symbiosis. *Proc. R. Soc. Edinburgh*, **85b**, 215–237.

Sprent, J.I., Sutherland, J.M., and Faria, S.M. de (1987). Structure and function of root nodules from woody legumes. In *The Biology of Legumes*. Eds. C.H. Stirton and J.L. Zarucchi. Missouri Botanical Garden, St. Louis.

Stone, E.L. (1955). Observations on forest fertilization in Europe. *Proc. 31st Annu. Meeting of the National Joint Commission on Fertilizer Application*. pp. 81–87.

Subba Rao, N.S., Yadava, D., Anantha Padmanabha, Nagaveni, Singh, C.S., and Kavimandan, S.K. (1990). Nodule haustoria and microbiol features of *Cajanus* and *Pongamia* parasitized by Sandal (Sandal wood). *Plant and Soil*, **128**, 249–256.

Trinick, M.J., and Hadobas, P.A. (1989). Biology of the *Parasponia-Bradyrhizobium* symbiosis. In *Nitrogen Fixation with Non-legumes*. Eds. F.A. Skinner, R.M. Boddey and I. Fendrik. Kluwer Academic Publishers, London. pp. 25–33.

Wickens, G.E. (1967). A study of *Acacia albida* Del (Mimosoideae). *Kew Bull.*, **23**, 181–198.

White, G. (1978). Legumes a silvicultural tool? In *Nitrogen Fixation in Southern Forestry*. Ed. S.G. Haines. International Paper Company, Bainbridge, Georgia. pp. 112–119.

12

Frankia Inoculant for Some Non-leguminous Trees

Soil organic matter or humus is the primary source of nitrogen to the plant kingdom, especially tree species in forests which do not ordinarily receive any chemical fertilizers. It has been estimated that, depending on the climatic and soil conditions, species, and age of stands, the annual nitrogen uptake by trees varies from 34 to 123 kg/ha. Of this, 22 to 79 kg is returned to the soil in litter fall and 8 to 44 kg is retained in the tree biomass (Duvigneand and Denaeyer-DeSmet, 1970). The nitrogen content of organic matter varies from 1.5 to 3.0 per cent and the available nitrogen for absorption by trees depends upon the extent of mineralization of organic nitrogen. In warmer regions of the world, mineralization may be so rapid that some nitrogen is lost though nitrification and leaching, whereas the reverse is true of colder regions. Raw humus is burned in some Scandinavian countries, which gives ash to fertilize the soil through mineralization. One way to accelerate mineralization is to add fertilizer nitrogen to raw humus sites. This practice of fertilizer application (50–200 kg N/ha/yr) has to be repeated periodically, which not only becomes expensive but also causes eutrophication of waterways. Burning of tree stands to clear the land followed by cultivation of food crops for one season on the cleared land and after harvesting the crop, letting the land develop a natural stand of fresh forest has been an age-old practice in temperate regions. This practice of 'shifting cultivation', which is also practised in the *térai* (hilly) areas of tropical countries such as India, is prone to ecological hazards.

In developing countries, deforestation for fuel has rendered the land barren and continuous deforestration of the same land in overpopulated regions of such countries has resulted in soils which remain deficient in nitrogen, the most important element for the normal growth of plants. One of the least expensive and non-polluting ways to replenish the lost soil nitrogen for reafforestation is to plant self-supporting nitrogen-fixing trees. In Pennsylvania, USA, reafforestation of mine spoils has been done by planting nitrogen-fixing red alder (*Alnus rubra*) inoculated with nodule-forming *Frankia* (Tarrant and Trappe, 1971). In New Quebec, Canada, *Alnus* spp. have been planted on a large scale to fill dam dykes (Tarrant, 1983). In Senegal, Egypt, India, and the coastal region of China nitrogen-fixing *Casuarina* spp. have been planted on a large scale to contain and stabilize sandy tracts which have made inroads into agricultural land (Andeke-Lengui and Dommergues, 1981; El-Lakany, 1981; Kondas, 1981).

This chapter particularly addresses root nodulating trees collectively designated as 'actinorhizal plants'. They do not belong to the large botanical family Leguminoseae but are nervertheless important in tropical as well as temperate sylviculture.

The Importance of Actinorhizal Plants

There are 24 genera from eight angiosperm families which have been reported to possess actinorhizal root nodules (Dixon and Wheeler, 1986). These genera, with families mentioned in parenthesis, from most primitive to most advanced orders, are *Coriaria* (Coriariaceae), *Cerocarpus, Chamaebatia, Cowania, Dryas, Purshia, Rubus* (Rosaceae), *Datisca* (Dastiscaceae), *Comptonia, Myrica* (Myricaceae), *Alnus* (Betulaceae), *Elaeagnus, Hippophae, Shepherdia (Elaeagnaceae), Coenothus, Colletia, Discaria, Kentrothamnus, Retamnilla, Talguenea, Trevoa* (Rhamnaceae), *Allocasuarina, Casuarina,* and *Gymnostoma* (Casuarinaceae). The genera *Casuarina* for tropical and subtropical regions and *Alnus (A. rubra, A. glutinosa, A. crispa, A. jorullensis, A. Acuminata)* for temperate regions stand out as excellent examples for the benefits they provide to the ecosystems by way of nitrogen inputs. They can adapt themselves to grow under most diverse environmental conditions and geographical zones. *Casuarina* species (*C. equisetifolia, C. cunninghamiana, C. littoralis, C. stricta, C. junghuhniana, C. glauca,* and *C. torulosa*) provide substantial fuel and building materials in tropical countries, while alders provide the most often used hard wood as well as bark for paper industries in temperate

regions. The microsymbiont in actinorhizal root nodules is an actinomycete and has been collectively designated as *Frankia* (see Table 45).

Table 45: Classification of non-leguminous dinitrogen-fixing angiosperms with
Frankia symbioses

Order	Family	Tribe	Genus	Number of nodulated species (in parentheses, total number of species)[1]
Casuarinales	Casuarinaceae		*Casuarina*	24 (45)
Myricales	Myricaceae		*Myrica*	26 (35)
			Comptonia	1 (1)
Fagales	Betulaceae	Betuleae	*Alnus*	33 (35)
Rhamnales	Elaeagnaceae		*Elaeagnus*	16 (45)
			Hippophae	1 (3)
			Shepherdia	3 (3)
	Rhamnaceae	Rhamneae	*Ceanothus*	31 (55)
		Colletieae	*Discaria*	6 (10)
			Colletia	3 (17)
			Trevoa	1 (6)
Coriariales	Coriariaceae		*Coriaria*	13 (15)
Rosales	Rosaceae	Rubieae	*Rubus*[2]	1 (250) (429)
		Dryadeae	*Dryas*	3 (4)
			Purshia	2 (2)
		Cercocarpeae	*Cercocarpus*	4 (20)
Cucurbitales	Datiscaceae		*Datisca*	2 (2)

Source: Becking, 1982.

[1] Taxonomic estimates mainly based on Willis (1973).

[2] According to Focke (1894) 429 *Rubus* species occur worldwide, but Willis (1973) gives
as estimate 250 *Rubus* species.

The importance of alders in sole cropping or mixed cropping
systems as nitrogen-fixing trees is well known (Tarrant and Trappe,
1971). Miller and Murray (1978) have demonstrated the benefits of
interplanting four-year-old Douglas fir with red alder in the
northwestern United States. In this long-term experiment, beginning
from 30 years after mixed planting, Douglas fir gave more yields when
mixed in the cropping system with red alder. Similar response by five
hardwoods and five conifers to mixed cropping with black alder has
been observed in the United States by Plass (1977). Observations on
productivity increases of *Populus, Fraxinus, Acer, Liriodendron,
Liquidambar, Platanus, Pseudotsuga, Pinus, Picea,* and other genera
have been made by several workers (Lawrence, 1958; Tarrant, 1961;

Silvester *et al.*, 1979; Courier and Garbaye, 1981; Dawson, 1983; Lawrence, 1958). An alder stand can provide 2–3 t/ha of leaf fall annually and *Elaeagnus* can provide 14 t/ha. These leaves contain 1.8 to 3.0 per cent nitrogen and mineralize in 1 to 4 years, which is well above the average leaf nitrogen content of pine needles, which may take 7–10 years to mineralize (Silvester, 1977; Cromack *et al.*, 1979; Kikuzawa *et al.*, 1984; Radwan *et al.*, 1984; Daniere *et al.*, 1986). Dommergues (1963) pointed out that *Casuarina equisetifolia* in sand dunes of the Cape Verde islands can contribute up to 58 kg N/ha/yr. *Casuarina* plantations in sea coasts of India and other countries are common and many contributions on the sylvicultural value of this versatile plant have been documented (Midgley *et al.*, 1983). Nitrogen accretion by *Alnus* spp. amounts to 40 to 360 kg N/ha/yr (Tarrant, 1983). Accurate estimates by way of measuring acetylene reduction activity under field conditions by intact plants have been made but the values were dependent on photosynthetic activity (Huss-Dannel *et al.*, 1989). Very few studies have addressed the problem of quantifying the nitrogen contribution by actinorhizal plants for lack of appropriate non-nodulating reference plants to measure nitrogen fixation by the use of ^{15}N. Domenach *et al.* (1989) measured annual nitrogen fixation in virgin alder forest using a ^{15}N natural abundance procedure and compared it with the result obtained from the ^{15}N-labelled fertilizer isotopic dilution method. These authors found that the results from both the methods were comparable and that alders maintained a high nitrogen-fixing capacity in a sequence ranging from first stage of establishment of climactic formation.

Actinorhizal plants (*Alnus*, *Dryas*, and *Shepherdia*) have been planted in deglaciated areas of the world rendering the barren, stony new substratum fertile for other plants (Crocker and Major, 1955). *Alnus viridis* has been found valuable due to its cold tolerance in reclaiming Swiss alpine zones (Moiround and Campellano, 1979). *Alnus* and *Myrica gale* have been planted in abandoned acidic peat-lands after excavation of usable peat deposits in Sweden and Canada in afforestation programmes where native *Frankia* strains capable of tolerating acidic pH nodulate and enhance the fertility status of such spoiled sites (Schwintzer, 1979, 1984; Faure-Raynaud *et al.*, 1986). Coastal areas inundated by salty water in the Netherlands are planted with salt-tolerating actinorhizal plants such as *Hippophae rhamnoides*, *Elaeagnus umbellata*, *E. angustifolia*, *Myrica pennsylvanica*, *M. asplenifolia*, and *M. faya*. The ability of these species to withstand high salinity is reflected by the fact that salty winds can deposit as much as 3 mg NaCl/ cm^2/day (Midgley et al., 1983). Casuarina equisetifolia is known to grow well up to a height of 20 m by the seaside and tolerate salinity levels up to 950 mol NaCl/m^3 along the Indian ocean (Aswathappa and Bachelard, 1986). The above examples serve to illustrate the fact that the macro- as well as the microsymbionts in actinorhizal symbiosis are versatile and suitable for pioneer colonization of extremely harsh and derelict land.

Isolation of Frankia

From time to time attempts have been made to isolate Frankia in pure culture, often with success, but the indisputability of such isolates was not achieved because the isolated culture did not reproduce nodules on new plants. Earlier accounts of such abortive attempts beginning from 1910 are given by Becking (1982) and Diem and Dommergues (1988). The first successful demonstration of the reproducibility of nodulation upon reinoculation of an isolated endophyte was from Callaham and associates in the United States (1978). These authors used cellulase and pectinase enzymes to separate active cells from nodules. Subsequently, several reports have appeared describing isolation methods, but for practical purposes, the protocol described by Diem and Dommergues (1988) can be taken into consideration. The different steps in the procedure are as follows:

1) Clear the nodule of extraneous organic matter, soil, and dirt under a stream of running water.

2) Fragment the nodule into small lobes.

3) Sterilize the outer layers of nodule lobes by immersing in a 3 per cent aqueous solution of osmium tetroxide for 1–4 minutes depending on the size of the lobe. Extreme care has to be taken due to the toxic nature of osmium tetroxide.

4) Wash in sterile distilled water several times and cut the nodule lobes into 0.1–0.5 mm^3 pieces (approximate) with the help of a sterile scalpel.

5) Transfer these nodule pieces into a bottom layer of 1.5 per cent of nutrient medium in a petri dish (see Appendix for composition of the medium; addition of cycloheximide at 50 μg/ml may be helpful in preventing fungal contamination).

6) Pour 3 ml of the same medium over the layer containing nodule pieces to provide micro-aerophilic condition (less oxygen) for Frankia growth.

7) Seal the petri dishes with paraffin and incubate at 28°–30°C. After 4 weeks, colonies of *Frankia* appear at the edge of nodule pieces.

Other methods of isolation of *Frankia* are also available (see Elkan, 1987). A filtration technique using nylon screens (Benson, 1982) consists of the following steps:

1) Wash root nodules with stream of distilled water.
2) Remove nodule lobes 1 mm from the tip of the nodule.
3) Wash nodule lobes with distilled water.
4) Place 4 to 15 nodule lobes in a polypropylene microfuge tube (1.5 ml capacity).
5) Add 1 ml of 20 per cent (vol./vol.) laundry bleach [1.05 per cent (wt/vol.) sodium hypochlorate] and agitate for 5 minutes.
6) Decant bleach and wash four times with 1 ml of sterile distilled water.
7) Homogenize nodule lobes in 5 ml of *Frankia* medium with a tissue homogenizer (7.5 ml capacity).
8) Gravity-filter homogenate through nylon screens of 50 and 20 μm pore size.
9) Collect nodule debris on the 52 μm filter and wash with 30 ml of *Frankia* medium.
10) Collect *Frankia* on the 20 μm filter and wash twice with 30 ml of *Frankia* medium.
11) Remove *Frankia* from the 20 μm filter with a Pasteur pipetter and place in sterile test tubes.
12) Dilute suspension and pour-plate the endophyte.
13) Incubate until visible colonies are observed.
14) Remove colonies aseptically and homogenize.
15) Inoculate 1 ml of *Frankia* medium containing 0.3 per cent (wt/vol.) filter-sterilized sodium pyruvate with a single homogenized colony.

Infection and Nodule Development

Deformation of root hairs is the first visible symptom upon inoculation of roots with *Frankia* strains. The occurrence of infection by thread-like structures has been demonstrated in *Alnus glutinosa, Comptonia perigrina, Casuarina cunninghamiana,* and *Myrica gale* (see Quispel and Burggraaf, 1988). The thread penetrates the cortical cells and under its influence, cell divisions are initiated in the cortex. These new cells also get infected and radial growth begins. Sooner or later, the cells are filled with starch. Further growth of the resulting primordial nodule is confined to the peripheral layers of cells which contain tannin-like substances (Torrey and Callaham, 1979). Up to this stage, similarities between the development of legume root nodules and actinorhizal root nodules can be seen. Very soon, differences set in during subsequent stages of development. Root initials develop near the primary root nodule. Such root primordia which develop from the pericycle of the main root are far greater in number in nodulated roots than in nodule-free roots. Furthermore, such roots are formed at sites where normally roots do not develop and hence this type of rooting may be attributed to auxins produced by the nodule. These roots, which may be called 'nodule roots' also get infected by *Frankia* resulting in a nodule mass (Callaham *et al.*, 1979). Further development of the nodule mass is confined to apical meristems of infected laterals. The entire structure is often referred to as 'rhizothamnion', which in some cases (as in *Casuarina*) may regenerate normal non-infected roots which show negative geotrophy.

In the infected nodular tissue of *Comptonia perigrina*, the hyphae pass through the walls of cells, parallel to cell walls or in the wall itself. The *Frankia* hyphae have cytoplasmic membranes, cell wall, the host-produced capsule, and the host cell plasmalemma. The nucleus becomes lobed, the vacuoles fuse, the number of mitochondria increases, the amyloplasts and proplastids degenerate, and free ribosomes predominate in infected cells (Gardner, 1976; Newcomb *et al.*, 1978, 1979). Barring *Casuarina,* vesicles are generally formed by *Frankia* in actinorhizal root nodules. Effectiveness is usually associated with vesicle formation. The shape of these vesicles varies from globular to club-shaped. It is possible that vesicles (Plate 8) may be the site of nitrogen fixation in the same way as bacteroids are in legume root nodules or heterocysts in cyanobacteria. In actinorhizal nodules and in pure cultures of *Frankia*, sporangia (Plate 8) are also formed which serve as initial cells for other colonies of the organism to develop.

Like legume root nodules, some actinorhizal nodules contain haemoglobin and others do not have the pigment or, if they do, have it in minute amounts. In nodules of *Casuarina* and *Myrica*, haemoglobin is found at high levels, whereas in *Alnus* and *Elaeagnus*, the pigment is present in low levels. *Datisca* nodules have no haemoglobin but still they fix nitrogen. This situation in nodules lacking haemoglobin can be explained by the existence of other mechanisms for protecting the oxygen-sensitive nitrogenase.

Growth of *Frankia* in Culture

Frankia has a long lag phase of nearly 14 days, a slow exponential phase, no stationary phase, and autolysis of most vegetative structures. These characteristics render *Frankia* unsuitable for mass multiplication. Besides being micro-aerophlic, it has temperature requirement of 28°–30°C and a pH optimum of 6.0 to 7.0. Among the carbon sources, succinate and tween 80 appear to be good sources (Diem and Dommergues, 1988). Spores are produced by the endosymbiont in culture as well as nodules. Two types of nitrogen-fixing nodules have been recognized based on spore formation: spore (−) are nodules where spores are absent or few and spore (+) are nodules containing many spores (Van Dijk, 1978). These spores are produced in sporangia. Besides these spores, vesicles and torulose hyphal propagules are also produced in cultures as well as nodules in *Casuarina*. Therefore, it is not clear whether hyphal propagules, spores, or vesicles give rise to cultures of *Frankia* when nodule lobes are used. In liquid cultures, growth results in ellipsoidal or spherical colonies of 0.5–1 mm diameter, often clustering together and sticking at the bottom of the glass containers. Addition of activated charcoal greatly stimulates the growth of reproductive structures of *Frankia* into new colonies (Diem and Dommergues, 1988).

Classification — Prior to the isolation of *Frankia* in pure culture, nodule suspensions were used in inoculation experiments to classify the endosymbiont of actinorhizal plants in the same way as rhizobia have been classified based on the ability of strains to infect and nodulate particular species of host plants. Some generalizations were made from results obtained by such studies which are not currently valid for the obvious fact that nodule suspensions may carry multiple strains (Van Den Bosch and Torrey, 1983). On the other hand, experimental results which are being obtained in recent years using pure cultures cf *Frankia* to infect and cause nodulation of aseptically grown plants have also the limitation that *Frankia* strains have not been isolated from all actinorhizal plants. Nevertheless, the following tentative conclusions can be made from recent experiments: *Frankia* strains isolated from genera *Alnus* of the family Betulaceae and *Myrica* and *Comptonia* of Myricaceae appear to be highly promiscuous and are interchangeable with the species of the three genera. On the other hand, *Frankia* isolates of *Alnus, Myrica*, and *Comptonia* do not appear to nodulate the tested species of other genera such as *Elaeagnus, Hippophae, Shepherdia, Coenothus, Colletia, Purshia, Datisca,* and *Coriaria,* all belonging to different divergent families. These results point to the existence of a cross-inoculation group covering the three genera *Alnus, Myrica,* and *Comptonia. Frankia* strains isolated from nodules of *Casuarina* species exhibit specificity which also suggests the existence of cross-inoculation groups within *Frankia* strains of actinorhizal plants (Zhang *et al.,* 1984). Hence, three groups could be made out as matters stand at present — group I, which includes the genera *Alnus* of Belulaceae and *Myrica* and *Comptonia* of Myricaceae; group II comprising nodulated members of Elaeagnaceae and Rhamnaceae; and group III comprising strains of Casuarinaceae (Rodriguez-Barrueco and Subramaniam, 1988). In recent years, however, new biochemical and molecular biological methods for classifying *Frankia* strains and understanding their phylogeny have been used in the taxonomy of *Frankia* (Simonet *et al.,* 1990). **Method of preparing nodule suspensions** — Most of the earlier studies on actinorrhizal plants, prior to the availability of pure cultures of *Frankia,* were made with suspensions of nodules. Bond (1957) and Torrey (1976) followed the method described hereunder for *Casuarina*: Fresh nodule material was ground in distilled water at a ratio of 1 g/20 ml water, filtered through muslin cloth, and the nodule suspension brushed onto seedlings previously raised in sand. During the process of grinding nodules, toxic polyphenols or tannins are released when the suspension changes colour from brown to grey. These polyphenols may damage the actinomycete in such suspensions. It has been found that the use of polyvinylpyrrolidone (PVP) at 1 per cent level retards the blackening of suspension. Similarly, 10 per cent (wt/vol.) of activated charcoal in distilled water keeps the suspension clear (Torrey 1981). The use of 1 per cent salt solution (NaCl) has been recommended for grinding nodules which keeps the filtrate clear, as has been shown in the case of *Alnus* (Lalonde, 1979). Normand and Lalonde (1982) took 1–2 g nodule (fresh weight) of alders, homogenized with the help of a blender, and repeatedly washed the homogenate by centrifugation with a saline phosphate buffer containing 2 per cent PVP for the elimination of phenols. The suspension was diluted in tap water and sprayed directly on the seedlings in nursery stocks. However, no systematic comparative studies have been made on the use of these different methods.

Nodule suspensions have to be made separately for each species forming actinorhizal nodules bacause systematic classification of *Frankia* isolates is yet incomplete and some information is already available on the specificity between *Frankia* strains and *Casuarina* spp. (Torrey, 1981).

Fresh nodules can be kept in a dry state over a layer of silica gel in containers and used as inoculum by grinding in saline solution without losing viability. The spores can remain viable for long periods (BOSTID report, 1984).

Method for using pure culture of *Frankia* — The size of the inoculum is critical in the mass multiplication of *Frankia*. When nodule suspensions are used, different types of colonies are formed. These colonies may contain a diffuse net work of hyphae around the centre or a dense network of hyphae with a number of sporangia. Sometimes starfish-shaped colonies arise. This polymorphism (Diem and Dommergues, 1988) is characteristic of *Frankia*. When nodule lobes are used instead of nodule suspensions, polymorphism can be minimized. Even after 4 weeks incubation time, the amount of biomass obtained is small. Hence, turbidimetry cannot be used for estimating the growth of *Frankia* but total protein or organic carbon estimations are sufficient to measure growth accurately, which can be done with a small amount of material (Burggraff and Shipton, 1983).

Selection of efficient strains for a given species needs careful evaluation under a given set of environmental conditions. For this purpose, strains are grown initially in test tubes on a suitable medium (see Appendix for the composition of the medium) incubated at 28°C for 4 weeks. These strains are first transferred to aliquots of 25 ml broth and when growth takes place, the contents are transferred to bottles containing 100 ml broth. The mycelia formed in such bottles are packed in a known small volume of the nutrient under aseptic conditions. This packed volume of mycelia produced by the procedure described above has been used at the rate 0.1 to 1.0 µl per plant for inoculating red alder (*Alnus glutinosa*) seedlings in containers (Stowers and Smith, 1985). Extensive mat formation by *Frankia* strains isolated from nodules of *Alnus rubra* on a yeast extract medium in 4–6 weeks has been reported by Berry and Torrey (1985). In extensive studies on large-scale inoculation with *Frankia* in Quebec, Canada, Perinet *et al* (1985) used the following procedure for actinorhizal plants: *Frankia* cultures were grown on QMod medium (see Appendix) for 4–8 weeks at 27°C. They were washed with nitrogen-free

Crone's mineral solution (see Appendix) and then homogenized by sonication. *Frankia* cells intended for nodulating 100,000 seedlings were suspended in nitrogen-free Crone's solution as one litre of concentrated inoculant. The stock solution was prepared prior to inoculation and stored at 4°C until use. One way of inoculation was by injection of the suspension into the substrate using standrad disposable 5 ml plastic syringes. The other was by pouring the 1000 ml suspension to another quantity of 2000 litres of Crone's solution and spraying the entire quantity on to 100,000 plants. The inoculum was agitated continuously and sprayed uniformly using a pump. Different types of automatic equipments could be designed for different nurseries depending upon the cost involved. In this way, nearly 7 million seedlings of actinorhizal plants were inoculated between 1979 and 1984. Pure culture inoculants were found superior to nodule homogenates. Both methods of injection and spraying followed by watering appeared to be equally efficient with regard to *Alnus crispa, A. rugosa, Elaeagnus angustifolia, E. commutata, Hippophae rhamnoides, Myrica gale,* and *Shepherdia argentea* (Perinet *et al.*, 1985). Diem and Dommergues (1988) have used polymeric gels such as polyacrylamide or calcium alginate beads to entrap *Frankia* cells and such preparations can be used for inoculation.

While more innovations are called for in future to standardize mass production of *Frankia* inoculum, the present limitations for *Frankia* growth in culture are the long lag phase and the poor growth of the organism. It is essential to disrupt the inoculum to fine propagules by the use of magnetic stirrers or by forcing the *Frankia* colony fragments through a syringe fitted with a fine needle.

Nitrogen Accretion to Soil by Actinorhizal Trees

Over 200 plants possess actinorhizal nodules on roots and all these are trees except *Datisca* species. In temperate conditions mineral nitrogen applications to forest stands bring more profits with attendant loss through leaching, denitrification, and volatilization because approximately 10 per cent of the added fertilizer nitrogen is taken up during juvenile stages of plant growth (Tarrant, 1983). For instance, about 150 kg N/ha are added in five to nine applications in Finland forests (Mikola *et al.*, 1983). Unlike non-nodulating trees such as *Quercus, Tilia, and Ulmus* which lock up nitrogen in their biomass, nodulating trees, especially *Alnus* spp., put back nitrogen into soil through leaf fall. It has been estimated that 2–3 t/ha of alder and 14 t/ha of *Elaeagnus orientalis* leaves fall annually to soil and contain

1.8–3.0 per cent nitrogen (Silvester, 1977; Kikuzawa *et al.*, 1984; Radwan *et al.*, 1984; Daniere *et al.*, 1986) Moreover, unlike pine needles, which take 10 years to decompose, alder leaves decompose and mineralize in one to four years (Cromack *et al.*, 1979). It has been shown by experiments using isotopic nitrogen that more than 85 per cent of leaf nitrogen from *A. incana* originates by actinorhizal symbiosis (Domenach, 1987). Experiments with *Casuarina* and *Ceanothus* by Stewart and Bond (1961) have shown that actinorhizal nodules continue to fix nitrogen whatever be the availability of mineral nitrogen in the rooting medium. These facts exphasize that fertilizer nitrogen and generation of actinorhizal nitrogen are quite compatible but what needs the attention of foresters in advanced countries is the practice of integrated fertilizer management to avoid eutrophication of water ways by the indiscriminate use of only chemical sources of nitrogen in forestry. This contention is amply justified when it is known that alders contribute a sizeable amount of nitrogen to the forest ecosystem; for example, in terms of kg N/ha/yr the contribution by *Alnus* spp. is as follows: *A. glutinosa*, 125; *A. rubra*, 142–209; and *A. rugosa*, 170.

Mixed plantations of non-nodulating *Populus, Fraxinus, Acer. Liriodendron, Liquidambar, Platanus, Pseudotsuga, Pinus,* and *Picea* and actinorhizal plants have increased the productivity of non-nodulating perennial trees (Tarrant, 1961; Silvester 1977; Miller and Murray, 1978; Courier and Garbaye, 1981; Dawson, 1983). For instance, young trees of *Populus* associated with *Alnus crispa* reached a biomass 22.5 times higher than that of a pure plantation of the same age (Lawrence, 1958).

Johnson (1982) classified Casuarinaceae into four genera — *Casuarina* (11 species), *Allocasuarina* (37 species), *Gymnostoma* (17 species), and yet undescribed genera (two species) — totalling more than 60 species. The taxonomic position of Casuarinaceae is in flux and many species of the family are still being described under the geneus *Casuarina*. The genus *Casuarina* comprises, shrubs and trees. It is a native of the southern hemisphere. In Australia, *Casuarina* speoies are dominant in tropical, subtropical, temperate coastal, and arid inland regions. *Casuarina equisetifolia* has been used as an ornamental tree and to stabilize coastal sand dunes because it can withstand saline situations. Two other species are equally popular — *C. cunninghamiana* and *C. glauca* — but there are more species which are harvested as firewood crops. Besides their ability to form actinorhizal nodules, they also have ectomycorrhizal and VAM fungal associations which help the plant in both phosphorus and nitrogen nutrition (Torrey, 1981). Approximately 30 of the 60 species appear to have nodules. They are *C. cunninghamiana, C. equisetifolia, C. fraserana, C. glauca, C. huegeliana, C. lepidophloia, C. littoralis, C. montana, C. muellerana, C. muricata, C. nodiflora, C. pusilla, C. quadrivalvis, C. stricta, C. sumatrana, C. tenuissima, C. torulosa, C. cristata, C. decussata, C. deplanchei, C. distyla, C. junghuhniana, C. nana, C. rigida, C. rumphianum, C. decaisneana, C. obesa, C. oligodon, C. papuana,* and *C. suberosa.* These species are cultivated in different parts of the world. *Casuarina cunninghamiana* is grown in Argentina, Egypt, Israel, Ceylon, Zimbabwe, and Australia whereas *C. equisetifolia* is predominantly grown in China, India, Egypt, the Philippines, Sri Lanka, and Florida (USA). The morphology of nodules developing on roots of *C. equisetifolia* is shown in plate 9. In Thailand, *C. junghuhniana* is grown in various types of soil even though *C. equisetifolia* is a native species. Therefore, the worldwide distribution of different species depends on the nature of uses to which the species has been introduced. Dommergues (1963) quantified the amount of nitrogen fixed by *C. equisetifolia* in dunes of the Cape Verde islands and found a value equivalent to that of 58 kg N/ha/yr.

Janse (1897) reported the presence of nodules on roots of *Casuarina* for the first time followed by Kamerling (1915), Narasimhan (1918), Mcluckie (1923), Rao, (1923), Chaudhuri (1931), Aldrich-Blake (1932), Parker (1932), Mowry (1933), Miehe (1981). Diem *et al.* (1982) isolated and cultivated an infective and effective strain of *Frankia* from nodules of a hybrid of *C. junghuhniana* and *C. equisetifolia.* The beneficial effect of a VAM fungus *Glomus mosseae* and *Frankia* were shown by Gauthier *et al.* (1983). Bamber *et al.* (1980) have shown the occurrence of an ectomycorrhizal association in *C. distyla,* the fungus probably being *Pisolithus tinctorius. Frankia* capable of effectively nodulating *C. equisetifolia* and *C. cunninghamiana* were isolated from *Allocasuarina lehmanniana* by Zhang and Torrey (1985).

There have been a number of studies on sylvicultural practices of *Casuarina* spp. in different countries the results of which have found place in departmental reports. Critical studies on nodulation and nitrogen fixation by the same species or different species under various agroclimatic conditions to pinpoint beneficial aspects of *Casuarina* plantations are lacking. It is undeniable, however, that *Casuarina* is a cash crop for developing nations, being a multipurpose plant for paper, for fuel, and for building huts.

Mycorrhizae and Actinorhizal Plants

One or more species of the following genera of actinorhizal plant species are known to possess either ectomycorrhiza or VAM or both (Hall *et al.*, 1979; Trappe, 1979; Rose, 1980; Rose and Youngberg, 1981; Daft *et al.*, 1985): *Alnus, Casuarina, Comptonia, Myrica, Elaeagnus, Shepherdia, Purshia, Cerocarpus, Dryas, and Coriaria* (both ectomycorrhiza and VAM), and *Discaria, Hippophae, Ceanothus, Rubus, Datisca, and Colletia* (VAM). In general the VAM symbionts belong to the genera *Glomus, Gigaspora,* and *Acaulospora* and have been recorded by Rose (1980). The ectomycorrhizal associations have been summarized by Molina (1981) and Harley and Smith (1983).

Gigaspora sp. and *Glomus* sp. seem to be associated with *Casuarina equisetifolia* and *C. cunninghamiana* in Florida and Japan (Rose, 1980).. When *Glomus mosseae* and crushed nodule suspensions of *Casuarina equisetifolia* were co-inoculated (Diem *et al.*, 1982) the plants contained twice as much nitrogen (96 mg/plant) as seedlings inoculated with nodule homogenates (51 mg/plant). The fresh weight of seedlings also differed and dual inoculation almost doubled the biomass. The following genera of ectomycorrhizal fungi have been recorded to be symbiotic with *Casuarina: Cenococcum, Pisolithus, Hymenogaster, Thelephora, Rhizopogon* and *Amanita*. Ectomycorrhiza was artificially established on *Allocasuarina distyla* by inoculating with *P. tinctorius* (Bamber *et al.*, 1980).

Molina (1979, 1981) found that only three species of fungi, *Alpora diplophloeus, Astraeus pteridis,* and *Paxillus involutus,* formed ectomycorrhizal association in pure culture synthesis with five species of *Alnus,* whereas a number of other mycorrhizal fungi associated with natural stands of *Alnus* (Trappe, 1962; Horak 1963) did not do so. Among these three fungi, *A. diplophloeus* formed a prominent mantle and Hartig net. Subsequently, Godbout and Fortin (see Tarrant, 1983) carried out experiments on artificial synthesis of ectomycorrhizae of *A. rugosa* and *A. crispa* and found that many more species could establish mycorrhizal associations. These results may show that some sort of specificity in *Alnus* and ectomycorrhizal association might exist, but Gardner (1986) has cautioned that any such generalization must be corroborated with field observations under natural conditions.

The influence of VAM association on roots of actinorhizal plants on nutrient uptake and plant growth has been studied in *Ceanothus velutinus* (Rose and Youngberg, 1981), *Casuarina equisetifolia*

(Gauthier *et al.*, 1983), and *Hippophae rhamnoides* (Gardner *et al.*, 1984). All these investigators found enhanced phosphorus uptake and better nodulation and nitrogen fixation. The added benefits by way of nutrients may provide resistance to disease but investigations on the direct role of mycorrhiza in minimizing the severity of diseases of actinorhizal plants, unlike the innumerable instances shown in other plants (see Zak, 1964; Marx, 1975; Powell and Bagyaraj, 1984), have not progressed rapidly. Trappe (1972) noticed that when *Alnus rubra* was intermixed with Douglas fir, the mycorrhizal fungi of alder influenced the population of *Poria weirii*, a root pathogen of Douglas fir.

Tripartite relations between *Glomus* spp. and *Frankia* have been reported previously in actinorhizal shrubs by Rose and Trappe (1980). In *A. acuminata* seedlings, a tripartite symbiosis was established under three different phosphorus levels. Nitrogen fixation was measured by way of acetylene reduction and found to be 150 per cent higher in plants inoculated with *Frankia* and *Glomus intraradices* than the mean values of plants treated otherwise with either one of the two symbionts (Russo, 1980). Similarly, when *A. incana* seedlings were inoculated with *G. fasciculatus* (VAM), *Paxillus involutus* (ectomycorrhizal fungus), and an isolate of *Frankia*, they were found to successfully estabilsh nodulation as well as the two types of mycorrhizal development on test plants. In terms of actual benefits of this tetrapartite association on 10-week-old seedlings, dry weight measurements showed that plants with no symbionts registered a value of 1.72 g, while the tetrapartite seedlings showed 5.11 g (mean of eight replicates). Both ecto- and endomycorrhizal fungi established well on nodulated seedlings and per cent infections were as high as 65.0 (ecto) and 8.5 (endo) in the triple inoculated series (Chatarpaul *et al.*, 1989).

In legumes, nodules appear to resist VAM fungal colonization but this does not seem to be the case in actinorhizal nodules since VAM association with nodules has been described in *Alnus* sp. and *Ceanothus* sp. (Rose, 1980; Rose and Youngberg, 1981). Apart from the enhancement of phosphorus uptake by VAM fungi in actinorhizal plants (Mejstrik and Benecke, 1969), increase in nitrogenase activity of nodules and consequent improvement of nitrogen nutrition of plants have also been attributed to VAM association (Rose and Youngberg, 1981).

Interaction of Microbes Other Than *Frankia* with Actinorhizal Symbiosis

Quite often, efforts to achieve root nodulation of *Alnus* spp. and *Comptonia* under axenic conditions with pure cultures of *Frankia* isolated from the host have met with no success (Uemura, 1964; Lalonde *et al.*, 1975; Knowlton *et al.*, 1980) However, under sand, water, or aeroponic cultures, nodulation invariably occurred and the suggestion was that associative effects of other microorganisms could influence actinorhizal nodulation under non-aseptic conditions. Therefore, Knowlton *et al.*, (1980) carried out experiments to demonstrate the role of rhizosphere microorganisms in the infection process of *A. rubra* seedlings inoculated with a homologous *Frankia* strain with different bacteria, one of which was identified as *Pseudomonas cepacia*. Aseptically grown seedlings of *A. rubra* did not show root hair curling with its homologous *Frankia* strain but did so in association with these helper bacteria, especially *P. cepacia*, which helped *Frankia* to initiate root nodulation. More studies are needed to confirm the role of rhizobacteria in influencing actinorhizal symbiosis (Akkermans *et al.*, 1989).

Hydrogen-consuming *Nocardia autotrophica* have been isolated from the roots and nodules of *A. glutinosa*. A novel tripartite relationship has been put forward by Dobritsa and Sharaya (1986) involving *Frankia*, *N. autotrophica*, and *A. rubra*. The hydrogen evolved by nodules is used by *Nocardia* and it is not unlikely that such a scavenging mechanism of hydrogen by associated microorganisms could be helpful where nodulation is caused by uptake hydrogenase-negative strains of *Frankia* unable to utilize hydrogen evolved by nitrogenase reaction (Akkermans *et al.*, 1989).

Some observations on fungal interactions in actinorhizal symbiosis need further study. For instance, we do not know how certain penicillia cause nodule-like structures on roots of *A. glutinosa* in certain soils (Capellano *et al.*, 1987).

Frankia strains excrete antifungal and antibacterial compounds and the ecological role of this phenomenon is unknown (Akkermans *et al.*, 1989). The exudation of bactericides by *A. glutinosa* is known (Seidel, 1972). Red alder (*A. rubra*) is resistant to infection by *Poria weirii*, a major pathogen of conifers in North America (Wallis and Reynolds, 1962, 1965). As already explained, ectomycorrhizal association with alder may be one of the reasons behind the observed resistance of alder to *P. weirii* infection (Trappe, 1979). The soil supporting alder is rich in nitrates which the pathogen *P. weirii* is unable to utilize and added to this the polyphenol oxidases in alder tissue may be fungitoxic (Li *et al.*, 1968). Obviously, these findings have to be followed up to their logical conclusions and the missing links fixed to explain why alder stands are resistant to *P. weirii*.

Azospirillum spp. have been isolated from the roots of many tropical trees (Subba Rao, 1983). In a recent study, normal as well as proteoid roots of *Casuarina* spp. from Kenya and Spain yielded *Azospirillum*. Seedlings of *Casuarina cunninghamiana* responded to *A. brasilense* inoculation and plants in inoculated pots increased in growth by 90 per cent over uninoculated controls. A similar significant trend was observable when both *Azospirillum* and *Frankia* were inoculated in combination but the increment was less than that obtained with *Azospirillum* treatment alone (Rodriguez-Barrueco *et al.*, 1991). *Azospirillum* is known to secrete growth-promoting phytohormones (Tien *et al.*, 1979) and fix nitrogen (Burris, 1977). However, it is now generally recognized that biomass improvement obtained by *Azospirillum* inoculation is attributable more to the phytohormones which the bactrium secretes than to the minimal amount of nitrogen fixation *in situ* so often observed (Okon *et al.*, 1988).

Genetics of *Frankia*

The *nif* structural genes *(nif HDK)* encode the nitrogenase enzyme, the *nif H* coding for polypeptides of Fe protein and *nif DK* coding for the alpha and beta subunits of MoFe protein. Extensive similarities have been found between *nif K, D,* and *H* genes of *Klebsiella pneumoniae* and those of *Frankia* (Ruvkun and Ausubel, 1980) and these structural genes appear to be contiguous in *Frankia* strain Ar 13 (Simonet *et al.*, 1988), but investigations so far are incomplete.

The location of *nif HDK* genes in fast-growing *Rhizobium* is on large Sym plasmids as one operon. In slow-growing *Bradyrhizobium*, they are borne on the chromosome even though in some species *nif H* is located on a separate operon 13 Kb away from *nif DK* (see Prakash and Atherley, 1986). In *Frankia*, some strains have been tested and *nif D* and *H* appear to be linked. Such a generalization for all *Frankia* strains is still premature (Simonet *et al.*, 1990).

Large plasmids (8 to 190 Kb) have been detected in *Frankia* strains but the information so far generated does not lend itself to any generalization whether *nif* genes are present on smaller plasmids

(14 to 80 Kb) such as Sym plasmids of rhizobia (Simonet *et al.*, 1990), even though plasmid as well as chromosome location of *nif* gene has been reported for a *Frankia* strain (Simonet *et al.*, 1986).

Nod genes are no doubt present in *Frankia* but their isolation and characterization have not yielded conclusive results (Simonet *et al.*, 1990), largely because of the lack of good cloning systems. No phages for *Frankia* have been detected so far and conjugation systems have not been standardized. However, attempts are underway to introduce DNA into *Frankia* through protoplast transformation with plasmid vectors. Different methods of producing *Frankia* protoplasts have been described.

Conclusions

It would be ambitious to think that we can qualify, understand, and quantify the very many complex interactions taking place in a forest ecosystem among plants, microflora, and microfauna. Even though certain symbiotic relationships between plants and some specialized microorganisms in soil have been fairly well understood, much remains to be done in extending this knowledge to other species of the plant kingdom as exemplified by the *Parasponia-Rhizobium* association (Trinick, 1973). There is also room for a greater under-standing of the role of non-symbiotic microorganisms in forest man-agement and of the interactions of mycorrhizae with these nitrogen fixers. An appraisal of microbial inhabitants of nodules and roots other than *Frankia* or rhizobia and their functioning in the operation of symbiotic events is called for since we are now aware that for successful consummation of symbiosis, many helper organisms in soil may be of importance, especially in the pre-penetration stages of the microsymbiont (Knowlton and Dawson, 1983).

There is a well-meant question whether biological nitrogen fixation is economical in the long run in forestry management in comparison with the application of chemical fertilizers. There are many gaps in our knowledge and as Turvey and Smethurst (1983) state, "many of these gaps are filled by common truths which pervade the subject with notions that biologically fixed nitrogen must be a good thing". No doubt the question of economics is not relevant to countries which can afford fertilizer nitrogen towards forest manage-ment. Isotopic measurements are needed to accurately quantify the amount of nitrogen fixed by trees and there is the need to define non-fixing control tree to achieve this objective. Assuming that we have on hand an accurate system to measure the input of biologically fixed nitrogen by forest trees, the transfer of fixed nitrogen to the companion or succeeding vegetation depends on denitrification losses, leaching, volatilization effects, and other factors. It is not easy to measure these effects under diverse ecological conditions. Nevertheless, the benefits in quantitative terms of the overall growth of vegetation succeeding a nodulated tree over the years would certainly provide a useful yardstick to measure the impact of biological nitrogen fixation in forest management. Such a consideration would also take into account the benefits derived by the improvement of soil structure and consequent better root growth. Indeed, the results so far obtained with *Robinia* and *Alnus* stand testimony to the sort of cumulative and long-range benefits offered by litter accumulation in soil followed by mineralization of the organic debris. To make biological nitrogen fixation a potent tool, genetically superior varieties of nitrogen-fixing plants can be evolved to equal the merits offered by chemical fertilizer inputs.

The situation in third world countries is entirely different where fertilizer nitrogen can be spared only to a few cash crops and staple rice and wheat. Management of quick-growing and high-yielding trees for fuel on zero input land is the prime goal of many motivated government as well as privately fostered agencies. Microbial technologies hold great promise in the operation of nurseries of plantation crops in a scientific way by inoculating containers with nitrogen-fixing and phosphate-solubilizing bacteria; if the species is mycorrhizal, proper inoculation with mycorrhizal fungi can help the plants to scavenge a variety of scarce nutrients in soil including phosphorus and also afford protection against root pathogens and drought.

REFERENCES

Akkermans, A.D.L., Hahn, D., and Zoon, F. (1989). Interactions between root symbionts, root pathogens and actinorhizal plants. In *Forest Tree Physiology*. Ed. E. Dreyer Elsevier/INRA, Paris. pp. 764–771.

Aldrich-Blake, R.N. (1932). On the fixation of atmospheric nitrogen by bacteria living symbiotically in root nodules of *Casuarina equisetifolia*. Oxford For. Mem. 14.

Andeke-Lengui, M.A., and Dommergues, Y. (1981). Coastal sand dune stabilization in Senegal. In *Casuarina Ecology Management and Utilization*. Eds. S.R. Midgley, J.W. Turnbull and R.D. Johnson. CSIRO, Melbourne. pp. 158–166.

Aswathappa, N., and Bachelard, E.P. (1986). Ion regulation in the organs of *Casuarina* species differing in salt tolerance. *Austral. J. Plant Physiol.*, 13, 533–545.

Atkinson, G.F. (1892). The genus *Frankia* in the United States. *Bull. Torrey Bot. Club*, 19, 171–177.

Bamber, R.K., Mullette, K., and Mackowski, C. (1980). Mycorrhizal studies. In Research Report 1977–1978 (Forest Communications W.S.W. Sydney). pp. 70–72.

Becking, J.H. (1982). Nitrogen fixation in nodulated plants other than legumes. In *Advances in Agricultural Microbiology*. Ed. N.S. Subba Rao. Oxford and IBH Publixhing Co., New Delhi and Butterworths, London. pp. 89–110.

Benson, D.R. (1982) Isolation of *Frankia* from alder actinorhizal root nodules. *Appl. Environ. Microbiol.,* **44,** 461–465.

Berry, A.M., and Torrey, J.G. (1985). Seed germination, seedling inoculation and establishment of *Alnus* spp. in containers in greenhouse trails. *Plant and Soil,* **87,** 161–173.

Bond, G. (1957). The development and significance of the root nodules of *Casuarina. Ann. Bot.* (Lond.) N.S., **21,** 373–380.

BOSTID (1984). *Casuarinas: Nitrogen-fixing Trees for Adverse Sites.* BOSTID report. National Academy Press, Washington, 1984.

Burris, R.H. (1977). A synthesis paper on non-leguminous N2- fixing systems. In *Recent Developments in Nitrogen Fixation.* Eds. W.E. Newton, J.R. Postgate and C. Rodriguez- Barrueco. Academic Press. London. pp. 487–511.

Burggraff, A.J.P., and Shipton, W.A. (1983). Studies on the growth of *Frankia* isolates in relation to infectivity and nitrogen fixation (acetylene reduction) *Can. J. Bot.* **61,** 2774–2782.

Callaham, D., Del Tredici, P., and Torrey, J.G. (1978). Isolation and cultivation *in vitro* of the actinomycete causing root nodulation in *Comptonia. Science,* **199,** 899–902.

Callaham, D., Newcomb, W., Torrey, J.G., and Peterson, K.L. (1979). Root hair infection of actinomycete-induced root nodule initiation in *Casuarina, Myrica* and *Comptonia. Bot. Gaz.,* **140,** 81–89.

Capellano, A., Dequatre, B., Valla, G., and Moiroud, A. (1987). Root nodule formation by *Penicillium* sp. on *Alnus glutinosa. Plant and Soil,* **104,** 45–51.

Chatarpaul, L., Chakravarty, P., and Subramaniam, P. (1989). Studies in tetrapartite symbioses. I. Role of ecto and endomycorrhizal fungi and *Frankia* on the growth performance of *Alnus incana. Plant and Soil,* **118,** 145–150.

Chaudari, H. (1931). Researcher sur la bacterie des nodosites radicularies du *Casuarina equisitifolia* (Fort.) *Bull. Soc. Bot. France,* **79,** 447–452.

Courier, G., and Garbaye, J. (1981). A propos de la sylviculture des peuplements melanges: Un example de l' effect benefique de l' aune sur la croissance des peupliers. *Rev. Forestiere Francaise,* **33,** 289–292.

Crocker, R.L., and Major, J. (1955). Soil development in relation to vegetation and surface age at Glacier Bay. *J. Ecol.,* **43,** 427–448.

Cromack, K., Delwiche, C., and McNabb, D.H. (1979). Prospects and problems of nitrogen management using symbiotic nitrogen fixers. In *Symbiotic Nitrogen Fixation in the Management of Temperate Forests.* Eds. J.C. Gordon, C.T. Wheeler and D.A. Perry. Forest Res. Lab. Oregon State University, Corvallis, Ore. pp. 210–223.

Daft. M.J., Clelland, D.M., and Gardner, I.C. (1985). Symbiosis with ectomycorrhizas and nitrogen-fixing organisms. *Proc. R. Soc. Edinburgh,* **85B,** 283–298.

Daniere, C., Capellano, A., and Moiroud, A. (1986). Dynamique de l'aazote dans un peuplement naturel d *Alnus incana* (L.) Moench. *Acta Oecol. Plant.,* **7,** 165–175.

Dawson, J.O. (1983). Dinitrogen fixation in forest ecosystems. *Can. J. Microbiol.,* **29,** 979–992.

Dazzo, F.B. and Hubbell, D.H. (1975). Cross-reactive antigens and lectin as determinants of symbiotic specificity in the *Rhizobium*-clover association. *Applied Microbiology*, **30**, 1017–1033.

Diem, H.G., and Dommergues, Y.R. (1988). Isolation, characterization and cultivation of *Frankia*. In *Biological Nitrogen Fixation — Recent Developments.* Ed. N.S. Subba Rao. Oxford and IBH Publishing Co. New Delhi. pp. 227–254.

Diem, H.G., Gauthier, D., and Dommergues, Y. (1982). Isolement et culture *in vitro* d'une souche infective et effective de *Frankia* isolee de nodules de *Casuarina* sp. *C.R. Acad. Sci., Paris*, t **295**, 759–763.

Dixon, R.O.D., and Wheeler, C.T. (1986). *Nitrogen Fixation in Plants*. Blackie and Son Ltd., Glasgow.

Dobritsa, A.V., and Sharaya, L.S. (1985). Gemome identity of different *Nocardia autotrophica* isolates from *Alnus* spp. root nodules and rhizosphere. In *Proc. 6th Intl. Symp. Actinomycetes Biology*. Eds. G. Szabo, S. Biro and M. Goodfellow. Acad. Kiado, Budapest. pp. 735–737.

Domenach, A.M. (1987). Estimation de la fixation symbiotique chez de plantes herbacees et ligneuses: Utilisation et validite de la methode basee sur la mesure d'abondances isotopiques naturelles de l'azote. Ph.D. thesis, Univ. Lyons. 193 pp.

Domenach, A.M., Kurdali, F., and Bardin, R. (1989). Estimation of symbiotic dinitrogen fixation in alder forest by the method based on natural ^{15}N abundance. *Plant and Soil*, **118**, 51–59.

Dommergues, Y.R. (1963). Evaluation du taux de fixation de l' azote dans un sol dunaire reboise en Filao (*Casuarina equisetifolia*) *Agrochem.*, **7**, 335–340.

Duvigneand, P., and Denaeyer-Desmet, S. (1970). Biological cycling of minerals in temperate deciduous Forests. In *Analysis of Temperate Forest Ecosystems*, Ed. D.E. Reichle., Springer Verlag, Berlin. pp. 452–461.

Elkan, G.H. (Ed.) (1987). *Symbiotic Nitrogen Fixation Technology*. Marcel Dekker Inc., New York.

El-Lakany, M.H. (1981). Breeding and improving of Casuarina: A promising multipurpose tree for arid regions of Egypt. In *Casuarina Ecology Management and Utilization*. Eds. S.R. Midgley, J.W. Turnbull and R.D. Johnston. CSIRO, Melbourne. pp. 58–65.

Faure-Raynaud, M., Bonnefoy-Poirier, M.A., and Moiround, A. (1986). Influence of pH acides sur la viabite d'isolats de *Frankia. Plant and Soil*, **96**, 355–375.

Focke, W.O. (1894). *Die Naturlichen Pflanzenfamilien*. Eds. A. Engler and P. Prantl, Teil 111, 3. *Abteilung Rosaceae*. Verlag W Engelmann, Leipzig. pp. 1–61.

Gardner, I.C. (1976). Ultrastructural studies of non-leguminous root nodules. In *Symbiotic Nitrogen Fixation in Plants*. Ed. P.S. Nutman. Cambridge University Press, Cambridge. pp. 485–495.

Gardner, I.C. (1986). Mycorrhizae of actinorhizal plants *MIRCEN J.*, **2**, 47–160.

Gardner, I.C., Clelland, D.M., and Scott, A. (1984). Mycorrhizal improvement in non-leguminous nitrogen-fixing associations with particular reference to *Hippophae rhamnoides* L. *Plant and Soil*, **78**, 189–199.

Gauthier, D., Diem, H.G., and Dommergues, Y. (1983). Preliminary results of research on *Frankia* and endomycorrhizae associated with *Casuarina equisetifolia*. In *Casuarina Ecology Management and Utilization*. Eds. S.J. Midgley, J.W. Turnbull and R.D. Johnston. CSIRO, Melbourne. pp. 211–217.

Hall, R.B., McNabh, H.S., Maynard, C.A., and Green, T.L. (1979). Toward development of optimal *Alnus glutinosa* symbioses. *Bot. Gaz.*, **140**, 120–126.

Harley, J.L., and Smith, S.E. (1983). *Mycorrhizal Symbiosis*. Academic Press, New York.

Horak, V.E. (1963). Pilzokitogische Untersuchungen in der subalpinen stufe (*Picetum subalpinum* and *Rhodoreto vaccinietum*) der Ratischen Alpen. *Milteilungen Schweiz. Anstalt Forsttiche Versuchswesen*, 39, 1–112.

Huss-Dannel, K., Lundquist, P., and Ekblad, A. (1989). Growth and acetylene reduction by intact cells of *Alnus incana* under field conditions. *Plant and Soil*, 118, 61–73.

Janse, J.M. (1897). Les endophytes radicaux de quelques plantes Javanaises. *Ann. d. Jard. bot. d. Buitenzorg*, 14, 53–201.

Johnson, L.A.S. (1982). Notes on Casuarinaceae II. *J. Adelaide Bot. Gardens*, 73–78.

Kamerling, Z. (1915). Overhet voorkomen van wortelknolletjes bij *Casuarina equisetifolia*. *Naturk. Tijdschr. Nederl, India*, 71, 73–75.

Kikuzawa, K., Asai, T., and Fukuchi, M. (1984). Leaf litter production in a plantation of *Alnus inokumae*. *J. Ecol.*, 72, 993–999.

Knowlton, S., and Dawson, J.O. (1983). Effects of *Pseudomonas cepacia* and cultural factors on the nodulation of *Alnus rubra* roots by *Frankia Can. J. Bot.*, 61, 2877–2882.

Knowlton, S., Berry, A., and Torrey, J.G. (1980). Evidence that associated soil bacteria may influence root hair infection of actinorhizal plants by *Frankia*. *Can. J. Microbiol.*, 26, 971–977.

Kondas, S. (1981). Casuarina equisetifolia—A multipurpose cash crop in India. In *Casuarina Ecology Management and Utilization*. Eds. S.R. Midgley, J.W. Turnbell and R.D. Johnston. CSIRO, Melbourne. pp. 66–76.

Lalonde, M. (1979). Techniques and observations of the nitrogen fixing Alnus root nodule symbiosis. In *Recent Advances in Biological Nitrogen Fixation*. Ed. N.S. Subba Rao. Oxford and IBH Publ. Co., New Delhi. pp. 421–444.

Lalonde, M., Knowles, R., and Fortin, J. (1975). Demonstration of the isolation of the non-infective *Alnus crispa* var. *mollis* Fern. nodule endophyte by morphological immunolabelling and whole cell composition studies. *Can. J. Microbiol.*, 21, 1901–1920.

Lawrence, D.B. (1958). Glaciers and vegetation in southeastern Alaska. *Amer. Sci.*, 46, 89–122.

Li, C.Y., Lu, K.C., Trappe, J.M., and Bollen, W.B. (1968). Enzyme systems of alder and Douglas-Fir in relation to infection by *Poria weirii*. In *Biology of Alder*. Ed. J.M. Trappe USDA Forest Service, Portland, Oregon. pp. 241–250.

Marx, D.H. (1975). Role of ectomycorrhizae in the protection of pine from root infection by *Phytophthora cinnamoni*. In *Biology and Control of Soil-borne Plant Pathogens*. Ed. J.W. Bruehl. American Phytopathological Society, Wisconsun.

McLuckie, J. (1923). Studies in symbiosis. IV. The root nodules of *Casuarina cunninghamiana* and their physiological significance. *Proc. Linn. Soc. N.S.W.*, 48, 194–205.

Mejstrick, V., and Benecke, U. (1969). The ectotrophic mycorrhizae of *Alnus viridis* (chaix) DC and their significance in respect to phosphorus uptake. *New Phyto.*, 68, 141–149.

Midgley, S.J., Turnbull, J.W., and Johnson, R.D. (Eds.) (1983). *Casuarina: Ecology, Management and Utilization*. CSIRO, Melbourne.

Miehe, H. (1981) Anatomische Undersuchung der Pilz-symbiose bei *Casuarina equisetifolia*. *Flora*, 111/112, 431–449.

Mikola, P., Uomala, P., and Malkonen, E. (1983). Application of biological nitrogen fixation in European sylviculture. In *Biological Nitrogen Fixation in Forest Ecosystems: Foundations and Applications*. Eds. J.C. Gordon and C.T. Wheeler. Martinus Nijhoff/Dr.W. Junk Publishers, The Hague. pp. 279–294.

Miller, R.E., and Murray, M.D. (1978). The effect of red alder on growth of Douglas-fir. In *Utilization and Management of Alder*. USDA Forest Service General Technical Report PNW-70. pp. 283–306.

Moiround, A., and Capellano, A. (1979). Etude de la dynamique de l'azote a haute altitude fixation (reduction de C_2H_2) per *Alnus viridis* Chair et etude ultrastructurale des nodules. In *Symposium Physiol. Racines et Symbioses*. Ed. A. Riedaccer, INRA-CNRF, Nancy, France. pp. 365–371.

Molina, R. (1979). Pure culture synthesis and host specificity of red alder mycorrhizae. *Can. J. Bot.*, **57**, 1223–1228.

Molina, R. (1981). Ectomycorrhizal specificity in the genus *Alnus*. *Can. J. Bot.*, **59**, 325–334.

Mowry, H. (1933). Symbiotic nitrogen fixation in the genus *Casuarina*. *Soil Sci.* **36**, 409–426.

Narasimhan, M.J. (1918). A preliminary study of root nodules of *Casuarina*. *Indian Forester*, **44**, 265–268.

Newcomb, W., Callaham, D., Torrey, J.G., and Peterson, R.L. (1979). Morphogenesis and fine structure of the actinomycetous endophyte of nitrogen-fixing root nodules of *Comptonia perigrina*. Botanical Gazette. **140**, 522–534.

Newcomb, W., Peterson, R.L., Callaham, D., and Torrey, J.G. (1978). Structure and host actinomycete interactions in developing root nodules of *Comptonia perigrina*. *Can. J. Bot.*, **56**, 502–531.

Normand, P., and Lalonde, M. (1982). Evaluation of *Frankia* strains isolated from provenances of two *Alnus* species. *Can J. Microbiol.* **28**, 1133–1142.

Okon, Y., Kapulnik, Y., and Sarig, S. (1988). Field inoculation studies with *Azospirillum* in Israel. In *Biological Nitrogen Fixation — Recent Developments*. Ed. N.S. Subba Rao. Oxford and IBH Publishing Co., New Delhi. pp. 267–276.

Parker, R.N. (1932). Casuarina root nodules. *Indian Forester*, **58**, 362–364.

Perinet, P., Brouillette, J.G., Fortin, J.A., and Lalonde, M. (1985). Large scale inoculation of actinorhizal plants with Frankia. *Plant and Soil*, **87**, 175–183.

Plass, W.T. (1977). Growth and survival of hardwoods in pine interplanted with European alder. USDA Forest Service Research Paper NE-376.

Powell, C. Li., and Bagyaraj, D.J. (Eds.) (1984). *VA Mycorrhiza*. CRC Press, Florida.

Prakash, R.K., and Atherley, A.G. (1986). Plasmids of *Rhizobium* and their role in symbiotic nitrogen fixation. *Intl. Rev. Cytol.*, **184**, 1.

Quispel, A., and Burggraaf, A.J.P. (1988). Infection, Initiation and structure of actinorhizal nodules. In *Biological Nitrogen Fixation* — Recent Developments. Ed. N.S. Subba Rao, Oxford and IBH Publishing Co., New Delhi. pp 255–281.

Radwan, M.A., Harrington, C.A., and Kraft, J.M. (1984). Litter fall and nutrient returns in red alder stands in Western Washington. *Plant and Soil*, **79**, 343–351.

Rao, K.A. (1923). Casuarina root nodules and nitrogen fixation (preliminary contribution). In *Yearbook of the Madras Agric. Dept. 1923*. pp. 60–67.

Rodriguez-Barrueco, C., and Subramaniam, P. (1988). Host-endophyte specificity in Frankia symbiosis. In *Biological Nitrogen Fixation — Recent Developments* Ed. N.S. Subba Rao. Oxford and IBH Publishing Co., New Delhi. pp. 283–310.

Rodriguez-Barrueco, C., Cervantes, E., Subba Rao, N.S., and Rodriguez Caceres, E. (1991). Growth Promoting effect of *Azosprillum brasilense* on *Casuarina cunninghamiana* Miq. *Plant and Soil*, **129**, 211–213.

Rose, S.L. (1980). Mycorrhizal associations of some actinomycete nodulated nitrogen fixing plants. *Can. J. Bot.*, **58**, 1449–1454.

Rose, S.L., and Trappe, J.M. (1980). Three new endomycorrhizal *Glomus* spp. associated with actinorhizal shrubs. *Mycotaxon*, **10**, 413–420.

Rose, S.L., and Youngberg, C.F. (1981). Tripartite associations in snowbrush (*Ceanothus velutinus*): Effect of vesicular arbuscular mycorrhizae on growth, nodulation and nitrogen fixation. *Can. J. Bot.*, **59**, 34–39.

Russo, R.O. (1980). Evaluating alder endophyte (*Alnus acuminata-Frankia*-mycorrhizae) interactions. I. Acetylene reduction in seedlings inoculated with *Frankia* strain Ar13 and *Glomus intraradices*, under three phosphate levels, *Plant and Soil*, **118**, 151–155.

Ruvkun, G.B., and Ausubel, F.M. (1980) Interspecies homology of nitrogenase genes *Proc. Natl. Acad. Sci. USA*, **77**, 191.

Schwintzer, C.R. (1979). Nitrogen fixation by *Myrica gale* root nodules in a Massachusets watland. *Oecologia*,**43**, 283–294.

Schwintzer, C.R. (1984). Production, decomposition and nitrogen dynamics of *Myrica gale* litter. *Plant and Soil*, **78**, 245–258.

Seidel, K. (1972). Exsudat-effekt der rhizodamnien von *Alnus glutinosa* Gaertner. *Naturwissenshaften*, **69**, 366–367.

Silvester, W.S. (1977). Dinitrogen fixation by plant associations excluding legumes. In *A Treatise on Dinitrogen Fixation. IV. Agronomy and Ecology*. Eds. A.H. Gibson and R.W. Hardy. John Wiley and Sons, New York. pp. 141–190.

Silvester, W.B., Carter, D.A., and Sprent, J.I. (1979). Nitrogen input by *Lupinus* and *Coriaria* in *Pinus radiata* Forest in New Zealand. In *Symbiotic Nitrogen Fixation in the Management of Temperate Forests*. Eds. J.C. Gordon, C.T. Wheeler and D.A. Perry, Forest Research Laboratory, Oregon State University, Corvallis, Oreg. pp. 253–265.

Simonet, P., Haurat, J., Normand, P., Bardin, R., and Moirund, A. (1986). Localization of *nif* genes on a large plasmid in Frankia sp strain ULQ0132105009. *Mol. Gen. Genet.*, **204**–492.

Simonet, P., Normand, P., Hirch, A.M., and Akkermans, D.L. 1990. The genetics of the Frankia-actinorhizal symbiosis. In *Molecular Biology of Symbiotic Nitrogen Fixation*. Ed. P.M. Gresshoff. CRC Press, Florida. pp. 77–109.

Simonet, P., Normand, P., and Bardin, R. (1988). Heterologous hybridization of *Frankia* DNA to *Rhizobium meliloti* and *Klebsiella pneumoniae nif* genes. *FEMS Microbiol. Lett.* **55**, 141.

Stewart, W.D.P., and Bond, G. (1961). The effect of ammonium-nitrogen on fixation of elemental nitrogen in *Alnus* and *Myrica*. *Plant and Soil*, **14**, 347–359.

Stowers, M.D., and J.E. Smith, (1985) Inoculation and production of container-grown red alder seedlings. *Plant and Soil*, **87**, 153–160.

Subba Rao, N.S. (1983). Nitrogen fixing bacteria associated with plantation and orchard plants. *Can. J. Microbiol.*, **29**, 863–886.

Tarrant, R.F. (1961). Stand development and soil fertility in Douglas-fir red alder plantation. *Forest Sci.*, **7**, 238–246.

Tarrant, R.F. (1983). Nitrogen fixation in North American forestry: Research and applications. In *Biological Nitrogen Fixation in Forest Ecosystem: Foundations and Applications* Eds. J.C. Gordon and C.T. Wheeler. Nijhoff/Junk Publ., The Hague. pp. 261–277.

Tarrant, R.F., and Trappe, J.M. (1971). The role of Alnus in improving the forest environment. *Plant and Soil*, special volume, 335–348.

Tien, T., Gaskins, M.H., and Hubbell, D.M. (1979). Plant growth substances produced by *Azospirillum brasilense* and their effect on the growth of pearl millet (*Pennisetum americanum* L.) *Appl. Environ. Microbiol.*, **37**, 219–226.

Torrey, J.G. (1976). Initiation and development of root nodules of *Casuarina* (Casuarinaceae). *Amer. J. Bot.* **63**, 335–344.

Torrey, J.G. (1981). Casuarina: Actinorhizal dinitrogen-fixing tree of the tropics. In *Casuarina Ecology Management and Utilization*. Eds. S.J. Midgley, J.W. Turnbull and R.D. Johnston CSIRO, Melbourne. pp. 193–204.

Torrey, J.G., and Callaham, D. (1979). Early nodule development in *Myrica gale. Bot. Gaz.*, **140**, 110–114.

Trappe, J.M. (1962). Fingus associates of ectotrophic mycorrhizae *Bot. Rev.*, **28**, 538–606.

Trappe, J.M. (1972). Regulation of soil organisms by red alder: A potential biological system for the control of *Poria weirii. Oregon State Univ. Forestry Symp.*, **3**, 35–51.

Trappe, J.M. (1979). Mycorrhiza-nodule-host interrelationship in symbiotic nitrogen fixation: A quest in need of questers. In *Symbiotic Nitrogen Fixation in the Management of Temperate Forests*. Eds. J.C. Gordon, C.T. Wheeler and D.A. Perry. Oregon State University. Corvallis, Ore. pp. 276–287.

Trinick, M.J. (1973). Symbiosis between *Rhizobium* and the non-legume *Trema (Parasponia) aspera Nature*, London, **244**, 459–460.

Turvey, N.D., and Smethurst, P.J. (1983). Nitrogen fixing plants in forestry management. In *Biological Nitrogen Fixation in Forest Ecosystems: Foundations and Applications*. Eds. J.C. Gordon and C.T. Wheeler. Dr. W. Junk Publishers. The Hague. pp. 232–259.

Uemura, S. (1964). Isolation and properties of microorganisms from root nodules of non-leguminous plants. A review with extensive bibliography. Bull. Govt. Forest Exp. Stn. No. 167, Tokyo.

Van Den Bosch, K.A., and Torrey, J.G. (1983). Host endophyte interactions in effective and ineffective nodules induced by endophytes of *Myrica gale, Can. J. Bot.*, **61**, 2898–2909.

Van Dijk, C. (1978). Spore formation and endophyte diversity in root nodules of *Alnus glutinosa* (L.) Vill. *New Phytol.*, **81**, 601–615.

Wallis, G.W., and Reynolds, G. (1962). Inoculation of Douglas-fir roots with *Poria weirii. Can. J. Bot.*, **40**, 637–645.

Wallis, G.W., and Reynolds, G. (1965). The initiation and spread of *Poria weirii* root rot on Douglas-fir. *Can. J. Bot.*, **43**, 1–9.

Willis, J.C. (1973). *A Dictionary of the Flowering Plants and Ferns*, 8th Ed. (Revised by H.K. Airy Shaw). Cambridge University Press, Cambridge.

Zak, B. (1964). Role of mycorrhizae in root disease. *Annu. Rev. Phytopathol.*, **2**, 377–392.

Zhang, Z., and Torrey, J.G. (1985). Studies of an effective strain of Frankia from *Allocasuarina lehmanniana* of the casuarinaceae. *Plant and Soil*, **87**, 1–16.

Zang, Z., Lopez, M.F., and Torrey. J.G. (1984). A comparison of cultural characteristics and infectivity of *Frankia* isolates from root nodules of *Casuarina* species. *Plant and Soil*, **78**, 79–90.

13

Outlook for the Future

Industrial nitrogen fixation is heavily dependent on energy derived from fossil fuel which is getting depleted at a very fast rate. On the contrary, biological nitrogen fixation requiring approximately half the quantum of energy needed for industrial fixation is dependent on energy from renewable resources such as products of photosynthesis and organic matter in soil. In recent years, several possibilities have been examined to augment the benefits of this unique process of biological nitrogen fixation.

The Key to Specificity of Nitrogen-fixing Microorganisms to Selected Plants

Bacteria of the genus *Rhizobium* are very selective in choosing roots of particular legume species to infect, invade, and form root nodules. For instance, *R. trifolii* can only infect roots of clover but not the roots of soybean and the reverse is also true. It is not clear how the recognition of bacteria and host roots takes place. Of late, a plant protein called 'trifoliin', which is a lectin, has been isolated from the roots of clover. Plant lectins are carbohydrate-binding proteins which can agglutinate cells (Fig. 20). It has been shown that the attachment of *R. trifolii* to clover root hairs is inhibited by 2-deoxyglucose, which indicates that carbohydrate-binding receptor sites are involved. This lectin can be removed from root surface of clovers by solutions containing 2-deoxyglucose. Therefore, it has been suggested that a lectin may be involved in the recognition process. In fact, trifoliin has been shown to agglutinate 34 strains of *R. trifolii*, but not strains of other species of *Rhizobium*. Immunofluorescence techniques have confirmed that trifoliin is actually present on root surfaces of clovers

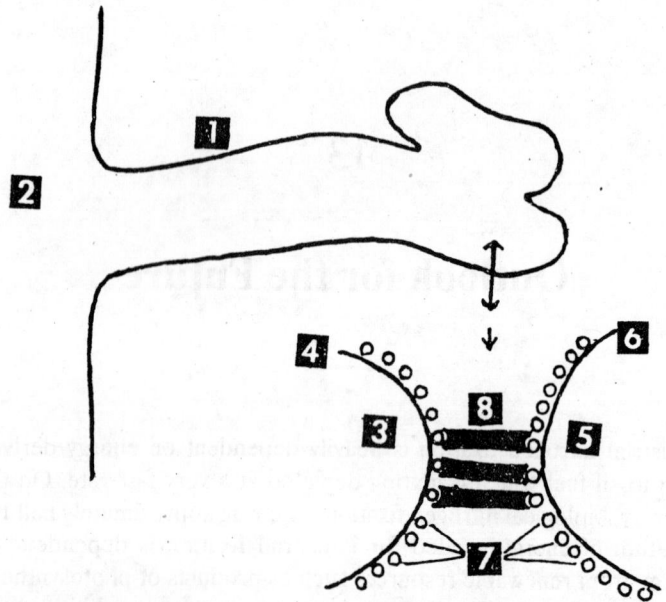

Fig. 20. Lectin (trifoliin — mediated binding of *Rhizobium trifolii* cells to the wall of
root hair of clover seedling — (1) enlarged diagram of a root hair of clover
seedlings; (2) root cortex; (3) root hair cell interior; (4) root hair cell wall;
(5) interior of *R. trifolii* cell; (6) *Rhizobium* cell wall; (7) cross-reactive antigens, one
of which is carbohydrate receptor on bacterial cell wall; (8) clover lectin, trifoliin
(Not to scale. Modified from Dazzo and Hubbell, 1975).

but not on roots of other representative legumes (Bohlool and
Schmidt, 1974; Dazzo and Brill, 1977; Bauer and Bhuvaneswari,
1979).

Researches on lectins may lead to breaking cross-inoculation
barriers in legumes. Eventually, It may be possible that *Rhizobium*
inoculants can be prepared with one efficient strain of *Rhizobium* for
all leguminous crops. It is not unlikely that lectins specific for a given
legume-*Rhizobium* attachment may be responsible for increasing sites
for nodulation on roots when preparations of such lectins are added
to seed inoculants.

Can Other Non-nitrogen-fixing Microorganisms Acquire the Property of Nitrogen Fixation?

Some of the recent major advances relate to a greater understanding of the genes controlling nitrogen fixation and assimilation.

The entire *nif* gene cluster in *K. pneumoniae* has now been sequenced and appears to contain 21 genes. It has served as a model for the analyses of *nif* genes in other nitrogen-fixing bacteria such as *Azotobacter, Azospirillum, Rhizobium, Enterobacter,* cyanobacteria, and *Frankia*. From the present knowledge on the *nif* cluster of genes in nitrogen-fixing microorganisms, it has been concluded that the basic genes are common to all of them and are highly conserved in nature.

In many nitrogen-fixing microorganisms, extrachromosomal genetic elements known as plasmids have also been shown to contain genes involved in N_2 fixation. They have been characterized in species of *Azospirillum, Azotobacter,* and *Rhizobium*. In *R. meliloti, R. leguminosarum,* and *Bradyrhizobium japonicum,* these plasmids are big and are known as megaplasmids and are known to carry Sym (symbiosis), *nod* (nodulation), and *nif* genes. Besides the plasmids, the *Rhizobium* cell has a single molecule of chromosomal DNA. However, the question whether all or part of the genes responsible for legume symbiosis are located on the rhizobial chromosomes or extra-chromosomal plasmids has not been entirely resolved since there have been reports that certain mutants of *R. meliloti* are known to have nitrogen-fixation genes on the chromosome (Evans *et al.*, 1985; Bothe *et al.*, 1988; Postgate, 1989).

One remarkable recent observation is that some of the genes necessary for nodulation (as many as 15 genes for nodulation have been characterized) are barely expressed by some *Rhizobium* species in a free-living condition. However, some of these genes can be induced to express by root exudate compounds coming from the host's metabolism. A group of common nodulation genes (*nod ABC*) have been identified in all *Rhizobium* and *Bradyrhizobium* species so far investigated. These gene products, one of which has been recently identified as 'Nod Rm^1' factor, is a sulphated and acylated gluco-samine oligosaccharide. This product specifically elicits root hair deformation in *R. meliloti*-alfalfa interaction. In lucerne (*Medicago sativa*) root exudate, the inducing compound is a flavone called 'luteolin'. The *nif D* gene in *Rhizobium* interacts with the flavonoid compounds secreted by the root. This interaction activates *nod ABC* genes involved in root hair curling. In this way, the two symbionts appear to signal to each other at the molecular level (Fig 21). Many different types of flavonoid compounds have been identified in root exudates of clover and soybean. There are two types of flavonoid compounds, some of which induce nodulation and others suppress it.

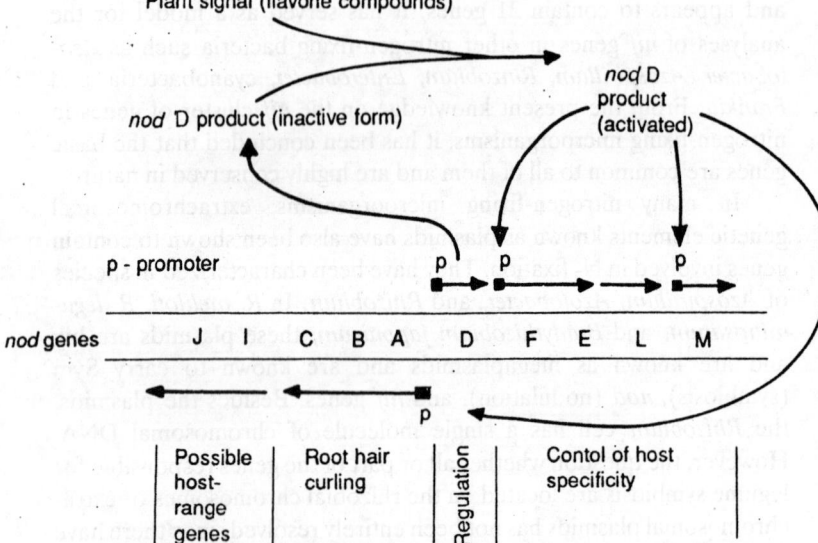

Fig. 21. A schematic diagram of events at the molecular level at the root region in *Rhizobium*-legume interaction. The protein product of *nod D* gene in *Rhizobium* is activated by contact with plant signal by way of flavonoid compounds. This then interacts on the promotor gene which controls *nod ABC* genes action to induce nodule formation.

It is believed that a critical balance of the inducer and anti-inducers is needed for successful nodulation. Other host gene-controlled proteins (about 100 of them) have been shown to regulate nodule functions. They are collectively known as nodulins. Leghaemoglobin, the red pigment in nodules which regulates the oxygen supply to nodules, is a nodulin. Other examples of nodulins are the enzymes uricase and glutamine synthetase which regulate translocation of ammonia from the nodule (Evans *et al.*, 1985; Bothe *et al.*, 1988).

Can We Evolve Nitrogen-fixing Plants?

Nitrogen-fixing nodulated plants are now confined to those species of leguminoseae which bear nodules and to members of diverse families of the plant kingdom whose root nodules are inhabited by species of actinomycetes tentatively classified under the genus *Frankia*. These nodulated plants are nearly self-sufficient with regard to their nitrogen nutrition and therefore a question has been posed whether it is possible to convert as many other land plants as possible into nitrogen fixers, more particularly cereals, so as to harness atmospheric nitrogen to a greater degree. In other words, can the *nif* genes from nitrogen-fixing microorganisms be transferred to a higher plant? This involves the nuclear recombination between a prokaryote and a eukaryote which poses a host of problems including compatibility of genomes. Nevertheless, through molecular cloning techniques, certain possibilities or strategies have been outlined.

Agrobacterium tumefaciens (crown gall bacterium) is a common soil bacterium. It infects dicotyledonous plants and forms cancerous outgrowths (tumours). This bacterium harbours a large plasmid Ti which is responsible for the formation of the tumour. A segment of the Ti plasmid which carries the genetic information for tumour gets implanted in the host cell genome and thus gets replicated. Therefore, once initiated, the crown gall can go on indefinitely without the need for fresh *A. tumefaciens* infection. This is possible because the tumour inducing principle in Ti plasmid genes is transferred from a bacterium to a higher plant. Here is an instance of how nature has overcome genetic barriers between a lower plant (prokaryote) and a higher plant (eukaryote). It has been envisaged that *nif* genes could be transferred to a Ti plasmid by molecular cloning and the latter used as a vehicle to implant *nif* genes into higher plants (Ausubel, 1979).

Other possible vehicles for molecular cloning of *nif* genes are plant viruses like cauliflower mosaic virus DNA (Hull and Howell, 1978) and chloroplast DNA. Of the two, the chloroplast approach is likely to offer least resistance. The strategy is to construct bacterial plasmids carrying *nif* genes and integrate them into chloroplasts. Later, the *nif* chloroplast plasmid is introduced into isolated chloroplasts. This is followed by introduction of 'transformed' chloroplasts into isolated plant protoplasts (Bedbrook and Bogorad, 1976).

Uptake of nitrogen-fixing bacteria and blue-green algae into higher plant protoplasts has been attempted as a possible method of modifying higher plants cells to fix nitrogen. In a similar way, cells and tissues of plants have been shown to take up nitrogen-fixing bacteria. Regeneration of such calluses into intact plants capable of fixing nitrogen is a distinct possibility although not seriously attempted up to seedling stage in recent years (Holsten *et al.*, 1971; Davey and Cocking, 1972; Ranga Rao and Subba Rao, 1976). Cells of *Azotobacter vinelandii* have been intgrated into the mycelium of *Rhizopogon*, a mycorrhizal fungus on roots of pine (Giles and Whitehead,

1976). If this approach is successful, then we can have nitrogen-fixing mycorrhizal roots.

Recently, novel approaches to breaking the cell wall barrier in root hairs of white clover (*Trifolium repens*) by treating seedlings with cellulase and pectolyase followed by treatment with polyethylene glycol (PEG) and calcium chloride have been successful. By these treatments, the protoplasts of root hairs were exposed for reception to rhizobia which normally do not invade white clover root hairs due to the cell wall barrier. For instance, *R. loti*, which can only infect species of *Lotus*, was able to enter the root hairs of white clover and cause nodules under axenic experimental conditions. The success of this experiment depended on the critical levels and combinations of cellulase, pectinase, and PEG. In fact nodules on white clover roots induced by heterologous *R. loti* fixed nitrogen, were pink in colour, and were comparable to nodules normally induced by *R. metiloti*, a homologous *Rhizobium* (see Cocking *et al.*, 1990).

Similary, pretreatment of seedlings of rice (*Oryza sativa*) and wheat (*Triticum aestivum*), both monocots, also resulted in root nodulation when they were inoculated with *R. trifolii* or *R. loti* or their mixture. The nodules were structurally sparsely infected and exhibited feeble nitrogenase activity (see Cocking *et al.*, 1990).

Nodulation of rape seedlings (*Brassica napus*) by *R. leguminosarum* and *Bradyrhizobium* has also been observed by following similar procedures adopted for rice. Interestingly *nod*+ strain of *R. leguminosarum* induced nodules on a variety of rape but no such response was seen on inoculation with *nod*− strain. The nodules had ultrastructural details similar to normal nodules and exhibited respectable amount of nitrogenase activity (see Cocking *et al.*, 1990).

What appears to be intriguing is the formation of nodules on the roots of rape seedlings even without enzyme and PEG treatment when inoculated with *R. Parasponium*, a strain which produces nodules on roots of a non-leguminous tree genus, *Parasponia*. Unlike temperate legumes such as clovers which are normally infected by rhizobia through root hairs, infection in tropical *Parasponia* and other genera such as *Aeschynomene, Sesbania,* and *Stylosanthes* is through wounds and points of lateral root emergence. While explaining these observations, due cognizance of different modes of entry of rhizobia have to be taken into consideration. As Cocking *et al.,* (1990) say, these researches 'may have important consequences for both basic and applied aspects of nitrogen fixation'.

Exploiting Other Plant-Microorganisms Associations

Blue-green algae are known to form a variety of symbioses in bryophytes, pteridophytes, and angiosperms. *Nostoc punctiforme* is an endophyte in glands or nodules of *Gunnera* (Silvester and Smith, 1969). Within the cells, there is a 10-fold increase in heterocyst frequency and hence ability to fix molecular nitrogen. Many plants of cycadeae are known to harbour *Nostoc* sp. in their coralloid roots. Leaf nodules of some members of the family Rubiaceae contain *Klebsiella* sp. It is imperative that we should exploit these already existing symbioses for the benefit of mankind (Table 46).

Table 46: Hitherto less emphasized plant-microorganism symbioses which can be exploited to greater degree in future

Higher plant	*Microorganism*
Anthoceros	*Nostoc* sp.
Blasia, Clavicularia	*N. sphaericum*
Sphagnum	*Hapalosiphon* sp.
Cycas, Encephalartos, Zamia,	*Nostoc* sp.
Ceratozamia, Macrozamia,	
Stangeria, Gunnera	
Tree legumes	*Bradyrhizobium* sp.
Pavetta, Chomelia, Psychotria, Dioscorea,	*Klebsiella* sp.
Calluna vulgaris, Neottia nidusavis	

Proper Utilization of Fertilizer Nitrogen by Means of Slow-release Nitrogen Fertilizer and Nitrification Inhibitors

Slow-release nitrogen fertilizers and nitrification inhibitors are sold as urea-form, isobutylidenediurea (IBDU), and sulphur-coated urea. Urea-form or urea formaldehyde fertilizer contains at least 35 per cent N largely in a slowly soluble form. In soil, it undergoes mineralization gradually and thus nitrogen is made available to plants evenly over the entire growth period.

Isobutylidenediurea is a condensation product of urea and isobutyraldehyde in a 2:1 ratio containing 31.8 per cent N and the product is mixed with fertilizers. It is sparingly soluble. Experiments in India have shown that a mixture of urea and IBDU is superior to urea alone in rice cultivation.

Certain chemicals which are made in Japan inhibit the nitrification processes in soil. They are 2-chloro-6-(trichloromethyl)-pyridine (trade name N-serve) and 2-amino-4-chloro-6-methylpyridine (trade name AM), which have been field tested in India and abroad. These chemicals inhibit the nitrification of fertilizer nitrogen and reduce nitrogen losses (Prasad et al., 1971). It is necessary to popularize the above-mentioned fertilizers by marketing them inexpensively. There are also many other materials made in India which are helpful in conserving fertilizer nitrogen. They are lac-coated urea, neem cake-coated urea, and coal acids. The Indian Lac Research Institute, Ranchi, has developed lac-coated urea containing 33 per cent N. The product comes in the form of brown prills. Neem cake-coated urea is obtained by mixing 1 kg coaltar, 2 liter kerosene, and 100 kg urea and 10–15 kg neem cake. Recovery of urea in rice cultivation can be substantially increased by mixing or coating urea with sulphur or neem cake obtained from seeds of *Azadarichta indica* (Table 47). Alternately, solid fertilizers may be blended with powdered cake or treated with acetone extract of the neem cake. The Central Fuel Research Institute, Dhanbad, is making organic fertilizers and other products which can work as nitrification inhibitors. Claims have also made on inhibition of urea hydrolysis to reduce losses due to volatilization of ammonia. Such inhibitors (e.g., pyridine-3-sulphonic acid, desthiobiotin) ought to be tested on a large scale and their economic feasibility understood (Prasad et al., 1971).

Table 47: Influence of rates and sources of nitrogen on the apparent recovery (%) of applied nitrogen

Treatment	1974	1975	Mean
Rates of N (kg/ha)			
50	20.0	27.0	23.5
100	26.7	29.3	28.0
150	31.2	31.8	31.5
200	27.4	28.6	28.0
Sources of N (100 kg N/ha)			
Urea	26.7	29.3	28.0
Sulphur-coated urea	32.5	42.9	37.7
Urea treated with Nitrapyrin	38.0	45.4	41.7
Urea mixed with neem cake	38.3	38.6	38.5
Urea coated with neem cake	46.1	48.6	47.4

Source: Sharma and Prasad, 1980.

Domestication and Cultivation of Promising Nodulated Legume Species

There is an obvious need for worldwide use of some of the following less-known legumes which are at present grown in areas where they have been known traditionally (National Academy of Sciences, 1979).

Yam bean (*Pachyrhizus erosus; P. tuberosus*) produces brown tubers and is widely grown in Mexico, the Philippines and Indoneisa, yielding 40–90 t/ha, The tuber is safe to eat but the remainder of the plant can be toxic to humans.

African yam bean (*Sphanostylis stenocarpa*) is an important crop of Western Africa. The underground tubers (rich in protein) and seeds are edible. The yield potential is 1,860 kg/ha.

Winged bean (*Psophocarpus tetragonolobus*) is a native of New Guinea and South east Asia. The protein content of tubers of this legume is approximately 20 per cent. It has a yield potential of over 11,000 kg/ha.

Wild mung (*Vigna vexillata*) grows wildly in the Himalayas and hills of eastern and northeastern India (1200–1500 m altitude) and is eaten by tribesmen (Chandel *et al.*, 1972). Other tuber-bearing species of *Vigna* which are eaten by tribesmen around the world which need further investigation are *V. lanceolata, V. lobatifolia, V. marina, V. ambacensis, V. fischeri,* and *V. reticulata.*

Soh-phlong (*Moghania vestita* or *Flemingia vestita*) is grown at altitudes of 1500 m and 1800 m in the Himalayan region. Its juicy tubers are much sought after in Meghalaya where a yield of 3000 kg/ha has been reported (Singh and Arora, 1973).

The prairie turnip (*Psoralea esculenta*) was a delicacy of North American tribesmen and needs to be domesticated. Two species of *Psoralea* grown in arid conditions in Central Australia bear edible tubers — *P. patens* and *P. cinerea.*

Indian potato (*Apios americana*), a north American native plant which produces tasty tubers, needs more consideration along with related species *A. priceana* and *A. fortunei.*

Other legumes with edible tubers which deserve domestication are *Periandra mediterranea, Phaseolus adenanthus, P. coccineus, P. heterophyllus, Pueraria lobata, P. phaseoloides,* and *P. tuberosa.*

Bambara groundnut (*Voandzeia subterranea*), is cultivated all over Africa. It resembles the groundnut plant in its growth habit and is suited to hot dry regions with poor soil.

Jack bean and sword bean (*Canavalia ensiformis* and *C. gladiata*) are widely consumed in Asia, can withstand drought, and are resistant to pests. The yields are fairly good (800–1000 kg/ha of seed). The vegetation (40–50 t/ha) serves as both a cover crop and an animal feed. The beans exhibit toxicity to humans and hence more research is needed to avoid toxic factors.

Lablab bean (*Dolichos lablab* or *Lablab purpurea* or *L. niger*) is very commonly grown in India with many cultivars in different regions. It provides not only food for human beings but also forage for animals. It is highly adaptable and hence needs intense research under diverse conditions (Joshi, 1971).

Marama bean (*Tylosoma esculentum* or *Bauhinia esculenta*), a native of Africa capable of tolerating extreme arid conditions, produces both tubers and seeds which are edible.

Moth bean (*Vigna aconitifolia*) is one of the most drought-tolerant edible leguminous crops of India and is mainly grown in Rajasthan. The crop requires little care.

Rice bean (*V. umbellata*) is an important crop in tribal areas of northern India and is grown in fallow rice fields. It can withstand the hottest climates and is drought resistant. However, the seeds contain toxic cyanogenic compounds and hence are eaten only after boiling (Chaudhuri and Prasad, 1973).

Tarwi (*Lupinus mutabilis* or *L. tauris*), a legume of South America (Peru), can fix 400 kg N/ha and produces protein-rich seeds. However, the toxic alkaloids in seed prevent its wider use.

Terpary bean (*Phaseolus acutifolius*) thrives well in Mexico, Guatemala, and the United States and can withstand arid situations. It has a good amount of protein in its seeds.

Tropical lima bean (*Phaseolus lunatus* or *P. limensis* or *P. inamoenus*) is suited to humid lowland tropical conditions. It is widely eaten but contains toxic compounds. Hence, the seeds must be thoroughly boiled before eating.

Ye-eb (*Cordeauxia edulis*) is a local bushy, semi-desertic plant (Somalia/Ethiopia) and produces a tasty nut.

Non-biological Systems

There has been no substitute for the Haber-Bosch method of ammonia production but the possibility of developing some novel non-biological systems for the reduction of N_2 to NH_3 which can be carried out at normal temperature and pressure are being examined. Such reactions are catalysed by model reductants (e.g., molybdothiol reductant). Alternatively, N_2-enriched gas is reduced to ammonia by means of a water-soluble catalyst contained in a selectively permeable membrane. Such innovations are designed to be installed *in situ* on the farm in the irrigation stream (Hardy *et al.*, 1975).

Recycling of Wastes for Nitrogen

Although collection, transportation, availability, and storage of wastes of agricultural products and urban refuse pose several problems including those relating to economic and social considerations, it is necessary to bear in mind that this vast perennial resource can yield some of the much-required plant nutrients through properly managed composting (Table 48).

Table 48: Wastes of plant and animal origin which offer potential resources for organic recycling in India (from various sources)

Type of material	Quantity (tons, approximate)	Nitrogen (%) (approximate)
Animal dung	778,000,000	0.4
Animal urine	450,000,000	0.8
Animal blood meal	60,000	10.0
Animal carcasses	15,000	10.0
Raw bones	500,000	3.0
Slaughterhouse waste	5,000	10.0
Crop residues	204,000,000	0.5
Bagasse, pressmud (sugarcane industry by-products)	300,000	0.25
Human faeces	29,000,000	1.3
Human urine	263,000,000	1.0
Urban compost	11,000,000	0.8

Nitrogen being a primary nutrient in agricultural production, management of soils for conserving this precious input calls for all-round effort by soil scientists, microbiologists, geneticists, molecular biologists, and physiologists to chalk out both short-term and long-term strategies to augment fixation of atmospheric nitrogen.

Plant Growth-promoting Rhizobacteria

The term 'rhizobacteria' describes the ability of certain bacteria to colonize the rhizosphere aggressively. *Pseudomonas* spp. are receiving worldwide attention under the broad general category known as plant growth-promoting bacteria (PGPR). The bacteria exhibit fluorescence under ultraviolet light and hence are also known as fluorescent pseudomonads. Initial observations were based on the ability of *P. fluorescence* and *P. putida* to improve the growth of potatoes when applied to potato seed pieces. Subsequent field studies have revealed that these species and similar bacteria increased the yield of potato (5.33 per cent), sugarbeet (4 to 8 t/ha), and radish (6 to

144 per cent of root weight) (Kloepper *et al.*, 1980a, 1980b; Schippers *et al.*, 1987; Weller, 1988).

Soil-borne pathogens may be distinguished as major and minor ones. The major pathogens include the well-known *Phytophthora* and *Fusarium* causing root rots and vascular wilts. The minor pathogens cause damage to young tissues of roots with no visual symptoms. The minor pathogens also include, according to recent thinking, certain non-parasitizing deleterious rhizosphere microorganisms (DRMO) which include deleterious rhizobacteria and deleterious rhizofungi. Some soils are conducive to soil-borne diseases, whereas others suppress diseases. The reasons behind these observations may lie in the soil structure or microbial composition (Schippers *et al.*, 1987; Weller, 1988).

Many genera of soil bacteria have shown great potential as biocontrol agents operating not merely by secreting antibiotics but also by other mechanisms. These genera include *Actinoplanes, Agrobacterium, Amarphosporangium, Arthrobacter, Cellulomonas, Bacillus, Azotobacter, Enterobacter, Erwinia, Flavobacterium, Micromonospora, Rhizobium, Bradyrhizobium, Serratia, Streptomyces,* and *Xanthomonas*. *Agrobacterium radiobacter* strain 84 is an excellent example of a biocontrol agent controlling crown gall disease caused by *A. tumefaciens*. *Bacillus subtilis*, capable of producing endospores and tolerant of heat, can suppress major and minor soil-borne diseases of carrots, oats, and groundnut (Baker and Cook, 1974; Kerr, 1982).

In the Netherlands, it has been shown that the frequency of potato cultivation in the same field has a bearing on the yield of potato tubers. When the crop was grown in the same field every third year, yields were reduced by 10–15 per cent from what would be expected if the crop were grown once in six years. The severity of decline in yield appeared to be progressive so that yield decrease reached 30 per cent if potato was cropped continuously in the field. Fluorescent pseudomonads are believed to improve the growth of plants by colonizing the root region aggressively and thus preempt the establishment of DRMO on roots, especially those which produce growth-inhibiting cyanide. No such growth promotion was possible in plots where no potato was cultivated probably due to the absence of factors which stimulated the production of toxic substances. Fluorescent pseudomonads have been shown to suppress major plant pathogens like the take-all, a root disease of wheat caused by *Gaeumannomyces graminis* var. *tritici*, by 11–17 per cent (Schippers *et al.*, 1987; Weller, 1988).

About 10 per cent of bacteria in the rhizosphere appear to be aggressive in reducing the population of DRMOs and there appears to be no relationship between *in vitro* inhibition and *in vivo* suppression effects. The field benefits are dependent on soil temperature, pH, moisture, and clay content, which influence the survival of PGPRs in the rhizosphere. This ecological competence may diminish by repeated sub-culturing *in vitro*, possibly related to loss of cell surface structure or reduction in antibiotic and siderophore production as explained below (Weller, 1988).

Three possible mechanisms have been suggested to explain the beneficial effects of PGPRs in enhancing production: competition for substrate and niche exclusion, siderophore production, and antibiotics. However, more than one mechanism may operate for mediating a biological control. Fluorescent pseudomonads 'mop up' nutrients in the rhizosphere because of their versatility in growth and nutrient absorption (Kloepper *et al.*, 1980a, 1980b). The points of emergence of lateral roots are favourite spots for deleterious rhizobacteria and PGPRs appear to compete for these spots very effectively. Siderophores are low molecular weight (500–1000 daltons), high affinity iron chelators that transport iron into bacterial cells. Fluorescent pseudomonads produce yellow-green, fluorescent siderophores which specifically recognize and sequester the limited supply of iron in the rhizosphere and thereby reduce the availability of this trace element for the growth of the pathogen. The availability of iron in soil decreases with increase in pH and therefore PGPRs function better in neutral and alkaline soils than in acid soils. The demonstration that siderophores minus mutants are less suppressive to pathogens in the rhizosphere than parental strains appears to evince the role of siderophores in pathogen suppression. As stated earlier, an example of the involvement of antibiotics is the role of Agrocin-84 produced by *Agrobacterium radiobacter* in controlling the crown gall symptoms of plants caused by *A. tumefaciciens*. The phenazin-type antibiotic produced by *Pseudomonas fluorescence* in the control of take-all disease of wheat has also been cited as an example.

Siderophore Production in the Rhizosphere

Many microorganisms respond to a fall in the availability of iron in soil by producing siderophores, which selectively complex with iron and supply it to the living cell. Siderophores also act as growth factors and/or antibiotics. Several investigations have shown that fluorescent pseudomonads in the rhizosphere produce yellow-green fluorescent pigment. Some strains, particularly B10, inhibit the growth of *Erwinia carotovora*, which causes the soft rot disease of potato. In the presence of iron, no beneficial effect of *Pseudomonas* inoculation was observed when the soil was amended with iron in the form of FeEDTA (Ethylenediaminetetra-acetatoferrate) in spite of effective colonization in the rhizosphere. A yellow-green pigment called 'pseudobactin' isolated from this fluorescent pseudomonad also did not exhibit beneficial effect when iron was sequestered (bound) in the form of 'red brown ferric pseudobactin', whereas pseudobactin by itself was effective. These results imply that the siderophore pseudobactin deprived *E. caratovora* of iron by scavenging the available element in the vicinity and thus reduced disease severity by minimizing the virulence of the pathogen (Leong, 1986).

In California, when FeEDTA was added to a *Fusarium*-suppressive soil where no inoculation was done to flax seedlings with the pathogen *F. oxysporum* f. sp. *lini*, 90 per cent of the seedlings survived. On the other hand, in the same suppressive soil with the pathogen in the presence of FeEDTA, only 47 per cent of the seedlings survived. However, the presence of the pathogen alone in the same soil resulted in the survival of only 47 per cent seedlings. These results reflect the possibility that microorganisms present in the soil produce siderophores which have the affinity for the limited available iron in the root milieu and thus deprive the pathogen of this vital element.

A similar experiment carried out in pathogen-conducive soil also proved that sequestering the limited iron was the reason behind the reduction in the severity of the disease. The experiment involved the addition of strain B10 of *Pseudomonas* sp. or siderophore pseudobactin to a pathogen-conducive soil infested with *F. oxysporum* f. sp. *lini* and growing flax seedlings. Pseudobactin is a linear hexapeptide requiring at least five gene clusters with a minimum of five genes for its biosynthesis. The addition of the PGPR or its siderophore pseudobactin increased the survival of flax seedlings to 87 to 90 per cent, whereas other treatments where ferric pseudobactin or FeEDTA plus *Pseudomonas* sp. strain B10 were added brought down seedling survival to 48 to 50 per cent. Similar results were also obtained with the take-all disease of wheat caused by *Gaeumannomyces graminis* var. *triticis* by the addition of *Pseudomonas* sp. strain B10. Some of these results obtained with either *Pseudomonas* or siderophores with and without EDTA have been summarized in Table 49.

Table 49: The influence of *Pseudomonas* sp. strain B10 or its siderophore with or without FeEDTA on the intersity of wilt of flax incited by *F. oxysporum* f. sp. *lini* or take-all disease of wheat incited by *Gaeumannomyces graminis* in disease-suppressive or disease-conducive soils of California
(summary of data from Leong, 1986)

Soil	Pathogen	Treatment	Per cent of seedling survival	
			Flax	Barley
Disease-suppressive	Present	H20	82	83
	Present	50 μm FeEDTA	47	38
	Absent	50 μm FeEDTA	90	85
Disease-conducive	Present	H20	48	27
	Present	50 μm FeEDTA	52	25
	Absent	50 μm FeEDTA	92	87
	Present	Strain B10	87	88
	Present	Strain B10 + 50 μm FeEDTA	48	25
	Present	50 μm pseudobactin (siderophore)	90	73
	Present	50 μm ferric pseudobactin	50	20

REFERENCES

Ausubel, F.M. (1979). Application of recombinant DNA technology to the study of nitrogen fixation, In *Recent Advances in Biological Nitrogen Fixation*. Ed N.S. Subba Rao. Oxford & IBH Publishing Co. Pvt. Ltd., New Delhi. pp. 257–280.

Baker, K.F., and Cook, R.J. (1974). *Biological Control of Plant Pathogens*. W.H. Freeman and Co., San Francisco.

Bauer, W.D., and Bhuvaneswari, T.V. (1979). The possible role of lectin in legume *Rhizobium* symbiosis and other plant microorganism interactions. In *Recent Advances in Biological Nitrogen Fixation*. Ed. N.S. Subba Rao. Oxford & IBH Publishing Co. Pvt. Ltd., New Delhi. pp. 244–279.

Bedbrook, J.R., and Bogorad, L. (1976). Endonuclease recognition sites mapped on *Zea mays* chloroplast DNA, *Proc. Natl. Acad. Sci.,* USA. **73**, 4309–4313.

Bohlool, B.B., and Schmidt, E.L. (1974). Lectins: A possible basis for specificity in *Rhizobium*-legume root nodule symbiosis. *Science,* **185**, 269–271.

Bothe, H., de Bruijn, F.J., and Newton, W.E. (Eds.) (1988). *Nitrogen Fixation: Hundred Years After,* Gustav Fischer, Stuttgart.

Chandel, K.P.S., Arora, R.K., and Joshi, B.S. (1972). *Vigna capensis* Walp (*V. vexillata*) —An edible root legume. *Curr.Sci.,* **41**, 537.

Chaudhuri, A.P., and Prasad, B. (1973). Grow rice bean —An excellent fodder legume for the scarcity period. *Indian Farmers Digest,* **6**, 27–30.

Cocking, E.C., Al-Mallah, M.K., Benson, E., and Davey, M.R. (1990). Nodulation of non-legumes by rhizodia. In *Nitrogen Fixation: Achievements and Objectives.* Eds. P.M., Greshoff, L.E., Roth, G., Stacey, and W.E. Newton, Chapman and Hall, New York. pp. 813–823.

Davey, M.R., and Cocking, E.C. (1972). Uptake of bacteria by isolated higher plant protoplasts, *Nature,* **239**, 455–456.

Dazzo, F.P., and Brill, W.J. (1977). Receptor site on clover and alfalfa for *Rhizobium*. *Appl. Environ. Microbiol.*, **33**, 132–136.

Evans, H.J., Bottomley, P.J., and Newton, W.E. (Eds.) (1985). *Nitrogen Fixation Research Progress*, Martinus Nijhoff Publishers, Boston.

Giles, K.L., and Whitehead, H.C.M. (1976). Uptake and continued metabolic activity of *Azotobacter* with fungal protoplasts. *Science*, **193**, 1125–1126.

Hardy, R.W.F., Burns, R.L., Stansy, J.T., and Parshall, G.W. (1975). The nitrogenase reaction, In *Nitrogen Fixation by Free-living Microorganisms*. Ed. W.D.P. Stewart. Cambridge Univ. Press, London. pp. 351–376.

Holsten, R.D., Burns, R.C., Hardy, P.W.F., and Herbert, R.R. (1971). Establishment of symbiosis between *Rhizobium* and plant cells *in vitro*. *Nature*, **232**, 173–176.

Hull, R., and Howell, S.H. (1978). Structure of the cauliflower mosaic virus genome. II. Variation in DNA structure and sequence between isolates. *Virology*, **86**, 482–493.

Joshi, S.N. (1971). Studies on genetic variability for yield and its components in Indian beans *Dolichos lablab* var. *lignosus*. *Madras Agric. Univ. J.*, **58**, 367–371.

Kerr, A. (1982). Biological control of soil-borne microbial pathogens and nematodes. In *Advances in Agricultural Microbiology*. Ed. N.S. Subba Rao. Butterworths, London. pp. 429–463.

Kloepper, J.W., Leong, J., Teintze, M., and Schroth, M.N. (1980a). *Pseudomonas* siderophores: A mechanism explanining disease-suppressive soils. *Curr. Microbiol.*, **4**, 317–320.

Kloepper, J.W., Leong, J., Teintze, M., and Schroth, M.N. (1980b). Enhanced plant growth by siderophores produced by plant growth-promoting rhizobacteria. *Nature*, **286**, 885–886.

Leong, J. (1986). Siderophores: Their biochemistry and possible role in biocontrol of plant pathogens. *Annu. Rev. Phytopathol.* **24**, 187–209.

Leroughe, P., Roche, P., Faucher, C., Mailet, F., Truchet, G., Prome, J.C., and Denarie, J. (1990). Symbiotic host specificity of *Rhizobium meliloti* is determined by a sulphated and acylated glucosamine oligosaccharide signal. *Nature*, **344**, 781–784.

National Academy of Sciences (1979). Tropical legumes: Resources for the future. Report of an ad hoc panel, National Academy of Sciences, Washington, DC.

Postgate, J. (1989). Trends and perspectives in nitrogen fixation research. In *Advances in Microbial Physiology*, Academic Press, New York. pp. 1–22.

Prasad, R., Rajale, G.B., and Lakhdive, B.A. (1971). Nitrification retarders and slow release nitrogen fertilizers, *Adv. Agron.*, **23**, 337–383.

Ranga Rao, V., and Subba Rao, N.S. (1976). Studies on the infection of legume root callus with *Rhizobium Z. Pflanzenphysiol.*, **80**, 14–20.

Schippers, B., Bakker, A.W., and Bakker, P.A.H.M. (1987). Interactions of deleterious and beneficial rhizosphere microorganisms and the effect of cropping practices. *Annu. Rev. Phytopathol.*, **25**, 339–358.

Sharma, S.N., and Prasad, R. (1980). Effect of rates of nitrogen and relative efficiency of sulphur-coated urea and nitrapyrin-treated urea in dry matter production and nitrogen uptake by rice. *Plant and Soil*, **55**, 389–396.

Silvester, W.B., and Smith, D.R. (1969). Nitrogen fixation by *Gunnera-Nostoc* symbiosis. *Nature*, London, **224**, 1231.

Singh H.B., and Arora, R.K. (1973). Soh phlong, *Moghania vestita*, a leguminous root crop of India, *Econ. Bot.*, **27**, 332–338.

Weller, D.M. (1988). Biological control of soil-borne plant pathogens in the rhizosphere with bacteria. *Annu. Rev. Phytopathol.*, **26**, 379–407.

Appendix on Media/Stains

Media for *Rhizobium* Studies

Yeast extract mannitol medium	g/l
K_2HPO_4	0.5
$MgSO_4.7H_2O$	0.2
NaCl	0.1
Mannitol[*]	10.0
Yeast extract	1.0
Distilled water	1000 ml
Agar	20.0
Congo red 1% solution	2.5 ml (only for solid medium during isolation)

Peptone-glucose agar	g/l
Glucose	5.0
Peptone	10.0
Agar	15–10
Distilled water	1000 ml

Hofers alkaline broth	g/l
K_2HPO_4	0.5
$MgSO_4$	0.2
NaCl	0.1
$CaCO_3$	0.05
Yeast extract	1.0
Mannitol	10.0
Distilled water	1000 ml

Carbol fuchsin stain	
Basic fuchsin	1.0 g
Ethyl alcohol	10.0 ml
5% phenol solution	100.0 ml

---

[*] May be replaced by sucrose or glucose

Gram stain (Vincent, 1970)

The following are the reagents

1) Crystal violet solution
Crystal violet	10.0 g
Ammonium oxalate	4.0 g
Ethyl alcohol	100.0 ml
Distilled water	400.0 ml

2) Iodine solution
Iodine	1.0 g
Potassium iodide	2.0 g
Ethyl alcohol	25.0 ml
Distilled water	100.0 ml

3) Iodinated alcohol
Iodine solution (2)	5.0 ml
Ethyl alcohol	95.0 ml

4) Counterstain
2.5% safranin in ethyl alcohol	10.0 ml
Distilled water	100.0 ml

Benedict reagent

173 g sodium citrate and 100 g anhydrous sodium carbonate are dissolved in 66 ml distilled water; 17.3 g crystalline copper sulphate is dissolved in 100 ml distilled water. The latter solution is added to the former with constant stirring, the mixture filtered if not clear and made up to 1000 ml with distilled water. The reagent may be stored indefinitely.

Nitrogen-free media for growing seedlings to test root nodulation of legumes

Jenesen's medium (1942)

	g/l
$CaHPO_4$	1.0
K_2HPO_4	0.2
$MgSO_4.7H_2O$	0.2
NaCl	0.2
$FeCl_3$	0.1
Water	1000.0 ml

Thornton's medium (1930)

	g/l
$Ca_3(PO_4)_2$	2.0
K_2HPO_4	0.5
$MgSO_4.7H_2O$	0.2
NaCl	0.1
$FePO_4$	1.0
$FeCl_3$	0.01
Water	1000.0 ml

Note:
1) Add agar 15 g/l when solid media are needed.
2) Prepare a stock solution of trace elements containing Bo, 0.05%; Mn, 0.05%; Zn, 0.005%; Mo, 0.005%; Cu, 0.002% (Gibson, 1963). Add 1 ml of the stock solution for every 1000 ml of the medium.
3) Adjust pH to 6.5–7.0.

Media for excised root nodulation studies
(Raggio *et al.*, 1957)

Substances (mg/l)	Plus nitrate	Nitrate-free	O
Inorganic constituents			
$Ca(NO_3)_2.4H_2O$	287.1	–	–
KNO_3	80.0	–	–
$CaCO_3$	–	–	3000.0
$CaCl_2.2H_2O$	–	–	300.0
$CaSO_4.2H_2O$	–	206.5	200.0
KCl	65.0	124.6	65.0
KH_2PO_4	–	–	200.0
$MgSO_4.7H_2O$	736.8	736.8	700.0
$NaH_2PO_4.H_2O$	19.0	19.0	–
$Na_2SO_4.10H_2O$	453.1	453.1	450.0
KI	0.75	0.75	0.75
$FeCl_3$	1.5	1.5	1.5
Micro-elements: H_3BO_3, 1.5; $MnSO_4$ H_2O, 4.5; Na_2MoO_4 $2H_2O$, 0.25; $CuSO_4$ $5H_2O$, 0.04; $ZnSO_4$ $7H_2O$, 1.5	+	+	+

Organic constituents

Glycine		3.0	3.0	3.0
Vitamins: nicotinic acid, 0.5; pyridoxine, 0.1; thiamin HCl, 0.1		+	+	+
Sucrose		20 g	20 g	5 g

Other constituents

Difco Bacto-Agar	15 g	15 g	15 g
Glass-distilled water to make one litre	+	+	+
Final pH	6.8	6.7	6.8

Tissue culture medium (Murashige and Skoog, 1962)

A) *Mineral salts*

Major elements (mg/l)		*Minor elements* (mg/l)	
NH_4NO_3	1650	H_3BO_4	6.2
KNO_3	1900	$MnSO_4\ 4H_2O$	22.3
$CaCl_2\ 2H_2O$	440	$ZnSO_4\ 4H_2O$	8.6
$MgSO_4.7H_2O$	370	KI	0.83
KH_2PO_4	170	$Na_2.MoO_4.\ 2H_2O$	0.25
Na_2-EDTA	37.3	$CuSO_4.\ 5H_2O$	0.025
$FeSO_4.7H_2O$	27.8	$CaCl_2.6H_2O$	0.025

B) *Organic constituents*

Sucrose	30 g/l	Agar	10 g/l
Edamin (optional)	1 g/l	Myo-inositol	100 mg/l
Glycine	2.0 mg/l	Nicotinic acid	0.5 mg/l
Indole-acetic acid	1–30 mg/l	Pyridoxin-HCl	0.5 mg/l
Kinetin	0.04–10 mg/l	Thiamin	0.1 mg/l

pH adjusted to 5.7–5.8 with HCl or KOH or NaOH

Media for Blue-green Algae

Pringsheim's medium (Pringsheim, 1964)

KNO_3	0.02%
$MgSO_4.\ 7H_2O$	0.001%
$(NH_4)_2HPO_4$	0.002%

| CaCl$_2$.6H$_2$O | 0.0005% |
| FeCl$_3$ | 0.00005% |

Chu's medium No. 10 (Chu, 1942)

Ca(NO$_3$)$_2$	0.004%
MgSO$_4$.7H$_2$O	0.0025%
K$_2$HPO$_4$	0.0005% to 0.001%
Na$_2$CO$_3$	0.002%
Na$_2$SiO$_3$	0.0025%
FeCl$_3$	0.0008%

Crone's plant nutrient medium	**g/l**
KCl or KNO$_3$	0.75
CaSO$_4$.2H$_2$O	0.50
MgSO$_4$.7H$_2$O	0.50
Ca$_3$(PO$_4$)$_2$	0.25
Fe$_3$(PO$_4$)$_2$5H$_2$O	0.25
Distilled water	1 litre

Trace element solution	**g/l**
LiSO$_4$	0.055
CuSO$_4$5H$_2$O	0.055
ZnSO$_4$	0.055
Al$_2$SO$_4$	0.055
NiSO$_4$7H$_2$O	0.055
H$_3$BO$_3$	0.62
SnCl$_2$	0.03
MnCl$_2$	0.40
CoCl$_2$6H$_2$O	0.055
TiO$_2$	0.055
KI	0.035
KBr	0.035
Na$_2$S$_2$O$_3$	0.43
Na$_2$MO$_4$2H$_2$O	0.03
KMnO$_4$	0.40

Media for *Azotobacter*

Ashby's medium	**g/l**
Mannitol	20.0
K$_2$HPO$_4$	0.2

$MgSo_4.7H_2O$	0.2
NaCl	0.2
K_2SO_4	0.1
$CaCO_3$	5.0
Agar	15.0
Distilled water	1000.0 ml

Jensen's medium

	g/l
Sucrose	20.0
K_2HPO_4	1.0
$MgSO_4.7H_2O$	0.5
NaCl	0.5
$FeSO_4$	0.1
$CaCO_3$	2.0
Agar	15.0
Distilled water	1000 ml

Burk's Medium

Prepare salt and trace element mixture as follows:

$MgSO_4$	20 g	⎫
K_2HPO_4	80 g	Burk's
KH_2PO_4	20 g	salt
$CaSO_4$	13 g	⎭
$FeCl_3$	1.45 g	Fe Mo
Na_2MoO_4	0.253 g	mixture
Distilled water	1000 ml	⎭

Then mix as under:

Burk's salt	1.3 g
Fe-Mo mixture	1.0 ml
Sucrose	20.0 g
Distilled water	1000 ml

Beijerinckia Medium (Becking, 1959)

	g/l
Sucrose	20.0
KH_2PO_4	0.8
K_2HPO_4	0.2
$MgSO_4.7H_2O$	0.5
$FeCl_3$	0.1
Na_2MoO_4	0.005
Agar	15.0
Distilled water	1000 ml
pH	6.5

Derxia medium
(Campelo and Dobereiner, 1969) g/l
   Starch 20.0
   K_2HPO_4 0.05
   KH_2PO_4 0.15
   $MgSO_4.7H_2O$ 0.20
   $CaCl_2$ 0.02
   $FeCl_3$ 0.01
   $Na_2MoO_4.2H_2O$ 0.002
   Bromothymol blue 0.5 ml
   (0.5% in absolute alcohol)
   $NaHCO_3$ 1.0
   Unrefined agar 20.0
   Distilled water 1000.0 ml

Medium for *Clostridium*

Ashby's medium for *Azotobacter* can be used but replace mannitol with glucose. Remove dissolved O_2 by steaming for 30 minutes, allow to cool, dispense in plates, inoculate, and incubate in an anaerobic jar for 7 days. Enrichment in liquid culture is recommended before plating on solid medium.

Media for *Azospirillum*

Okon et al., *(1977) medium as modified by Lakshmi Kumari* et al., *(1980)*

                         g/l
a) K_2HPO_4 6.0
    KH_2PO_4 4.0
    Distilled water 500.0 ml
b) $MgSO_4$ 0.2
    NaCl 0.1
    $CaCl_2$ 0.02
    NH_4Cl 1.0
    Malic acid 5.0
    NaOH 3.0
    Yeast extract 0.05
    Na_2MoO_4 0.002
    $MnSO_4$ 0.001
    H_3BO_3 0.0014
    $Cu(NO_3)_2$ 0.0004
    $ZnSo_4$ 0.0021

$FeCl_3$	0.002
Distilled water	500.0 ml
Bromothymol blue	2 ml
(0.5% alcoholic solution)	

The phosphate buffer portion of the medium was made in half of the total volume required and also contained enough agar (1.5 to 2.0%) for solidification. Part (a) and (b) were sterilized separately, mixed while hot, poured into plates, and allowed to set.

Nitrogen-free Bromothymol Blue (NFB) Medium
(Dobereiner *et al.*, 1976)

	g/l
Malic Acid	5.0
KOH	4.0
K_2HPO_4	0.5
$FeSO_4.7H_2O$	0.05
$MnSO_4.H_2O$	0.01
$MgSO_4.7H_2O$	0.10
NaCl	0.02
$CaCl_2$	0.01
Na_2MoO_4	0.002
Distilled water	1000.0 ml
Bromothymol blue	
(0.5% alcoholic solution)	2.0 ml
Agar	1.75
pH adjusted to 6.6–7.0	

Media for Isolation of Cellulolytic Microorganisms

Asparagine medium (for fungi)	g/l
$(NH_4)_2SO_4$	0.5
L-Asparagine	0.5
K_2HPO_4	1.0
KCl	0.5
$MgSO_4.7H_2O$	0.2
$CaCl_2$	0.1
Yeast extract	0.5
Cellulose (filter paper strips for enrichment)	10.0
Distilled water	1000.0 ml
pH	6.2

Hans medium (for bacteria)

	g/l
K_2HPO_4	0.5
KH_2PO_4	0.5
$(NH_4)_2SO_4$	1.0
$MgSO_4.7H_2O$	0.1
$CaCl_3$	0.1
NaCl	6.0
Yeast extract	0.1
Cellulose (filter paper strips for enrichment)	10.0
Distilled water	1000.0 ml

Ken Knight medium (for actinomycetes)

	g/l
K_2HPO_4	1.0
$NaNO_3$	0.1
KCl	0.1
$MgSO_4.7H_2O$	0.1
Cellulose (filter paper strips for enrichment)	10.0
Distilled water	1000 ml
pH	7.0–7.2

After enrichment, the following media are used for plating:

Martin's rose bengal medium
(for isolation of fungi)

	g/l
Glucose	10.0
Peptone	5.0
KH_2PO_4	1.0
$MgSO_4.7H_2O$	0.5
Rose bengal	0.33
Streptomycin sulphate (10% solution)	3 ml
Agar	15.0
Distilled water	1000 ml

Nutrient agar
(for bacteria and actinomycetes)

	g/l
Peptone	5.0
Beep extract	3.0
NaCl	5.0
Distilled water	1000 ml

Media for assaying cellulase

Czapek medium

	g/l
$NaNO_3$	2.0
KCl	0.5
$MgSO_4.7H_2O$	0.5
K_2HPO_4	1.0
$FeSO_4.7H_2O$	0.01
Cellulose	10.0
Distilled water	1000 ml
pH	6.4–7.0

Mandel and Reese medium
(Mandel and Reese, 1957)

	g/l
Proteose peptone	1.0
$(NH_4)_2SO_4$	1.4
KH_2PO_4	2.0
Urea	0.3
$MgSO_4.7H_2O$	0.3
$CaCl_2$	0.3
$FeSO_4.7H_2O$	0.05
$MnSO_4.H_2O$	0.016
$ZnCl_2$	0.017
$CaCl_2$	0.020
Cellulose	10.0
Distilled water	1000 ml
pH	5.3

Dickermann medium
(Dickermann and Staff, 1951)

	g/l
K_2HPO_4	0.8
KH_2PO_4	0.2
$MgSO_4.7H_2O$	0.2
NaCl	0.2
$NaNO_3$	0.1
Yeast extract	0.01
Cellulose	20.0
Distilled water	1000 ml

Medium to Measure Lignin Degradation
(Day *et al.*, 1949)

	g/l
NH_4NO_3	5.00
KH_2PO_4	1.50

$MgSO_4.7H_2O$	0.50
$CaCO_3$	0.20
Thiamine	0.01
Lignin	5.00
Mineral supplement*	1 ml/1000 ml
Agar	20.00
pH	7.0

Arnon's microelement solution   g/l

H_3BO_3	2.90
$MnCl_2.4H_2O$	1.80
$ZnCl_2$	0.11
$CuSO_4.5H_2O$	0.08
$(NH_4)_6Mo_7O_{24}.4H_2O$	0.018
Distilled water	1000 ml

Note: By ommitting agar, a liquid medium is prepared for colorimetric determination.

Media for Determining Phosphate Solubilization

Katznelson and Bose medium (1959)

Soil extract	100 ml
	(autoclave soil suspension, filter and use clear filtrate)
Glucose	1.0 g
Agar	2.0 g

Sterilize in 100 ml lots, cool and add 5 ml of 10% K_2HPO_4 and 10 ml of 10% $CaCl_2$ to each flask. Adjust pH to 7.0 with sterile N/10 NaOH. Pour plates immediately and allow to solidify.

Pikovskaya's medium (modified by
Sundara Rao and Sinha, 1963)   g/l

Glucose	10.0
$Ca_3(PO_4)_2$	5.0
$(NH_4)_2SO_4$	0.5
KCl	0.2
$MgSO_4.7H_2O$	0.1
$MnSO_4$	trace
$FeSO_4$	trace
Yeast extract	0.5
Agar	15.0
Distilled water	1000 ml

---

*Hoagland A–Z mineral supplement is replaced by Arnon's As micro-elements solutions.

Barton's Reagent

    A. Dissolve 25 g ammonium molybdate in 400 ml H_2O.

    B. Dissolve 1.25 g ammonium metavanadate in 300 ml of boiling water, cool and then add 250 ml concentrated HNO_3. Afterwards, mix A and B solutions and make up to a litre.

Media for *Frankia*

BAP medium (Murry et al., 1984)   g/l

K_2HPO_4	0.591
KH_2PO_4	0.952
NH_4Cl	0.267
$MgSO_4\ 7H_2O$	0.095
$CaCl_2\ 2H_2O$	0.010
FeNa EDTA	0.010
Na propionate[*]	0.480
Trace elements solution[**]	1 ml
Vitamin solution[***]	1 ml

pH adjusted to 6.7 (propionate) or 6.3 (pyruvate)

M6B medium (modified from Baker and Torrey, 1980)
                                        g/l

Yeast extract (Difco)	5
Dextrose	10
Casamino Acids (Difco)	5
KH_2PO_4	1
$MgSO_4.7H_2O$	0.1
$CaCl_2.2H_2O$	0.01
$CoCl_2$	0.001
FeNa EDTA	0.01
Trace elements solution (see BAP medium)	1 ml
Vitamin solution (see BAP medium)	1 ml

pH adjusted to 6.5

---

[*] Na propionate may be replaced by Na pyruvate (1.1 g/l). They are filter sterilized.

[**] Trace elements solution (g/l) H_3BO_3: 2.86; $MnCl_2.4H_2O$: 2.27; $ZnSO_4.7H_2O$: 0.22; $CuSO_4.5H_2O$: 0.08; $Na_2MoO_4.2H_2O$: 0.025; $CuSO_4.7H_2O$: 0.001.

[***] Vitamin solution (mg/l) thiamin HCl: 10; nicotinic acid: 50; pyridoxin HCl: 50; biotin: 225; folic acid: 10; Ca pantothenate: 10; riboflavin: 10. Phosphate was added after autoclaving.

Qmod medium (Lalonde and Calvert, 1979)

K_2HPO_4	300 mg/l	
NaH_2PO_4	200 mg/l	
$MgSO_4 7H_2O$	200 mg/l	
KCl	200 mg.l	
Yeast extract	500 mg/l	Lipid supplement:
Bacto-peptone (Difco)	5 g/l	Dissolve 500 mg of 1-a-lecithin in 50 ml
Glucose	10 g/l	absolute ethanol and
Ferric citrate (citric acid and ferric citrate 1% solution)	1 ml	add 50 ml distilled water. Add this at the rate of 0.5–50 mg.
Trace element solution (see BAP medium)	1 ml	
pH adjusted to	6.7–7.0	
Autoclave	20 minutes	
Agar if used	15 g	

Benson's medium (Benson, 1982)

K_2HPO_4, 3.0 g/l; KH_2PO_4, 2.0 g/l; $MgSO_4 . 7H_2O$, 0.2 g/l; NaCl, 0.3 g/l; ferric sodium EDTA, 0.16 g/l; 1 ml trace elements; and 1 ml vitamin mixture. Calcium carbonate is added to liquid cultures at 0.05 mg/ml. Carbon sources are added at 3 g/l.

REFERENCES

Baker, D., and Torrey, J.G. (1980). Characterization of an effective actinorhizal microsymbiont, *Frankia* sp. Arcll (Actinomycetales). *Can. J. Microbiol.*, **26**, 1066–1071.

Becking, J.A. (1959). Nitrogen fixing bacteria of the genus *Beijerinckia* in South African soil. *Plant and Soil*. .11, **193–206.**

Benson, D.R. (1982). Isolation of *Frankia* from older actinorhizal root nodules. *Appl. Environ. Microbiol.*, **44**, 461–465.

Campelo, A.B., and Dobereiner, J. (1969). Soil biology. *Intl. News Bull.*, **11**, 40–44.

Chu, S.P. (1942). The influence of the mineral composition of the medium on the growth of planktonic algae. I. Methods and culture media. *J. Ecol.*, **30**, 284–325.

Day, M.C., Palczar, H.J. Jr., and Gottlieb, S. (1949). The biological degradation of lignin I. *Arch Biochem.*, **23**, 360–369.

Dickermann, J.M., and Staff, T.J. (1951). A medium for the isolation of the pure cultures of cellulolytic bacteria. *J. Bacteriol.*, **62**, 133–134.

Dobereiner, J., Marriel, I.E., and Nery, M. (1976). Ecological distribution of *Spirillum lipoferum*, Beijerinck. *Can. J. Microbiol.*, **22**, 1464–1473.

Gibson, A.H. (1963). Physical environment and symbiotic nitrogen fixation. I. The effect of root temperature on recently nodulated *Trifolium subterraneum* L. plants. *Austral. J. Biol. Sci.*, 16, 28–42.

Hoagland, D.R., and Arnon, D.I. (195). The water culture method for growing plants without soil. *Calif. Agr. Expt. Stn. Circ.*, 347.

Jensen. H.L. (1942). Nitrogen fixation in leguminous plants, I. General characters of root nodule bacteria isolated from species of *Medicago* and *Trifolium* in Australia. *Proc. Linn. Soc., N.S.W.*, 66, 98–108.

Johnson, C.M., Stout, P.R., Broyer, T.C., and Carlton, A.B. (1957). Comparative chlorine requirements of different plant species. *Plant and Soil*. 8, 337–353.

Katznelson, H., and Bose, B. (1959). Metabolic activity and phosphate dissolving capability of bacterial isolates from wheat roots, rhizosphere and non-rhizosphere soil. *Can. J. Microbiol.*, 5, 79–85.

Lalonde, M., and Calvert, H.E. (1979). Production of *Frankia* hyphae and spores as an infective inoculant for *Alnus* sp. In *Symbiotic Nitrogen Fixation in the Management of Temperate Forests*. Eds. J.C. Gordon, C.T. Wheeler and D.A. Perry. Forest Research Laboratory, Corvallis, Ore. pp. 95–110.

Lakshmi Kumari, M., Lakshmi, V., Nalini, P.A., and Subba Rao, N.S. (1980). Reactions of *Azospirillum* to certain dyes and their usefulness in enumeration of the organism. *Curr. Sci.*, 49, 438–439.

Mandel, M., and Resse, R.T. (1957). Induction of cellulase in *Trichoderma viride* as influenced by carbon source. *J. Bacteriol.*, 37, 269–278.

Murashige, T., and Skoog, F. (1962). A revised medium for rapid growth and bioassay with tobacco tissue culture. *Physiol. Plant.*, 15, 473–497.

Murry, M.A., Fontaine, M.S., and Torrey, J.G. (1984). Growth kinetics and nitrogenase induction in *Frankia* sp. H F P ArI3 grown in batch culture. *Plant and Soil*, 78, 61–78.

Okon, Y., Albrecht, S.L., and Burris, R.H. (1977). Methods for growing *Spirillum lipoferum* and for counting it in pure culture and in association with plants. *J. Appl. Environ. Microbiol.*, 33, 85–88.

Pringsheim, E.G. (1964). *Pure Cultures of Algae: Their Preparation and Maintenance*. Hafner Publishing Co., New York and London.

Raggio, M., Raggio, N., and Torrey, J.G. (1957). The nodulation of isolated leguminous roots. *Amer. J. Bot.*, 44, 325–334.

Sundara Rao, W.V.B., and Sinha, M.K. (1963). Phosphate dissolving organisms in the soil and rhizosphere. *Indian J. Agric. Sci.*, 33, 272–278.

Thornton, H.C. (1930). The early development of the root nodule of lucerne (*Medicago sativa* L.). *Ann. Bot.*, 44, 385–392.

Vincent, J.M. (1970). *A Manual for the Practical Study of the Root Nodule Bacteria*. Blackwell Scientific Publications, Oxford and Edinburgh.

Index

The Plates

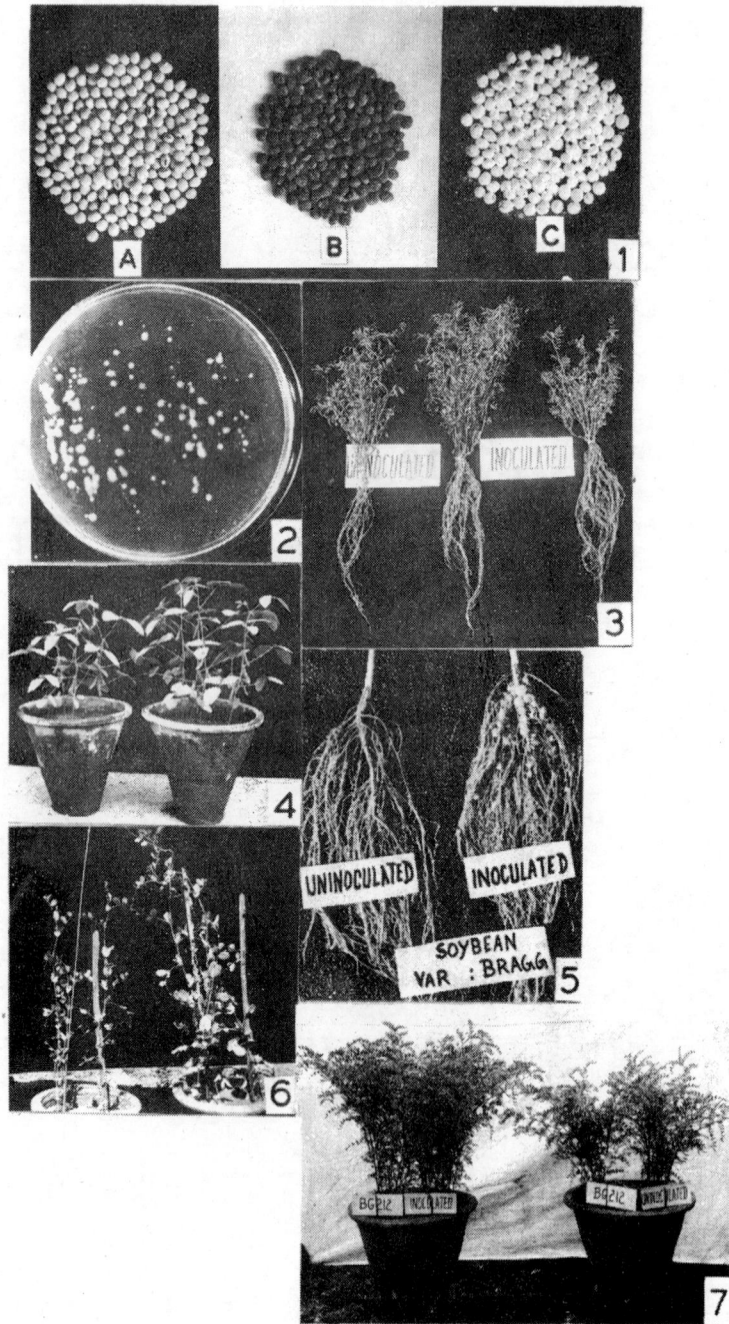

Plate 1.   *Rhizobium* and legume root nodulation: 1. Seed inoculation with *Rhizobium*—(a) uninoculated soybean seed; (b) soybean seed inoculated with peat-based *Rhizobium* culture; and (c) *Rhizobium*-inoculated seeds are again coated or pelleted with finely powdered and sieved lime for sowing in acidic soils. 2. Colonies of *Rhizobium* growing on nitrogen-free agar medium. 3. Bengal gram or chickpea (*Cicer arietinum*) plants—from left to right—uninoculated control plant, plant inoculated with an inefficient strain of *Rhizobium* and plant inoculated with an efficient strain of *Rhizobium*, (Courtesy, Dr. R.B. Rewari). 4. Soybean (*Glycine max*) plants—on the left is a pot with uninoculated plants while on the right is a pot with plants inoculated with an efficient strain of *R. japonicum*. 5. The root system of soybean plants from pots shown above—Note profuse nodulation in inoculated plants. 6. Pea (*Pisum sativum*) plants—on the left is a pot with uninoculated plants, while on the right is a pot with *Rhizobium*-inoculated plants. 7. Bengal gram of chickpea (*C. arietinum*) plants—on the left is a pot with plants inoculated with *Rhizobium*, while on the right is a pot with plants which have not been inoculated (Courtesy, Dr. R.B. Rewari).

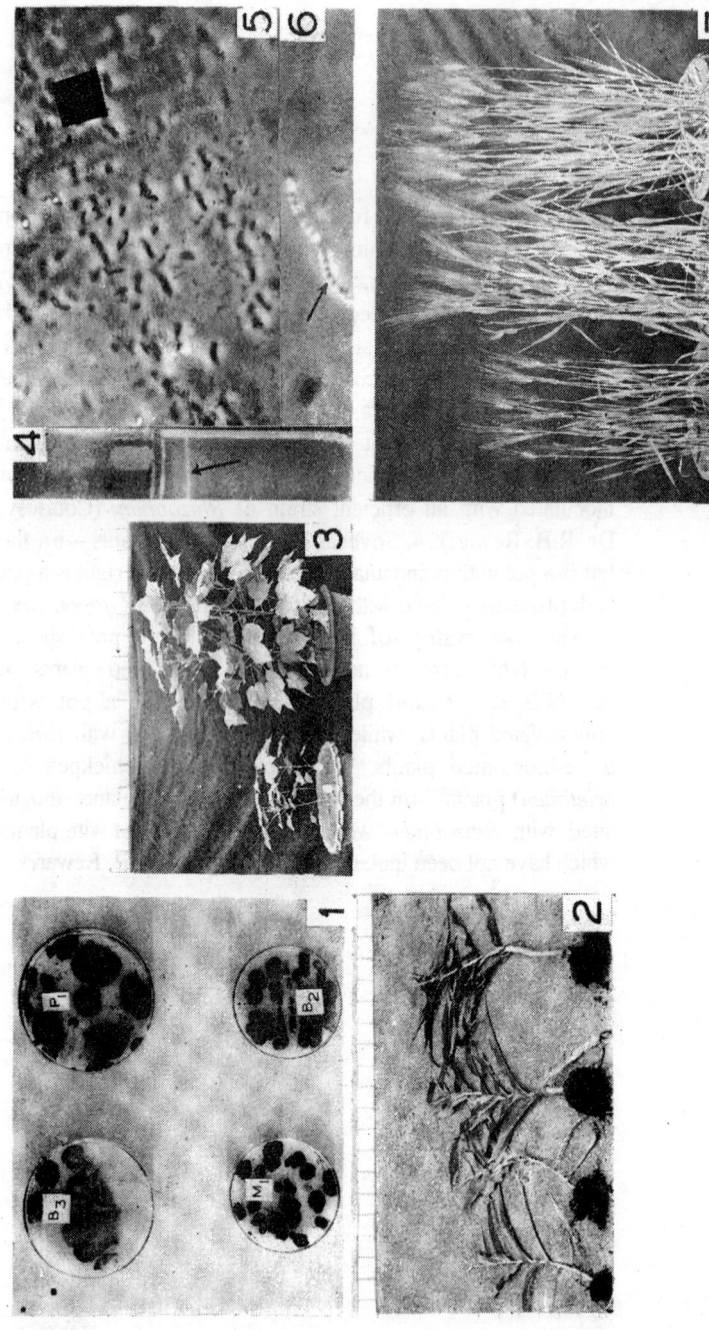

Plate 2. *Azotobacter* and *Azospirillum* effects of plants: 1. Colonies of different isolates of *Azotobacter chroococcum* grown on Jensen's nitrogen-free agar medium showing brownish-dark pigmentation. 2. Effect of *A. chroococcum* inoculation on sorghum (*Sorghum bicolor*)—from left to right—uninoculated plant, inoculated plant, plant receiving 40kg N/ha alone, plant receiving 40 kg N/ha with *Azotobacter* inoculation. 3. Effect of *A. chroococcum* inoculation on cotton (*Gossypium* sp.)—The potted plants on the left are uninoculated (control) and the potted plants on the right are inoculated with *A. chroococcum*. 4. A screw-capped test tube containing nitrogen-free semi-solid malate medium to which a drop of diluted plant extract has been added. After incubation for 3–5 days, note the formation of a thin 'pellicle' much below the surface layer of the medium. The pellicle (see arrow) is formed under micro-aerophilic conditions (low O$_2$ content) and contains *Azospirillum* cells. Further purification of *Azospirillum* is done by repeated transfer of portions of this pellicle into fresh tubes containing semi-solid malate medium, until a pure colony of *Azospirillum* develops. 5. Motile and spiral-shaped cells of *A. brasilense* isolated from roots of rice as seen under the low power of a compound microscope. 6. The same isolate as seen under the high power of a phase contrast compound microscope showing two spiral-shaped bacteria attached to each other and depicting the characteristic PHB granules (see arrow). 7. Effect of *A. brasilense* inoculation on oats (*Avena sativa*)—from left to right—potted plants which are not inoculated (control), potted plants which have been inoculated with *A. brasilense*, and potted plants which are not inoculated but have received fertilizer nitrogen (urea) at the rate of 40 kg N/ha. (Courtesy, Drs. Shende, Kavimandan, Lakshmi Kumari, Tilak, and Apte.)

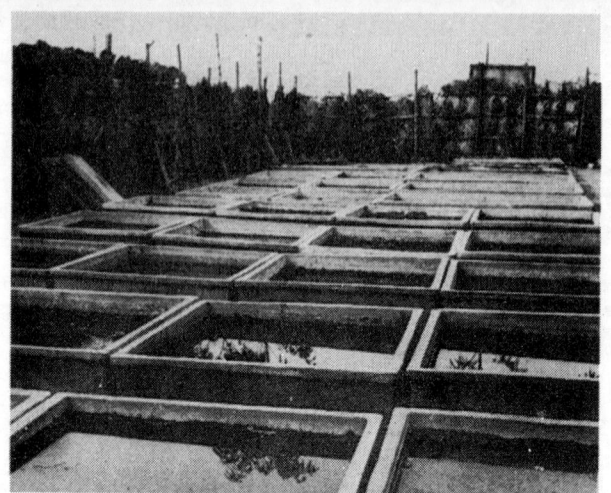

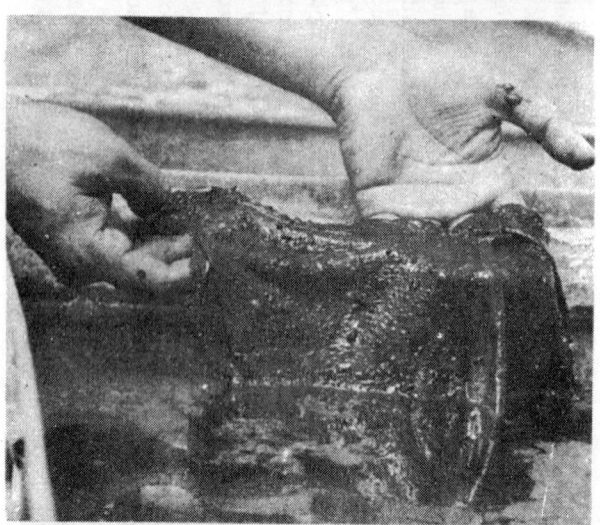

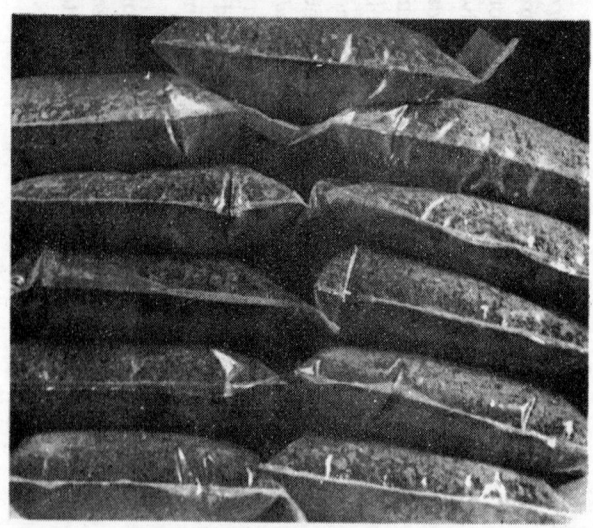

Plate 3. Farm-oriented low-cost technology for blue-green algal production (Courtesy, G.S. Venkataraman).

Top—Algal tanks in open air, having a soil-based blue-green algal culture.

Middle—After several days' growth, a mat of blue-green algae can be harvested.

Bottom—Dried flakes of algae stored in polythene bags.

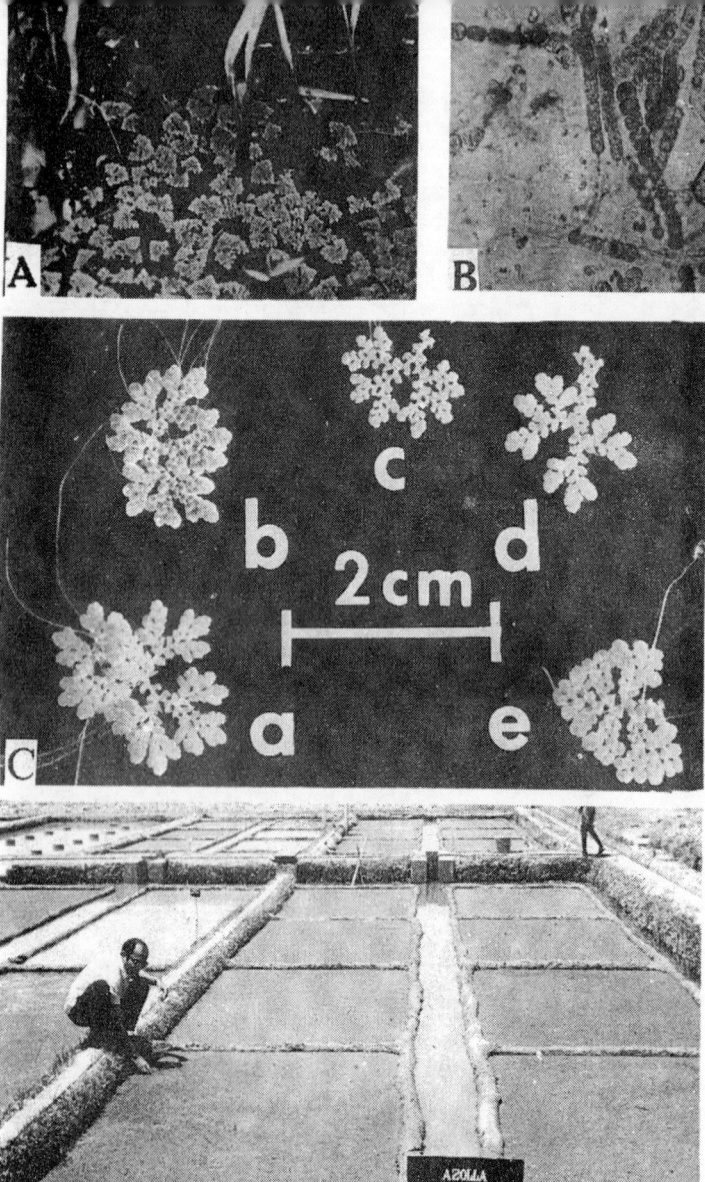

Plate 4. *Azolla* as a biofertilizer—A—*Azolla* fronds, growing in stagnant water among rice plants; B—A frond crushed to reveal filaments of nitrogen fixing *Anabaena azollae* (a view under a binocular microscope; C— Different species of *Azolla*—a) *A. mexicana*, b) *A. caroliniana*, c) *A. microphylla*, d) *A. filiculoides* and e) *A. pinnata*; D—Multiplication of *Azolla pinnata* in nurseries at.the Central Rice Research Institute, Cuttack, India (Courtesy, Charles Kettering Research Laboratory, Ohio and P.K. Singh CRRI Cuttack). All except C not to scale.

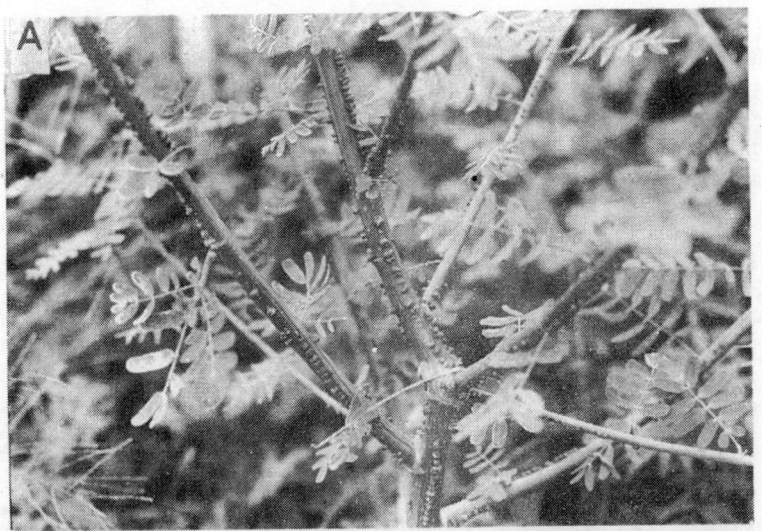

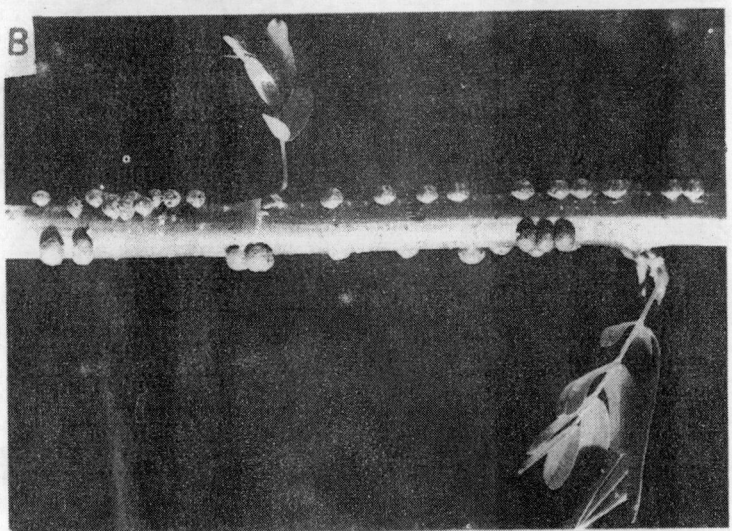

Plate 5.　*Sesbania rostrata*, a stem nodulating green manure plant—
(A) An adult plant bearing a number of outgrowths on the
shoot system which are nitrogen-fixing nodules on stem (Courtesy, N. Bonkerd, Thailand). (B)—An enlarged portion of a
stem showing the distinct pattern of stem nodulation (Courtesy, A.R.J. Eaglesham, U.S.A.).

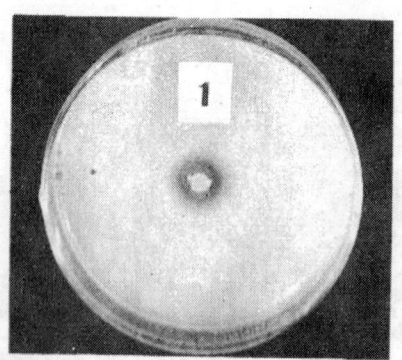

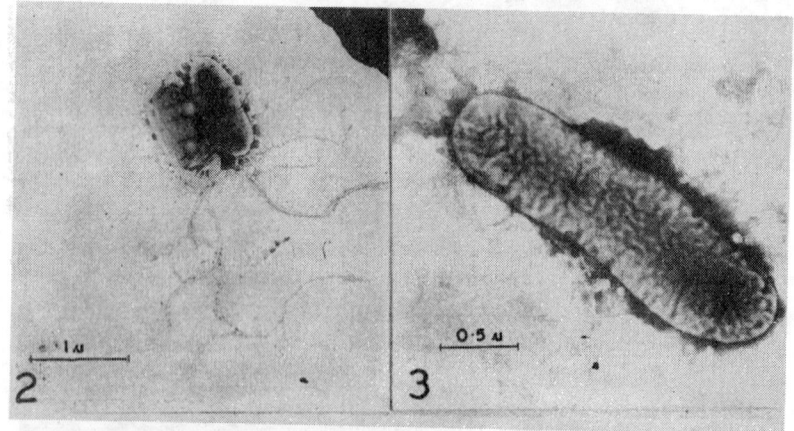

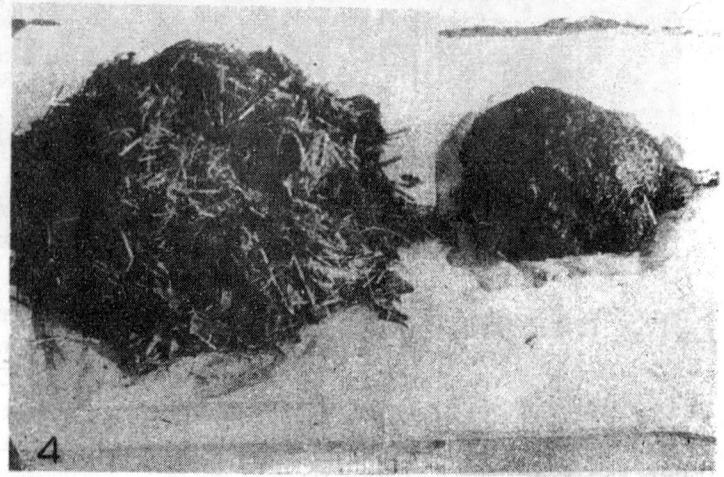

Plate 6. Phosphate-solubilizing and cellulolytic microorganisms. 1. A colony of *Pseudomonas striata* growing in the centre of tricalcium phosphate agar medium in a petri dish. Note the halo around the colony indicating the ability of the bacterium to secrete acid and solubilize the bound phosphate. 2. Cells of *P. striata* under electron microscope. 3. Cells of *Bacillus polymyxa* under electron microscope showing solubilization of bound phosphate (Courtesy, Dr. A.C. Gaur). 4. Acceleration of composting by the use of cellulolytic *Cellulomonas* sp. On the left is a heap of organic matter without any addition of cellulolytic cultures and on the right is a similar heap with *Cellulomonas* sp. added to it. Note the difference between the two heaps, indicating the cellulolytic activity of the bacterial culture (Courtesy, Dr. K.S. Yadav).

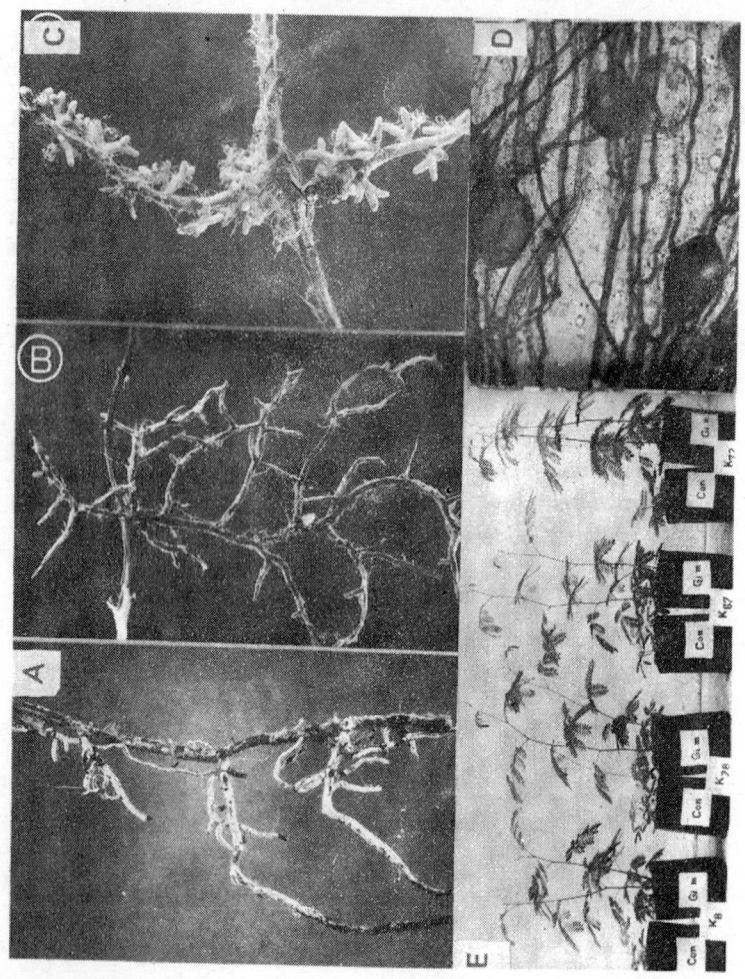

Plate 7. Mycorrhizal associations with plants. A, B, C—Ectomycorrhizal associations with three forest trees, namely *Larix* sp., *Tsuga* sp., and *Pinus* sp. Note the fungal mycelial mantle around the root system (Courtesy, R. Molina and J. Trappe, USA). D—Ramifications of fungal mycelia and vesicles of a typical VAM fungal association with plants (Courtesy, D.S. Hayman, UK). E—Beneficial response of inoculation of four cultivars of *Leucaena leucocephala* with a VAM fungus *Gigaspora margarita* in experimental plants raised in polythene pouches. Note that the uninoculated pouches on the left of the each of the four cultivars have smaller plants than the ones in VAM-inoculated pouches on the right (Courtesy, D.J. Bagyaraj, India).

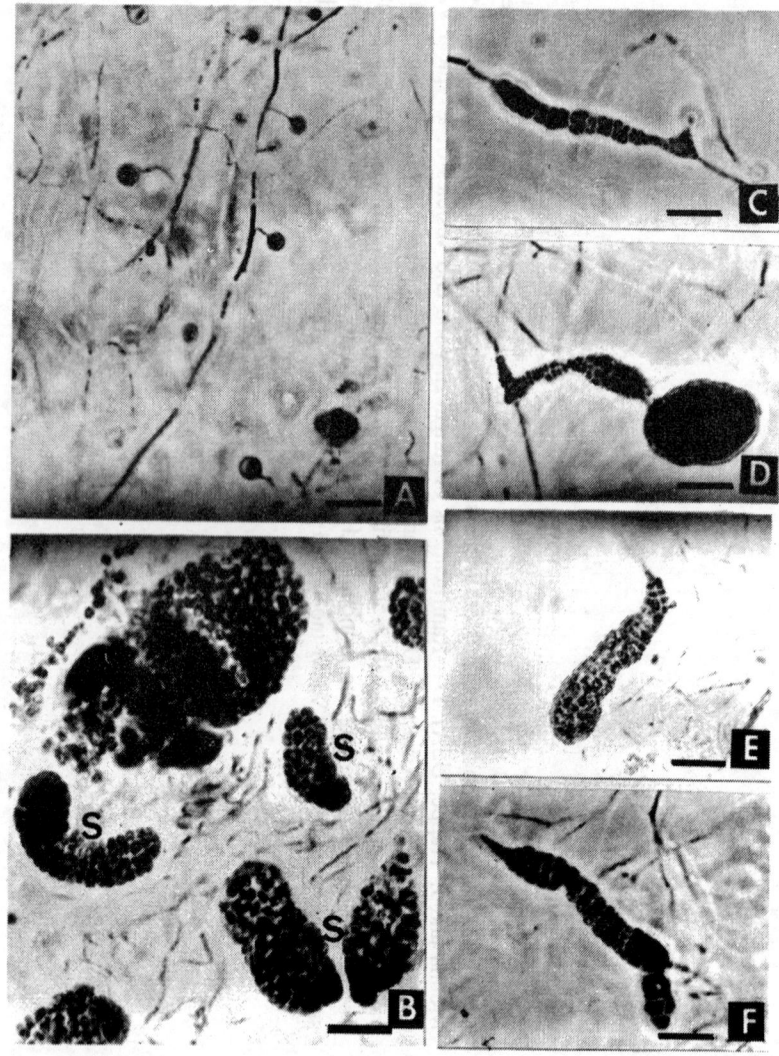

Plate 8. Vesicles and sporangia of *Frankia*

A—N$_2$-fixing septate vesicles produced by *Frankia* strain 020602(syn. D11) in Qmod agar medium. Vesicles are attached to vegetative hyphae by means of short parent hyphae. Bar = 100 μm.

B—Globose sporangia liberating mature sporangiospores. Note large size of sporangia and high number of sporangiospores produced by each sporangium. Bar = 10 μm.

C—Intercalary elongated sporangium. Bar = 10 μm.

D—Elongated sporangium connected to a globose sporangium. Bar = 10 μm.

E—Club-shaped sporangium. Bar = 10 μm.

F—Elongated terminal sporangium. Inside, the sporangium spores are arranged in transverse lines. Bar = 10 μm. (Courtesy, Diem and Dommergues, France).

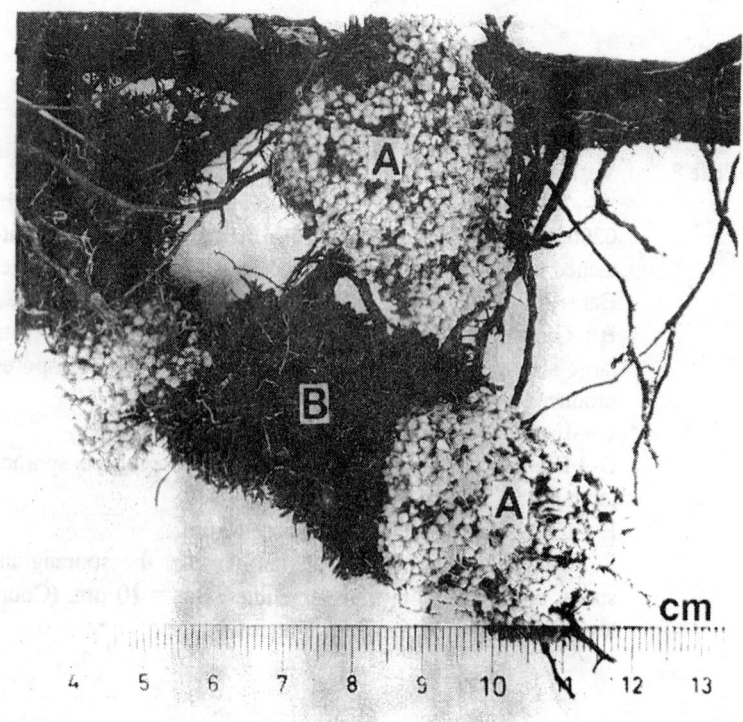

Plate 9.   Nodules formed on the roots of a 10-year-old *Casuarina equisetifolia* tree. A—Young nodule lobes; B—degenerating nodule lobes (Courtesy, Diem and Dommergues, France).